# Midwifery

## THE EFFICIENT MIDWIFE

**Lauren A. Dutton, MSN, CNM**
Easton, Maryland

**Jessica E. Densmore, MSN, CNM**
Keene, New Hampshire

**Meredith B. Turner, PhD, CNM**
Athens, Georgia

**JONES AND BARTLETT PUBLISHERS**
*Sudbury, Massachusetts*
BOSTON    TORONTO    LONDON    SINGAPORE

*World Headquarters*

| Jones and Bartlett Publishers | Jones and Bartlett Publishers | Jones and Bartlett Publisher |
| 40 Tall Pine Drive | Canada | International |
| Sudbury, MA 01776 | 6339 Ormindale Way | Barb House, Barb Mews |
| 978-443-5000 | Mississauga, Ontario L5V 1J2 | London W6 7PA |
| info@jbpub.com | Canada | United Kingdom |
| www.jbpub.com | | |

Jones and Bartlett's books and products are available through most bookstores and online booksellers. To contact Jones and Bartlett Publishers directly, call 800-832-0034, fax 978-443-8000, or visit our website www.jbpub.com.

Substantial discounts on bulk quantities of Jones and Bartlett's publications are available to corporations, professional associations, and other qualified organizations. For details and specific discount information, contact the special sales department at Jones and Bartlett via the above contact information or send an email to specialsales@jbpub.com.

**Production Credits**
Publisher: Kevin Sullivan
Acquisitions Editor: Emily Ekle
Acquisitions Editor: Amy Sibley
Associate Editor: Patricia Donnelly
Editorial Assistant: Rachel Shuster
Senior Production Editor: Carolyn F. Rogers
Marketing Manager: Rebecca Wasley
V.P., Manufacturing and Inventory Control: Therese Connell
Composition: Shawn Girsberger
Illustrator: Katrina Peterson Design
Cover Design: Scott Moden
Cover Image: © Cobalt Moon Design/ShutterStock, Inc.
Printing and Binding: Malloy, Inc.
Cover Printing: Malloy, Inc.

**Library of Congress Cataloging-in-Publication Data**
Dutton, Lauren A.
  A pocket guide to clinical midwifery : the efficient midwife / Lauren A. Dutton, Jessica E. Densmore, Meredith B. Turner.
     p. ; cm.
  Includes bibliographical references and index.
  ISBN 978-0-7637-6134-9 (pbk. spiral)
  1. Midwifery–Handbooks, manuals, etc. I. Densmore, Jessica E. II. Turner, Meredith B. III. Title.
  [DNLM: 1. Midwifery–Handbooks. WQ 165 D981p 2010]
  RG950.D88 2010
  618.2–dc22

                                    2009012325

6048

Printed in the United States of America
13 12 11 10 09   10 9 8 7 6 5 4 3 2 1

# CONTENTS

## C

## D

## E

# PREFACE

*A Pocket Guide to Clinical Midwifery* was conceived while the three authors were in midwifery school at Yale University School of Nursing. As new midwifery students we were instructed to create a "black book" that would provide a quick reference to critical topics in midwifery practice. As we entered clinical practice this resource proved to be invaluable, because it kept everything at our fingertips while seeing patients. While many obstetrical and gynecological reference guides are organized by patient care (prenatal, well-woman, etc.), this resource is presented alphabetically so that the topic of interest can be found quickly. Additionally, we have included with each topic the resources needed to practice evidenced-based medicine. Our goal is to consolidate information you need in one compact reference. We realize that information in midwifery and obstetrics will change, but this book provides a comprehensive overview of topics midwives commonly encounter. We hope that this guide will become a reference you keep in your bag wherever you go.

Without the guidance of our mentors in both midwifery school and clinical practice this book would not have been possible. We offer heartfelt thanks to those brilliant midwives who instilled in us the importance of practicing evidenced-based medicine each and every day.

You can contact the authors with comments or suggestions at efficientmidwife@gmail.com.

# ABDOMINAL PAIN

## Overview

*Acute Pain*
PID (GYN)
Ectopic pregnancy (GYN)
Spontaneous Ab (GYN)
Outflow obstruction (GYN)
Pelvic adhesions (GYN)
Ovarian cyst/mass (GYN)
Ovarian tumor (GYN)
Appendicitis
Urinary tract infection (GU)
Nephrolithiasis (GU)
Uteral obstruction (GU)
Abdominal mass (GI, GYN)

*Cyclic Pain*
Primary GYN cause
Endometriosis (GYN)
Uterine fibroids (GYN)
IUD (GYN)
Outflow obstruction (GI, GU, GYN)
Pelvic adhesions (GYN)
Ovarian cyst/mass (GYN)

*Sporadic Pain*
Irritable bowel (GI)
Inflammatory bowel (GI)
Lactose intolerance (GI)
UTI (GU)
Nephrolithiasis (GU)
Constipation (GU)
Abdominal mass (GU, GI, GYN)

*Chronic Pain*
PID (GYN)
Endometriosis (GYN)
Fibroids (GYN)
Outflow obstruction (GU)
Ovarian cyst/mass (GYN)
Appendicitis (GI, GU)
Inflammatory bowel (GI)
Lactose intolerance (GI)
Nephrolithiasis (GI)
Diverticulitis (GU)
Abdominal mass (GI, GU, GYN)
Scoliosis (musculoskeletal)
Arthritis (musculoskeletal)
Herniated disk (musculoskeletal)

## Diagnosis Tips

*Red Flags = Surgical Abdomen = Emergency Room*

1. Pain that changes location
2. Pain that awakens pt from sleep
3. Weight loss
4. Pain that persists for longer than 6 h or worsens
5. Pain followed by vomiting
6. Hypotension

*Symptoms Most Likely Related to Specific Conditions*

**Ectopic pregnancy** = amenorrhea, irregular vaginal bleeding, sharp, low, lateral pain
**Ruptured abdominal aortic aneurism** = pain + pulsatile mass + hypotension
**Gallbladder disease** = Murphy's sign (four fingers in RUQ at the midclavicular line of the costal margin, press downward as pt expires, pain will be felt with inspiration)
**Constipation and gastroenteritis** = frequent changes in position to find comfort
**Ischemia** = sudden onset, intense, continuous, progressive, not relieved by medication, emesis
**Obstruction** = high-pitched bowel sounds + exaggerated peristaltic rushes
**Peritoneal irritation** = painful percussion
**Peptic ulcer disease** = gnawing ache or emptiness in the epigastrum
**Psychogenic abdominal pain** = difficult to localize, nonprogressive in intensity or location, does not wake them from sleep, describes nonabdominal-related symptoms
**Inflammatory pain** = pt will get relief from staying still
**Appendicitis** = McBurney's sign (rebound tenderness over RLQ) and obturator sign (pain when rotating hip)
**Irritable bowel syndrome, Crohn's disease** = abdominal pain and changes in bowel patterns, bloating, flatulence, straining, passage of mucus in stool, feeling of incomplete evacuation
**Mesentery artery infarct** = general midabdominal pain, poorly localized, sudden and intense onset, continuous, progressive

## SOURCES

Stap, G. (2003). Menstrual disorders in adolescence. *Best Practice and Research Clinical Obstetrics and Gynecology, 17*(1), 75–92.
Schuiling, K. D., & Likis, F. E. (2006). *Women's gynecologic health.* Sudbury, MA: Jones and Bartlett.
Miller, S., & Alpert, P. (2006). Assessment and differential diagnosis of abdominal pain. *Nurse Practitioner, 31*(7), 38–47.

## ABORTION

### Types
Spontaneous
Medical
Surgical

### Counseling/Informed Consent
Risk and benefits must be reviewed
Patient must affirm that she understands the procedure and its alternatives and that she is not being coerced into her decision
The Ab must be performed as expeditiously as possible once consent is given (waiting period laws vary between US states)
Information about birth control must be given at the Ab facility
Patient confidentiality must be observed

### Preoperative Requirements
Pertinent medical history
Confirmation of pregnancy (urine hCG, B-hCG, or U/S)
Gestational age verified and documented
Ectopic pregnancy ruled out
Vital signs
HCT or Hb w/ significant anemia history
Contraceptive plan
Rh typing

### Surgical Risks
Blood clots accumulating in the uterus, requiring another suctioning procedure (< 0.2% of cases)
Infection (0.1–0.2% of North American cases)
Tear in the cervix (0.6–1.2% of cases)
Perforation of the uterus (< 0.4% of cases)
Missed Ab which does not end the pregnancy (< 0.3% of cases)
Incomplete Ab in which pregnancy tissues remain in the uterus requiring repeat suctioning (0.3–2.0% of cases)
Excessive bleeding requiring blood transfusion (0.02–0.3% of cases)
Death (0.0006% of cases)

### Procedure
Analgesic and other comfort measures should be offered unless contraindications exists
All instruments should be sterile
Vagina cleaned w/ bacteriocidal agent
Cervix dilated gently and gradually
U/S guidance for location of fetal parts, to aid in extraction, to verify completion, and to verify an intact uterus is recommended
Rhogam given if pt Rh neg

### Anesthesia Options
*Local (Paracervical Block)—Reduction of Sensation and Pain in Cervix*
Preparation of solution: 5 ml of 1% or 0.5% lidocaine w/ 2 units (0.1 ml) vasopressin, and 5 ml of 8.4% sodium bicarbonate to buffer the solution
May add 2 mg/50 ml of atropine to total of 20 ml of mixture per pt
Slow injection is less painful than rapid
Deep injections more anesthetizing than superficial injections
Inject 1–2 ml at desired site of tenaculum placement
Inject remaining at intervals of approx 5 ml at multiple locations around the cervix and the deep lower uterine segment

*Conscious Sedation*
Minimally depressing the level of consciousness
Pt able to maintain a patent airway independently
Pt able to respond to physical and verbal stimuli

*Common Sedation Regimens*
Lorazepam (Ativan) 0.5–2 mg sublingually 20–30 min prior
Midazolam (Versed) 1–3 mg IV followed by fentanyl 50–100 mcg IV
Ibuprofen (600–800 mg PO) should be given w/ or w/out antianxiety medication
Deep sedation or general anesthesia when medically indicated

## Postsurgical Ab Care
Rh negative women < 12 wks gestation 50 mcg Rhogam
Rh negative women > 12 wks gestation 300 mcg Rhogam
Methergine series (0.2 mg q 4 h × 6 doses) if excessive bleeding
Doxycycline 100 mg BID on day of evacuation or BID × 7 d, optional
Pelvic rest × 2 wks, advised
Birth control method, initiated the day of procedure if possible

**SOURCES**

Allen, R. H., Kumar, D., Fitzmaurice, G., Lifford, K. L., & Goldberg, A. B. (2006). Pain management of first-trimester surgical abortion: Effects of selection of local anesthesia with and without lorazepam or intravenous sedation. *Contraception, 74*(5), 407–413.

National Abortion Federation. (2007). *2007 clinical policy guidelines.* Washington, DC: National Abortion Federation. Retrieved May 20, 2008, from http://www.guidelines.gov

Paul, M., Lichtenberg, S., Borgatta, L., Grimes, D. A., & Abdalla, M. (1999). *A clinician's guide to medical and surgical abortion.* Washington, DC: National Abortion Federation. Retrieved May 25, 2008, from http://www.prochoice.org

## ABORTION: FOLLOW-UP

### Signs of Post-Ab Complications

Severe or persistent pain

Chills or fever w/ an oral temp > 100.4°F

Bleeding that is 2 × the pt's normal menstrual period *or* soaks through more than 1 sanitary pad per h × 2 h in a row

Malodorous discharge or drainage from the vagina

Continues symptoms of pregnancy

### Essential Elements of Post-Ab Care

Help pt receive appropriate and timely care for complications

Identify and respond to the pt's emotional and physical healthcare needs and concerns

Tx incomplete or unsafe Abs

Help prevent unwanted pregnancies

### Resources for Patients

*The Healing Choice: Your Guide to Emotional Recovery After an Abortion* by Candace De Puy and Dana Dovitch

Postabortion Care Consortium Community Task Force. (2002). *Essential elements of postabortion care: An expanded and updated model.* Washington, DC: National Abortion Federation. Retrieved May 25, 2008, from http://www.prochoice.org

**SOURCES**

National Abortion Federation. (2007). *2007 clinical policy guidelines.* Washington, DC: National Abortion Federation. Retrieved May 25, 2008, from http://www.guidelines.gov

Paul, M., Lichtenberg, S., Borgatta, L., Grimes, D. A., & Abdalla, M. (1999). *A clinician's guide to medical and surgical abortion.* Washington, DC: National Abortion Federation. Retrieved May 25, 2008, from http://www.prochoice.org

# ABORTION: MEDICATION

A

### Eligibility

Gestational age < 49–63 d depending on the regimen, confirmed by U/S

Pt should *not* have a hemorrhagic disorder, chronic adrenal failure, concurrent long-term systemic corticosteroid therapy, confirmed or suspected ectopic pregnancy, inherited porphyrias, IUD in place, history of allergy to medications used, or unwillingness to undergo a vacuum aspiration if indicated

Able to give informed consent and comply w/ Tx regimen

Must have access to a telephone and transportation to a medical facility equipped to provide emergency care

### Risks

Failure of medication to terminate pregnancy requiring a suction procedure (< 2% of cases)

Incomplete expulsion of pregnancy requiring a suction procedure (< 6% of cases)

Excessive bleeding requiring suction procedure and rarely transfusion (< 1% of cases)

Infection (0.09–0.6% of cases)

Death secondary to toxic shock following infection w/ *Clostridium sordellii* (< 0.001% cases in United States and Canada)

### Counseling Points

Bleeding usually begins within 4 h of taking misoprostol, but some pts may experience spotting after mifepristone administration

Protocol for completion of Ab at home

Need for multiple visits to a medical facility

Usual range of pain experienced and how to take pain medications

Amount and quality of bleeding throughout the Ab and the following 3–5 wks

Known side effects and possible complications

How to contact the on-call provider

After-care instructions

Contraception

Emotional support

### U/S Examination

TVU/S preferable to abdominal probe because it can detect pregnancy approx 1 wk earlier

Document gestational sac, yolk sac, embryonic pole, and presence of cardiac activity

If embryonic pole is visible, measure it instead of the gestational sac to increase accuracy

If intrauterine sac is not present, workup for ectopic pregnancy or early intrauterine pregnancy

### Lab Requirements

Confirm pregnancy via urine hCG, B-hCG, or U/S

Document Rh factor

Hb or HCT

B-hCG not required unless being monitored for completeness of Ab or ectopic pregnancy

#### SOURCES

National Abortion Federation. (2002). *Protocol recommendations for use of methotrexate and misoprostol in early abortion.* Washington, DC: National Abortion Federation. Retrieved May 20, 2008, from http://www.prochoice.org

National Abortion Federation. (2002). *Protocol recommendations for use of mifepristone and misoprostol in early abortion.* Washington, DC: National Abortion Federation. Retrieved May 20, 2008, from http:/www.prochoice.org

National Abortion Federation. (2008). *NAF protocol for mifepristone/misoprostol in early abortion.* Washington, DC: National Abortion Federation. Retrieved May 20, 2008, from http:/www.prochoice.org

National Abortion Federation. (2008). *Facts about mifepristone (RU-486).* Washington, DC: National Abortion Federation. Retrieved May 21, 2008, from http://www.prochoice.org

Paul, M., Lichtenberg, S., Borgatta, L., Grimes, D. A., & Abdalla, M. (1999). *A clinician's guide to medical and surgical abortion.* Washington, DC: National Abortion Federation. Retrieved May 25, 2008, from http://www.prochoice.org

## ABORTION: PROTOCOL

TABLE A-1   FDA and Evidence-Based Regimens for Medical Abortions

|  | **FDA Regimen (49 d gestation)** | **Evidence-Based Regimen (63 d gestation)** |
|---|---|---|
| Mifepristone | 600 mg orally | 200 mg orally |
| Misoprostol Dosage | 400 mcg orally | 800 mcg bucally or vaginally |
| Misoprostol Timing | 48 h after mifepristone | 6–72 h after mifepristone < 56 d gestation |
|  |  | 6–48 h after mifepristone < 63 d gestation |
| Misoprotol Location | At medical office | At home |
| All suggestion follow up within 14 d |  |  |

Source: Adapted from National Abortion Federation. (2008). *NAF protocol for mifepristone/misoprostol in early abortion.* Retrieved May 8, 2008, from http://www.prochoice.org/pubs_research/publications/downloads/professional_education/medical_abortion/protocol_mife_miso.pdf

### Supportive Care

*N/V, Diarrhea*

Eat a light meal before misoprostol administration

Take prescribed antiemetic before initiating mifepristone or misoprostol

Take prescribed antidiarrhea agent

*Pain/Cramping*

Ibuprofen 600–800 mg PO q 6 h, starting 1 h before misoprostol administration

Acetaminophen w/ codeine (Tylenol #3) 1–2 tabs PO q 4–6 h, max 12 tabs/24 h

Hot water bottle or heating pad to abdomen or lower back PRN

Abdominal massage

*Abnormal Bleeding*

Bleeding normally slows 1–2 h after passing the pregnancy

Soaking > 2 pads per h for less than 2 h, reassure pt that the bleeding should decrease soon

Encourage rest, use of a heating pad or hot water bottle, NSAIDs, hydration w/ nonalcoholic or noncaffeinated beverages, and rising from resting position slowly

Encourage pt to contact you again in 1–2 h

Send pt to hospital if heavy bleeding persists longer than 10–12 h, s/sx hemorrhage (soaking > 2 pads for > 2 h), s/sx of hypovolemia

*Infection*

Prophylactic antibiotics can be started d 1 w/ mifepristone administration, however this is not considered a routine adjunct to medication-induced abortions

### SOURCES

National Abortion Federation. (2008). *Management of side effects and complications in medical abortion: A guide for triage and on-call staff.* Washington, DC: National Abortion Federation. Retrieved May 25, 2008, from http://www.prochoice.org

Postabortion Care Consortium Community Task Force. (2002). *Essential elements of postabortion care: An expanded and updated model.* Washington, DC: National Abortion Federation. Retrieved May 25, 2008, from http://www.prochoice.org

# ABORTION: SPONTANEOUS—GRIEF/LOSS DURING 1ST TRIMESTER AND EARLY 2ND TRIMESTER

**A**

Acknowledge the loss of the potential of this baby
Be available to the family
Consider F/U visit in 1 wk regardless of outcome (expectant management or D&C)
Discuss w/ pt genetic testing of aborted tissue, especially important if × 2 SABs
Screen pt for depression at F/U visit

## Questions to Ask at Visit Regarding Pregnancy Loss

"What was the hardest part for you?"
"Have you had awkward encounters?"
"How have your family members responded?"
"Who is your main support person?"
*Also see* Demise
*Also see* Depression

## Resources to Refer Patients to for Support After a Loss

*Miscarriage: A Shattered Dream* by Sherokee Ilse & Linda Hammer Burns
A collection of Internet articles about miscarriage—www.borntolove.com/miscarriage.html
Guidelines for supporting families experiencing a perinatal loss from the Canadian Paediatric Society (CPS)— www.cps.ca/english/statements/FN/fn01-02.htm
A clearinghouse for grief resources—www.centeringcorp.com/catalog/resourses.php
March of Dimes—www.marchofdimes.com/pnhec/572_4150.asp

**SOURCE**
Turner, M., & Bridges, M. (2006). *Silent warmth: Midwifery management of stillbirth.* Unpublished manuscript.

## ABORTION: SPONTANEOUS—MISCARRIAGE

### Definition
Pregnancy that ends spontaneously before the fetus reaches viability
WHO: expulsion or extraction of an embryo or fetus weighing < 500 g
(corresponds to a gestational age of 20–22 wks)
IUFD if > 22 wk
10–20% of documented pregnancies < 20 wks gestation will undergo SAB; of
these 80% will occur in the first 12 wks of pregnancy
Recurrent defined as × 3 SAB

### Risk Factors for SABs
Maternal age
Gravidity
Previous SAB
Smoking
ETOH abuse
Fever
Trauma (CVS, amnio)
Caffeine intake
Teratogens (e.g., parvovirus B19, drugs, environmental toxins)

### Diagnosis of SAB
U/S absence of fetal cardiac activity in an embryo w/ crown-rump length > 5 mm
U/S absence of a fetal pole

### Management of SAB
**Expectant:** GA < 13 wks w/o evidence of infection; may be as long as 2–4 wks
until completion; F/U w/ U/S
**Medical:** prostaglandin E1 analogue (misoprostil 800 mcg PV × 1 dose or
400 mcg PV q 4h × 4 doses, not recommended in asthmatics and those w/
glaucoma); POC expelled w/in 5 d of tx
**Surgical:** D&C: usually done w/ sepsis, heavy bleeding or if a pt does not want to
wait for spontaneous or medication-assisted expulsion

### Postsurgical Ab Care
Methergine series (0.2 mg q 4 h × 5 doses)
Doxycycline 100 mg BID on day of evacuation
Pelvic rest × 2 wks, birth control methods reviewed
Give Rhogam 300 mcg if woman is Rh negative

### Recurrent SAB Workup
*Office Visit*
Detailed family hx
Detailed PE
Discuss recurrence risks
Discourage cigarettes and alcohol
Order lab tests

*Lab Tests*
Parental chromosomal studies—chromosomal balance, autosomal trisomy
Karyotype aborted fetuses—often difficult to obtain fresh tissue and very expensive
Luteal phase defects testing by timed endometrial biopsy—if biopsy reveals < 2 d
of expected cycle, then luteal phase defect dx can be made
Endocrine testing—diabetes, thyroid
Endometrial infection testing—culture for ureaplasma urealyticum or CT
Hysterosalpingography or hysteroscopy—detect uterine anomalies or submucosal
leiomyomas
Autoimmune disease testing—aPL and aCL antibodies

*Treatment Options Depend on Diagnosis*
Surgical removal of uterine anomalies
Endocrine level control

Antibiotics—doxycycline 100 mg BID × 10 d or CT tx

Progesterone therapy—17 alpha-hydroxyprogesterone produced during first 7 wks of pregnancy by the corpus luteum; lack of production can result in recurrent SABs

**A**

## SOURCE

Hatcher, R. A. (2007). *Contraceptive technology* (19th ed.). New York, NY: Ardent Media Inc.

Gabbe, S. G., Niebyl, J. R., & Simpson, J. L. (Eds.). (2002). *Obstetrics: Normal and problem pregnancies* (4th ed.). New York: Churchill Livingstone.

## ABUSE: INTIMATE PARTNER VIOLENCE

### Screening

"Have you ever been hit, slapped, kicked, or otherwise physically hurt by your partner?"

"Have you ever been forced to have sexual activities?"

"Many women have had unpleasant sexual experiences—being touched or forced into sex—or they have been physically abused. Have you ever experienced anything like that?" (Simkin & Klaus, 2006, p. 1)

*Cycle That Repeats*

Tension building phase

Acute battering incident

Calm or loving phase

*Clinician's Role*

Screen every pt for abuse

Provide a safe space to discuss abuse

Assess pt safety

Provide access to resources

Document report of abuse

*Emergency Bag*

Money

Clothing

Bank records

Immunization records

Birth certificates

Protective legal orders

Keys

***Call police before abuse occurs

***Set up a 24 hour safety net

### Resources

National Domestic Violence Hotline at 1-800-799-SAFE—www.ndvh.org

ChildHelp USA National Child Abuse Hotline: 800-4-A-CHILD

National Child Abuse Hotline: 1-800-25-ABUSE

Elder Abuse Hotline: 800-252-8966

Nationwide RAINN National Rape Crisis Hotline: 800-656-4673

National Youth Crisis Hotline: 800-442-HOPE

Local Hotline: _____

Local Shelter: _____

Crisis Intervention: _____

### SOURCES

McFarlane, J., Greenberg, L., Weltge, A., & Watson, M. (2008). Identification of abuse in emergency departments: Effectiveness of a two question screening tool. *Journal of Emergency Nursing*, *21*(5), 391–394.

Simkin, P., & Klaus, P. (2006). When survivors give birth: Childhood sexual abuse and its impact on the woman's later childbearing. In K. D. Schuiling, & F. E. Likis (Eds.). *Women's gynecologic health*. Sudbury, MA: Jones and Bartlett.

# ALCOHOL ABUSE

A

### Red Flags for Abuse

Frequent absences from school or work

History of frequent trauma or accidental injuries

Depression or anxiety

Labile hypertension

GI symptoms, such as epigastric distress, diarrhea, or weight changes

Sexual dysfunction

Sleep disorders

### C.A.G.E.

**C**ut Back/**C**oncern: "Have you ever tried to **c**ut back?"; "Are you **c**oncerned about your drinking?"

**A**nnoyance: "Are you **a**nnoyed by comments about your drinking?"

**G**uilty: "Have you ever felt **g**uilty about your drinking?"

**E**ye Opener: "Do you ever need an '**e**ye opener' when you get up in the morning?"

*Alcoholics Anonymous*

www.alcoholics-anonymous.com

**SOURCE**

Mersy, D. J. (2003). Recognition of alcohol and substance abuse [see comment]. *American Family Physician, 67*(7), 1529–1532.

## ALPHA FETAL PROTEIN (AFP)

AFP (a glycoprotein) is produced first in the fetal yolk sac and then by the liver and GI tract of the developing fetus

Excreted into the amniotic fluid through the urine

AFP can be measured in the maternal serum

### Maternal Serum AFP Screening

Performed as part of the quad screen (between 15 and 22 wks) and measured w/ 1st trimester screening for Down's syndrome

Most accurate measurement obtained between 16 to 18 wks

Measured as ng/ml in maternal serum; reported as a multiple of the median (MOM)

### Patient Education

Screens for possible fetal anomalies

Approximately 3–5% of pregnant women screened are abnormal

Of those positive results, only 2–6% are true positives for a fetal abnormality

There is a greater chance the screen will be positive, and no fetal abnormality will be present than that the positive result stems from an actual problem w/ the fetus

### Causes of Elevated AFP (≥ 2.0 to 2.5 MOM)

Underestimated gestational age

Multiple gestations

Neural tube defects

Gastrointestinal obstruction/abnormality

Renal anomalies or urinary obstruction

Osteogenesis imperfecta

Low birth weight

Oligohydramnious

Low maternal BMI

Placental abnormalities

Black race

### Causes of Decreased AFP

Overestimated gestational age

Down's syndrome/other trisomies

High maternal BMI

### When AFP Levels Are Abnormal

Ensure that gestational age is appropriate based on pt hx and early U/S

Abnormal AFP levels indicate the need for further testing (level II U/S, amniocentesis)

Patient guidance and reassurance are very important

**SOURCES**

American College of Obstetricians and Gynecologists. (2003). Neural tube defects: Clinical management guidelines for obstetricians and gynecologists. In *2006 compendium of selected publications* (p. 754). Washington, DC: Author.

Cunningham, G., Leveno, K. J., Bloom, S. L., Hauth, J. C., Gilstrap, L. C., Wenstrom, K. D. (2005). *Williams obstetrics* (22nd ed). New York: McGraw-Hill Professional.

Thomas, R. L., & Blakemore, K. J. (1990). Evaluation of elevations in maternal serum alpha-fetoprotein: A review. *Obstetrical & Gynecological Survey, 45*(5), 271–283.

# AMENORRHEA AND ANOVULATION

A

### Definition of Amenorrhea

No period by age 14 in the absence of growth or development of secondary characteristics

No period by age 16 regardless of the presence of normal growth and development w/ the appearance of secondary sexual characteristics

"In a woman who has been menstruating, the absence of periods for a length of time equivalent to a total of at least three of the previous cycle intervals or 6 months of amenorrhea." (Spearoff & Fritz, 2005, p. 402)

### Primary Amenorrhea

Pregnancy

Mullerian agenesis (absence of a uterus and vagina, normal secondary sex characteristics present)

Testicular feminization (absence of a uterus, blind ending vaginal pouch, normal breast development, scant pubic and maxillary hair)

Lower genital tract problems (labial agglutination, imperforate hymen, transverse vaginal septum)

Hypergonadotrophic hypogonadism (FSH > 40 mIU/l), gonadal dysgenesis, ovarian enzyme disorder, resistant ovarian syndrome

### Secondary Amenorrhea

Pregnancy

Asherman's syndrome

Cervical stenosis

Hormonal contraception

Hypothyroidism

Polycystic ovarian syndrome

Pituitary tumor

Premature ovarian failure

Menopause

Hypothalamic/CNS disorders (stress, eating disorder, extreme athleticism)

### Anovulation

S/Sx:
  Irregular menstrual bleeding
  Amenorrhea
  Infertility
Physiologic causes:
  Pregnancy
  Lactation
  Perimenarch
  Perimenopause
Pathologic causes:
  Hyperandrogenic disorder (PCOS)
  Hyperprolactinemia
  Extreme stress

### Diagnosis

*Hx and PE*
  (Note: Anovulation manifesting as irregular bleeding and/or infertility requires same workup)
  Bleeding: Ensure hx/o menstruation
  Lifestyle:
    Gain or loss of body fat
    Stress
    Illness
    Eating disorder
    New medications
    Contraception history

Health:
    Illness
    Medications
    Contraception hx
    Surgeries and procedures—D&C, Ab, endometrial infection, cervical procedures
    S/sx of menopause
    Headaches
PE:
    Ht
    Wt
    Fat distribution
    Hair pattern
    Thyroid
    Vital signs
    Skin changes
    Tanner staging
    Galactorrhea
    Pelvic exam

*Labs*
    Pregnancy test
    TSH & Free T4
    Prolactin level

*Progestin Challenge*

**FIGURE A-1**  Progestin Challenge Protocol

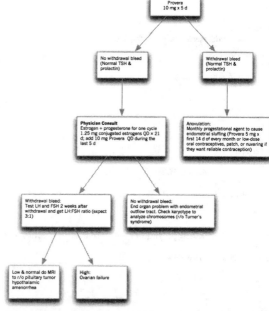

*Source:* Adapted from Speroff, L., & Fritz, M. A. (2005). *Clinical gynecology, endocrinology, infertility* (7th ed.). Philadelphia: Lippincott Williams & Wilkins.

# AMNIOINFUSION

## Facts

Amnioinfusion strikingly reduced the number of C/S, but had no significant effect on long-term neonatal outcomes (Hofmeyr, 1998)

Amnioinfusion is *not* indicated to dilute meconium-stained fluid

## Indications

Oligohydramnios

Repetitive variable fetal heart rate decelerations during labor

## Contraindications

Amnionitis

Polyhydramnios

Uterine hypertonus

Multiple gestation

Known uterine anomaly

Severe fetal distress

Non-vertex presentation

Fetal scalp pH < 7.2

Placental abruption

Placenta previa

## Procedure

\*\*\*Membranes must be ruptured\*\*\*

Place IUPC if not already in place

Apply internal fetal scalp lead or external Doppler

Obtain Ringer's lactate or sterile saline solution (warming the solution is not required)

Infused transcervically

Infused using gravity or IV pump

Bolus infusion: 500–800 ml in 30 min

Continuous infusion begins w/ 250 ml bolus then 10 ml/min for 1 h, maintenance at 3 ml/min

Monitor for polyhydramnios

Effects on FHR may not be noted for 20–30 min

## Risks

Umbilical cord prolapse

Uterine perforation

Placental abruption

Infection

Hypertonic contractions

Fetal heart rate abnormalities

Fetal malpresentation

Maternal cardiac or respiratory compromise

Maternal death

Amniotic fluid embolism

Uterine scar separation

### SOURCES

American College of Obstetricians and Gynecologists. (October 2006). *Amnioinfusion does not prevent meconium aspiration syndrome.* (No. 346). Washington, DC: Author.

Frye, A. (2004). *Holistic midwifery: A comprehensive textbook for midwives in homebirth practice.* Portland, OR: Labrys Press.

Hofmeyr, G. (1998). Amnioinfusion for potential and suspected umbilical cord compression in labour. *Cochrane Database of Systematic Reviews, 1*(CD000013).

Tharpe, N. (2006). *2006–2009 clinical practice guidelines for midwifery & women's health.* Sudbury, MA: Jones and Bartlett.

## AMNIOTOMY

### Weigh Risks and Benefits

"Evidence does not support the routine breaking the waters for women in spontaneous labour." (Smyth, Alldred, & Markham, 2007, p. 1)

### Indications for Amniotomy

To attach an internal fetal monitor electrode

Baby about to be born w/ membranes intact w/ possible meconium-stained fluid

Need to stimulate/augment labor

Best to AROM after active labor w/ well-established contraction pattern and cervix dilated to 4–5 cm

### Hazards/undesirable Effects:

Cord prolapse—especially if head is unengaged or w/ compound presentation, breech, or small baby (less than 2000 g)

Intrauterine infection if labor progression is slow

Cord compression

Uneven head compression w/ more extensive molding and caput succedeum may increase the risk of IVH

### Procedure

Have woman empty bladder

Check FHR

White pad or surface on which to view color of fluid

Ensure vertex presentation w/ head engaged

R/o cord presentation, vasa previa

Use an amnicot or amnihook to gently create a hole in the bag

Leave fingers in vagina through next ctx to evaluate effect on dilation of cvx, and to assess for cord prolapse

Evaluate FHR during and after procedure

**SOURCES**

Frye, A. (2004). *Holistic midwifery A comprehensive textbook for midwives in homebirth practice.* Portland, OR: Labrys Press.

Smyth R. M. D., Alldred S. K., & Markham C. (2007). Amniotomy for shortening spontaneous labor (review). *Cochrane Database of Systematic Reviews, 4*(CD006167).

Varney, H., Kriebs, J. M., & Gegor, C. L. (2004). *Varney's midwifery* (4th ed.). Sudbury, MA: Jones and Bartlett.

# ANEMIA

## Labs
Rule of thumb: HCT = Hb × 3; normal Hb = 12–16 g/dl
CBC w/ indices (MCV, MCHC, RDW, reticulocytes)
Normal MCV = 80–96
Reticulocyte count indicates the number of immature red blood cells; increases
   2–3 wks after initiation of iron therapy for anemia
RBC lifespan = 120 d

## Diagnosis
Microcytic anemia: MCV < 80, hypochromic, low MCHC
Macrocytic anemia: $B_{12}$/folate deficiency, MCV > 96, malabsorption of $B_{12}$ (possible
   lack of intrinsic factor; vegan diet)
Anemia can be related to overall blood volume/dilution, i.e., pregnancy,
   hemorrhage, dehydration

## Follow-Up
Recheck CBC w/ indices in 2 wks
Hb electrophoresis (test all women of Asian, Mediterranean, African descent)
Patient compliance
Parasites
Folate deficiency
Chronic disease

TABLE A-2   Cutoff Values for Anemia in Pregnant Women

| | Hemoglobin (<g/dl) | Hematocrit (<%) |
|---|---|---|
| *Trimester* | | |
| First | 11.0 | 33.0 |
| Second | 10.5 | 32.0 |
| Third | 11.0 | 33.0 |
| *Adjustment for smoking* | | |
| 0.5–<1.0 packs/day | +0.3 | +1.0 |
| 1.0–<2.0 packs/day | +0.5 | +1.5 |
| >2.0 packs/day | +0.7 | +1.0 |
| *Adjustment for altitude (feet)* | | |
| 3,000–3,999 | +0.2 | +0.5 |
| 4,000–4,999 | +0.3 | +1.0 |
| 5,000–5,999 | +0.5 | +1.5 |
| 6,000–6,999 | +0.7 | +2.0 |
| 7,000–7,999 | +1.0 | +3.0 |
| 8,000–8,999 | +1.3 | +4.0 |

*Source:* Reprinted with permission from Graves, B. W., & Barger, M. K. (2001). A "conservative"
approach to iron supplementation during pregnancy. *Journal of Midwifery & Women's Health, 46*(3), 159.

### ANEMIA PREVENTION BREW
½ oz dried nettle leaves
½ oz dried parsley leaves
½ oz dried comfrey leaves
½ oz dried yellow dock
¼ oz peppermint leaves

Place herbs into container and cover w/ 4 cups of water
Steep for at least 8 h
This brew is an excellent source of iron, folic acid, vitamin $B_{12}$, and vitamin C
The mint is for flavor
Drink up to 4 cups daily for 1 wk each month

## Treatment

Supplements are available as ferrous and ferric iron

TABLE A-3    Oral Iron Preparations

| Oral Iron Preparations | Dose | Elemental [Iron] |
|---|---|---|
| Ferrous sulfate | 325 mg TID | 65 mg |
| Ferrous sulfate | 200 mg TID | 65 mg |
| Ferrous gluconate | 325 mg TID | 36 mg |
| Ferrous fumarate | 325 mg BID | 106 mg |

*Source:* Adapted from Varney, H., Kriebs, J. M., & Gegor, C. L. (2004). *Varney's midwifery* (4th ed.). Sudbury, MA: Jones and Bartlett.

Ferrous forms are the most readily absorbed
Elemental iron content indicates the amount of iron that is available for absorption
Severity of anemia dictates amount of daily supplementation (60–120 mg of elemental iron QD)

*Side Effects*
Nausea
Constipation
Diarrhea
Cramping
Black stool

## Iron Absorption Tips

Take iron supplement between meals or 30 min before eating
Avoid calcium and magnesium ingestion w/ iron
Do take w/ vitamin C (orange juice, tomato juice)
Cook iron-rich foods in minimal amount of water, for shortest time needed
Iron from meat, poultry, and fish is absorbed most readily
*See also* Blood: Hemoglobin electrophoresis

### SOURCES

Burrow, G., Duffy, T., & Copel, J. (2004). *Medical complications during pregnancy* (6th ed.). Philadelphia: Elsevier Saunders.

Centers for Disease Control and Prevention. (2005). *Pediatric and pregnancy nutrition surveillance system health indicators.* Retrieved May 29, 2008, from http://www.cdc.gov/pednss/what_is/pnss_health_indicators.htm#Maternal%20Health%20Indicators

Desai, S. P. (2004). *Clinician's guide to laboratory medicine: A practical approach* (3rd ed.). Hudson, OH: Lexi-Comp.

Frye, A. (2004). *Holistic midwifery: A comprehensive textbook for midwives in homebirth practice.* Portland, OR: Labrys Press.

Graves, B. W., & Barger, M. K. (2001). A "conservative" approach to iron supplementation during pregnancy. *Journal of Midwifery & Women's Health, 46*(3), 159.

Varney, H., Kriebs, J. M., & Gegor, C. L. (2004). *Varney's midwifery* (4th ed.). Sudbury, MA: Jones and Bartlett.

Weed, S. S. (1985). *Wise women herbals for the childbearing year.* Woodstock, NY: Ash Tree Publishing.

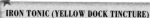

## IRON TONIC (YELLOW DOCK TINCTURE)

2 oz dried yellow dock roots
4 T honey
2 T brandy (optional)

Put yellow dock roots into a container; add 4 cups boiling water, cover
Infuse the tincture for at least 8 h or overnight
Strain and discard roots
Steam liquid over low heat until it is reduced to 1 cup, careful to not boil the tincture
Add honey; stir to dissolve
Now bring tincture briefly to a boil, pour into a clean container
Add brandy if desired. Take 1–2 T daily as an iron supplement

# ANTENATAL CARE

**TABLE A-4**   Antenatal Care Outline

| Gestational Age | Lab Tests | Education |
|---|---|---|
| 11–13 wks<br>Visits q month | 1st trimester screen<br>Cystic fibrosis<br>CVS (9–14)<br>New OB labs<br>Dating U/S | Prenatal care overview<br>Pregnancy progression<br>Diet, exercise, vitamins<br>Medications<br>Common discomforts |
| 15–20 wks<br>Visits q month | Anatomy U/S (18–20)<br>Quad screen (16–22)<br>Amniocentesis (15+) | Childbirth classes<br>Weight gain<br>Flu shot |
| 26–28 wks<br>Visits q 2 wks | Glucose screen<br>HCT/Hgb<br>HIV<br>Antibody screen/Rh | When to call<br>Danger signs<br>Kick counts |
| 32–34 wks<br>Visits q 2 wks | | Going to the hospital<br>Pediatrics, breastfeeding, circumcision<br>Anesthesia/analgesia<br>Traveling/work<br>Sexuality |
| 36 wks<br>Visits q week | GBS culture<br>Herpes prophylaxis | Labor talk<br>GBS |
| 37–40 wks<br>Visits q week | | Postpartum/going home<br>Support system<br>Contraception<br>Post dates (NST & induction) |

**TABLE A-5**   Antenatal Care: Common Initial Labs

| Lab Tests | Reason |
|---|---|
| Pap smear | Assess for overall health of cervical epithelia, no need to repeat if WNL within the last 6 mo |
| GC/CT culture | Infection with GC or CT increases the risk of PTL, PPROM, and neonatal sepsis |
| Hb/HCT | Assess for anemia; early intervention promotes better pregnancy outcomes |
| Blood type/Rh factor | Identify Rh neg pts |
| Antibody screen (Indirect Coombs') | Assess for previous exposure to Rh antibodies; pos screen requires MD consult |
| Syphilis | Assess for syphilis infection; positive result requires f/u with FTA-ABS to assess for current vs. previous infection |
| HIV | Consent must be given for this test to be performed<br>Treatment of infected mothers has been shown to decrease the risk of vertical transmission of HIV |
| Hepatitis B | Presence of core antigen indicates pos Hep B infection<br>Surface antibody only indicates Hep B immunity conferred by vaccination or previous infection<br>Infants born to pts pos for Hep B need to be treated with Hep B immunoglobulin |
| Rubella titer | Neonatal rubella infection can lead to severe birth defects<br>Mothers not immune to rubella need to be cautioned about exposure during the pregnancy and should be vaccinated postpartum |

/ continues

TABLE A-5    Antenatal Care: Common Initial Labs (continued)

| Lab Tests | Reason |
|---|---|
| Urinalysis | Asymptomatic bacturia should be treated to prevent pyelonephritis |
| PPD (Tuberculin test) | Assess for TB infection<br>Should *not* be performed if pt had previous positive test |
| Hb electrophoresis | Should be performed if pt's hx or ethnicity indicates the need |
| *Varicella* antibody titer | Assess for immunity to *Varicella*<br>Test if pt has no hx/o previous infection or vaccination |

Sources: Desai, S. P. (2004). *Clinician's guide to laboratory medicine: A practical approach* (3rd ed.). Hudson, OH: Lexi-Comp. Varney, H., Kriebs, J. M., & Gegor, C. L. (2004). *Varney's midwifery* (4th ed.). Sudbury, MA: Jones and Bartlett.

TABLE A-6    Antenatal Care: F/U Labs

| Lab/Test | Gestation | Reason |
|---|---|---|
| Quad screen | 15–20 wk | Screen for Down's syndrome, trisomy 18, NTDs |
| GCT/GTT | 24–28 wk | Assess for GDM. At risk pts should be tested earlier |
| Hb/HCT | 28 wk/36 wk | Assess for anemia |
| Antibody screen | 28 wk | To ensure no cross-reactivity in Rh neg pts with an Rh pos baby<br>Rhogam should be give to Rh neg pts.<br>Pos result requires MD consult |
| GBS screen | 36 wk | Screen for lower genital tract/rectal GBS colonization<br>Tx pos pts in labor |
| Urinalysis | Q visit | Screen for asymptomatic bacturia, proteinuria, and glycosuria |
| Syphilis/ HIV | 28 wk/36 wk | High-risk populations should be screened accordingly |
| GC/CT culture | 28 wk/36 wk | High-risk populations should be screened accordingly |
| Wet mount | Per pt c/o of s/sx of vaginitis | Assessment for c/o vaginitis<br>Current evidence is controversial, but some studies suggest a link between bacterial vaginosis and PTL |

Sources: Desai, S. P. (2004). *Clinician's guide to laboratory medicine: A practical approach* (3rd ed.). Hudson, OH: Lexi-Comp. Varney, H., Kriebs, J. M., & Gegor, C. L. (2004). *Varney's midwifery* (4th ed.). Sudbury, MA: Jones and Bartlett.

# ANTENATAL: NEW OB VISIT

**A**

### Intake Information
Planned vs. unplanned
Wanted vs. unwanted
Dating
OB/GYN hx
Med/Surg hx
Family hx
Genetic hx for mom and FOB
Social hx (relationship w/ FOB)
Allergies
Vaccine hx
Cats, seatbelts, guns, domestic violence
Vitamins

### Discussion Points
Outline prenatal care
Overview of practice
Initial OB info packet
Genetic testing (ethnicity for guidance)

### Baseline exam
BP
Ht
Wt
BMI

### Initial Labs
CBC
Platelets
Blood Type/Rh
Antibody screen
HCT/Hb
RPR
HIV
HBsAG
Rubella
Urine C/S

### P/E
Skin—assess for lesions
Thyroid—assess for enlargement, tenderness, nodules
Heart/lung—assess for breath sounds, heart rate/rhythm
Breast—assess for masses, tenderness, skin changes, nipple d/c
Abdomen—assess for masses, tenderness, bowel sounds
Extremities/DTRs—rate reflexes, assess for edema
Vagina—assess for rugae, discharge
Genitalia—assess for lesions, rashes
Cervix—assess for friability, lesions, motion tenderness
Uterus—assess for size, shape, position
Adenexa—assess for masses, tenderness

### Optional Labs
Cystic fibrosis
1st trimester screen
Pap—depending on date/results of last exam
GC/CT
Wet mount

# ANTIANXIETY/SEDATIVE AGENTS

TABLE A-7   Antianxiety/Sedative Agents

| Agent and Risk Categories | Half Life | Pharmacology |
|---|---|---|
| Ambien (zolpidem)<br><br>Preg C<br>Lact L3 | 2.5–2.8 hours | Liver metabolized<br>CYP450<br>Urine excretion<br>Class: Anxiolytic/Hypnotic<br>Non-BZD<br>Interacts with GABA-benzodiazepine receptor complexes |
| Benadryl (diphenhydramine)<br><br>Preg B<br>Lact L2 | 2–8 hours | Liver metabolized<br>CYP450<br>Urinary excretion<br>Class: Antihistamines, sedation, antitussives/expectorant, anaphylaxis, anti-Parkinsonians<br>Antagonizes central and peripheral H1 receptors and suppresses the medulla cough center, possesses anticholinergic properties, antiemetic and sedative effects |
| Phenergan (promethazine)<br><br>Preg C<br>Lact L2 | 7–14 hours | Liver metabolized<br>CYP450<br>Urine and feces excretion<br>Class: N/V<br>Antagonizes central and peripheral H1 receptors |

| Contraindications/Cautions | Side Effects |
|---|---|
| Hypersensitivity to class | Headache |
| Use of other depressants | Drowsiness |
| Alcohol use | Dizziness |
| Depression | Lethargy |
| Psychiatric disorders | Drugged feeling |
| Impaired respiratory and liver function | Back pain |
| | Allergic reactions |
| | Diarrhea |
| | Sinusitis |
| | Pharyngitis |
| | Dry mouth |
| | Palpitations |
| | Depression |
| | Rash |
| | Suicidal ideations |
| | Aggressive behavior |
| | Hallucinations |
| | Withdrawal symptoms |
| Hypersensitivity to class | Sedation |
| Newborns, premature infants | Dizziness |
| Breastfeeding | Coordination problems |
| Glaucoma | Thickened bronchial secretions |
| Increased IOP | Dry mucous membranes |
| GI obstruction | Blurred vision |
| Bladder neck obstruction | Paradoxical CNS stimulation |
| Asthma | Constipation |
| Cardiovascular dx | Palpitations/tachycardia |
| HTN | Urinary retention |
| Peptic ulcer | Epigastric discomfort |
| CNS depressant use | Anorexia |
| | Confusion |
| | Tremor |
| | Chest tightness |
| | Tinnitus |
| | Rash/urticaria |
| | Photosensitivity |
| Bone-marrow cardiovascular or liver dx | Drowsiness |
| Compromised respiratory function | Sedation |
| Glaucoma | Blurred vision |
| Stenosing peptic ulcer | Dizziness |
| Pyloroduodenal obstruction | Confusion |
| Bladder-neck obstruction | Extrapyramidal effects |
| Hx of seizure disorder | Dry mouth |
| Sulfite allergy | Dermatitis |
| | Photosensitivity |
| | Rhinitis |
| | Urinary retention |
| | Tissue damage |
| | Respiratory depression |
| | Seizures |
| | Leukopenia |
| | Agranulocytosis |
| | Hallucinations |
| | Brady/tachycardia |

/ continues

TABLE A-7  Antianxiety/Sedative Agents (continued)

| Agent and Risk Categories | Half Life | Pharmacology |
|---|---|---|
| Seconal (secobarbital)<br><br>Preg D<br>Lact L3 | 28 hours | Liver metabolized CYP450<br>Urine excreted<br>Anxiolytic/hypnotic<br>Non-BZD<br>Alters sensory cortex<br>Produced sedation<br>Hypnosis<br>Anesthesia |
| Versed (midazolam)<br><br>Preg D<br>Lact L3 | 2.5 hours | Liver metabolized<br>CYP450<br>Active metabolite<br>Urine excretion<br>BZD 1, short acting<br>Bind to benzodiazepine receptors<br>Enhances GABA effects |
| Vistaril (hydraxyzine)<br><br>Preg C<br>Lact L1 | 20–25 hours | Liver metabolized<br>CYP450<br>Active metabolites (cetirizine)<br>Urine excreted<br>Class: Anxiolytic/hypnotics<br>Non-BZD, Antihistamine, sedating<br>Antagonizes central and peripheral H1 receptors |

| Contraindications/Cautions | Side Effects |
|---|---|
| Hypersensitivity | Drowsiness |
| Severe respiratory distress | Lethargy |
| Porphyria | Respiratory depression |
| Liver impairment | Stevens-Johnson syndrome |
| Impaired renal function | Angioedema |
| Elderly | Dependency/abuse |
| | Hepatotoxicity |
| | Complex sleep-related behavior |
| Hypersensitivity to class | Nausea |
| Glaucoma | Vomiting |
| Shock | Sedation |
| CNS depression | Headache |
| Substance abuse | Hypotension |
| COPD | Agitation |
| CHF | Involuntary movements |
| Impaired renal and liver function | Retrograde amnesia |
| | Euphoria |
| | Hallucination |
| | Confusion |
| | Ataxia |
| | Dizziness |
| | Metallic taste |
| | Dry mouth |
| | Constipation |
| | Urticaria |
| | Rash |
| | Respiratory arrest |
| | Cardiac arrest |
| | Withdrawal symptoms |
| Hypersensitivity to class | Dry mouth |
| Pregnancy 1st trimester | Drowsiness |
| Asthma | Dizziness |
| | Ataxia |
| Never given IV | Weakness |
| | Slurred speech |
| | Headache |
| | Agitation |
| | Bitter taste |
| | Nausea |
| | Wheezing |
| | Dyspnea |
| | Seizures |

Sources: Adapted from Epocrates, I. (2008). Epocrates online. Retrieved May 27, 2008, from http://www.epocrates.com. Hale, T. W. (2008). Medications and mothers' milk (13th ed.). Amarillo, TX: Hale Publishing. Thompson Healthcare Inc. (2007). MICROMEDEX: Healthcare series. Retrieved May 27, 2008, from http://www.micromedex.com

## ANTIBIOTICS

TABLE A-8    Antibiotics

| Class | Antibiotic (Preg Cat; Lact Cat) | Clinical Use |
|---|---|---|
| Aminoglycosides | Gentamicin (C; L2)<br>Tobramycin (D; L3)<br>Amikacin (D; L2)<br>Kanamycin (D; L2)<br>Streptomycin (D; L3) | Gram neg<br>Most often used in combo with PCN, cephalosporins, and vancomycin |
| Antianaerobic agents | Metronidazole (B; L2)<br>Clindamycin (B; L2) | Anaerobic organisms<br>Metro—*C. diff*, BV, trich<br>Clinda—Gram pos, toxoplasmosis, *P. cainii* pneumonia, toxic shock, PID |
| Beta-lactam/ beta-lactamase inhibitors | Amoxicillin-clavulanic acid (B; L1)<br>Ampicillin-sulbactam (B; L1)<br>Piperacillin-tazobactam (B; L2)<br>Ticarcillin-clavulanic acid (B; L1) | Polymicrobial infections |
| Carbapenems | Imipenem-cilastatin (C; L2)<br>Meropenem (B; L3)<br>Ertapenem  (B;L2) | Polymicrobial infections<br>No oral bioavailability<br>Cilastin provides Imipenem with resistance to bacterial dehydropepidase |
| Cephalosporins | 1st gen: cefazolin, cephalexin, cefadroxil (all B; L1)<br>2nd gen: cefuroxime (B; L2), cefoxitin (B; L1), cefotetan (B; L2)<br>3rd gen: ceftriaxone (B; L2), cefotaxime (B; L2), ceftazidime (B, L1), cefdinir (B; L2)<br>4th gen: cefepime (B; L2) | 1st gen: gram pos skin infections, pneumococcal RTIs, UTIs, presurgery prophylaxis<br>2nd gen: CAP, RTIs, skin infections, meningitis<br>3rd gen: community acquired bacterial meningitis<br>Nosocomial infections: ceftazidime, cefepime (esp. *P. aeruginosa*) |
| Chloramphenicol | Chloramphenicol (C; L4) | Bacterial meningitis in PCN allergic pts<br>Rocky Mountain spotted fever and typhus in tetracycline-allergic pts or pregnant women<br>Tx VRE infection |
| Fluoroquinolones | Ciprofloxacin (C; L3)<br>Ofloxacin (C; L2)<br>Norfloxacin (C; L3)<br>Levofloxacin (C; L3)<br>Gatifloxacin (C; L3)<br>Moxifloxacin (C; L3, L2 ophthalmically)<br>Sparfloxacin (C; L3)<br>Trovafloxacin (C; L4) | UTIs<br>STIs<br>Soft tissue infections<br>GI infections<br>Osteomyelitis<br>Cipro for nosocomial RTIs; meningococcal prophylaxis |

/ continues

TABLE A-8   Antibiotics (continued)

| Class | Antibiotic (Preg Cat; Lact Cat) | Clinical Use |
|---|---|---|
| Lipopeptides | Daptomycin (B; L3) | Skin infections including MRSA<br>Gram pos microbes: *Staphalycoccus aureus, Streptococcus pyogenese, S. agalactiae, S. dysgalactiae, Enterococcus faecalis* |
| Macrolides | Erythromycin (B; L2, L3 early postnatal d/t risk of pyloric stenosis)<br>Clarithromycin (C; L1)<br>Azithromycin (B; L2)<br>Dirithromycin (C; L3)<br>Telithromycin (C; L3) | Skin infections<br>STIs<br>Chlamydia, Rickettsia, Legionellae |
| Monobactams | Aztreonam (B; L2) | RTIs; UTIs; gram neg organisms |
| Oxazolidinones | Linezolid (C; L3) | Community- and hospital-acquired pneumonia, skin structure infections, VRE, MRSA, PCN resistant strep |
| Penicillins | Penicillin G (B; L1)<br>Ampicillin (B; L1)<br>Amoxicillin (B; L1) | Upper and lower RTIs, UTIs, STIs<br>CNS infections |
| Rifampin | Rifampin (C; L2) | Tuberculosis; combine with cell wall-active agent to tx gram pos infections that fail to respond to other tx |
| Streptogramins | Quinuspristin/dalforpristin (B; L3) | Skin infections: VRE, MRSA |
| Sulfonimides | Trimethoprim-sulfamethoxazole (C, D 3rd tri; L3)<br>Sulfaslazine (B; L3) | 1st line for UTIs;<br>Ulcerative colitis (sulfasalazine) |
| Tetracyclines | Tetracycline (D; L2)<br>Doxycycline (D; L3, L4 if long-term use)<br>Minocycline (D; L2, L4 if long-term use) | Broad spectrum: gram neg, Rickettsia, Chlamydia, PID, acne<br>Typically used when beta-lactams are not an option<br>Doxycycline is tx of choice in early Lyme's disease dx |
| Vancomycin | Vancomycin (C; L1) | MRSA; *Clostridium* species |

*Sources:* Adapted from Arcangelo, V. P., & Peterson, A. M. (Eds.). (2006). *Pharmacotherapeutics for advanced practice: A practical approach* (2nd ed.). Philadelphia: Lippincott Williams and Wilkins. Hale, T. W. (2008). *Medications and mothers' milk* (13th ed.). Amarillo, TX: Hale Publishing.

See also Lactation Risk Categories
See also Pregnancy Risk Categories

## APGAR

****Apgar score alone cannot establish hypoxia or acidosis****

TABLE A-9 APGAR Score

| Sign | 0 | 1 | 2 |
|---|---|---|---|
| Color | Blue or pale | Acrocyanotic | Completely pink |
| Heart rate | Absent | < 100 minute | > 100 minute |
| Reflex irritability | No response | Grimace | Cry or active withdrawal |
| Muscle tone | Limp | Some flexion | Active motion |
| Respiration | Absent | Weak cry; hypoventilation | Good, crying |
| | | | **Total** |

Source: Reprinted with permission from American College of Obstetricians and Gynecologists, American Academy of Pediatrics, & Gynecologists and Committee on Obstetric Practice. (2006). The apgar score. Pediatrics, 117, 1444.

**Important Factors Affecting APGAR**
   Gestational age
   Timing
   Personnel training
   Maternal medications
   Resuscitation efforts

**1-Minute APGAR**
   Does *not* correlate w/ infant's future outcome

**5-Minute APGAR**
   If the 5-min APGAR < 7, additional scores should be obtained q 5 min until two scores > 8 are recorded; these scores indicate the effectiveness of resuscitative efforts

   0–3: correlates poorly w/ future neurological problems, low scores alone are "not conclusive markers of an acute intrapartum hypoxic event" (ACOG, 2006, pp. 1210–1211)

   4–6: "Scores of 4, 5, and 6 are intermediate and are not markers of increased risk of neurologic dysfunction. Such scores may be the result of physiologic immaturity, maternal medications, the presence of congenital malformations, and other factors." (ACOG, 2006, p. 1210–1211)

   7–10: considered normal

**10-Minute APGAR and Beyond**
   "The risk of poor neurologic outcomes increases when the Apgar score is 3 or less at 10, 15, and 20 minutes" (ACOG, 2006, p. 1210)

**SOURCES**

Frye, A. (2004). *Holistic midwifery: A comprehensive textbook for midwives in homebirth practice.* Portland, OR: Labrys Press.

American College of Obstetricians and Gynecologists, American Academy of Pediatrics, & Gynecologists and Committee on Obstetric Practice. (2006). The apgar score. *Pediatrics, 117,* 1444.

# ASTHMA CLASSIFICATION

TABLE A-10   Asthma Classification System

| Classification | Symptoms | Night Symptoms | Lung Function |
|---|---|---|---|
| Step 1: mild intermittent asthma | Symptoms occurring twice a week or less<br>No symptoms and normal PEF between exacerbations<br>Brief exacerbations (lasting a few hours to days) with variable intensity | Symptoms occurring no more than twice a month | $FEV_1/FVC$ is 80% or more of predicted<br>PEF variability of less than 20% |
| Step 2: mild persistent asthma | Symptoms occurring more than twice a week<br>Exacerbations may affect activity | Symptoms occurring more than twice a month | $FEV_1/FVC$ is 80% or more of predicted<br>PEF variability of 20 to 30% |
| Step 3: moderate persistent asthma | Daily symptoms<br>Daily use of inhaled short-acting beta agonist<br>Exacerbations affect activity<br>Exacerbations occur more than twice a week and may last for days | Symptoms occurring more than once a week | $FEV_1/FVC$ is greater than 60% but less than 80% of predicted<br>PEF variability of greater than 30% |
| Step 4: severe persistent asthma | Continual symptoms<br>Limited physical activity<br>Frequent exacerbations | Frequent symptoms | $FEV_1/FVC$ is 60% or less of predicted<br>PEF variability of greater than 30% |

PEF = peak expiratory flow; $FEV_1$ = forced expiratory volume in one second; FVC = forced vital capacity; $FEV_1/FVC\%$ = $FEV_1$ as percentage of FVC.

*Source:* Reprinted from National Heart, Lung, and Blood Institute. (2002). *Guidelines for the diagnosis and management of asthma* (No. 02-5075). Bethesda, MD: NIH.

TABLE A-11  Asthma Treatment

| | |
|---|---|
| Step 1: mild intermittent asthma | No daily medication needed |
| Step 2: mild persistent asthma | One daily medication:<br>Anti-inflammatory drug<br>Low-dose inhaled corticosteroid or cromolyn (Intal) or nedocromil (Tilade)<br>Children usually begin with a trial of cromolyn or nedocromil<br>Zafirlukast (Accolate), or zileuton (Zyflo) may also be considered in patients 12 years or older<br>*or*<br>Sustained-release theophylline to serum concentration of 5 to 15 µg per mL is an alternative but not preferred therapy |
| Step 3: moderate persistent asthma | One daily medication:<br>Medium-dose inhaled corticosteroid<br>*or*<br>Two daily medications:<br>Low- to medium-dose inhaled corticosteroid and long-acting bronchodilator, especially for nighttime symptoms (either salmeterol [Serevent], sustained-release theophylline or long-acting beta$_2$ agonist tablets) |
| Step 4: severe persistent asthma | Daily medications:<br>High-dose inhaled corticosteroid<br>*and*<br>Long-acting bronchodilator (salmeterol, sustained-release theophylline or long-acting beta$_2$ agonist tablets)<br>*and*<br>Oral corticosteroid in a dosage of 2 mg per kg per day with the daily dose generally not exceeding 60 mg |
| Quick relief | Short-acting inhaled beta$_2$ agonist as needed |

*Source:* Reprinted from National Heart, Lung, and Blood Institute. (2002). *Guidelines for the diagnosis and management of asthma* (No. 02-5075). Bethesda, MD: NIH.

TABLE A-12  Asthma Medications

| Agent | Low Dose (per day) | Medium Dose (per day) | High Dose (per day) |
|---|---|---|---|
| Beclomethasone (Beclovent, Vanceril): 42 and 84 µg per puff | Adults: 4 to 12 puffs at 42 µg per puff or 2 to 6 puffs at 84 µg per puff | Adults: 12 to 20 puffs at 42 µg per puff or 6 to 10 puffs at 84 µg per puff | Adults: more than 20 puffs at 42 µg per puff or more than 10 puffs at 84 µg per puff |
| Budesonide (Pulmicort): 200 µg per puff | Adults: 1 or 2 puffs Children: 1 puff | Adults: 2 or 3 puffs Children: 1 or 2 puffs | Adults: more than 3 puffs Children: more than 2 puffs |
| Flunisolide (AeroBid): 250 µg per puff | Adults: 2 to 4 puffs Children: 2 or 3 puffs | Adults: 4 to 8 puffs Children: 4 or 5 puffs | Adults: more than 8 puffs Children: more than 5 puffs |
| Fluticasone (Flovent): 44 µg, 110 µg, and 220 µg per puff | Adults: 2 to 6 puffs at 44 µg per puff or 2 puffs at 110 µg per puff | Adults: 2 to 6 puffs at 110 µg per puff | Adults: more than 6 puffs at 110 µg per puff or more than 3 puffs at 220 µg per puff |
| Triamcinolone acetonide (Azmacort): 100 µg per puff | Adults: 4 to 10 puffs Children: 4 to 8 puffs | Adults: 10 to 20 puffs Children: 8 to 12 puffs | Adults: more than 20 puffs Children: more than 12 puffs |
| Cromolyn sodium MDI (Intal), 800 mg per puff; nebulizer, 20 mg per 2-mL ampule | Adults: 6 puffs or 3 ampules in three divided doses Children: 3 puffs or 3 ampules in three divided doses | Adults: 9 to 12 puffs in three divided doses Children: 6 puffs in three divided doses | Adults: 16 puffs in three divided doses or 4 ampules in four divided doses Children: 8 puffs or 4 ampules in four divided doses |
| Nedocromil (Tilade), 1.75 mg per puff | Adults: 4 to 6 puffs in two to three divided doses | Adults: 9 to 12 puffs in two to three divided doses | Adults: 16 puffs in four divided doses |

Source: Reprinted from National Heart, Lung, and Blood Institute. (2002). Guidelines for the diagnosis and management of asthma (No. 02-5075). Bethesda, MD: NIH.

# AUTOIMMUNE DISORDERS IN PREGNANCY

## Antiphospholipid Syndrome (APS)
70% of cases are women
Usually serum positive for anticardiolipin antibody (aCL) and/or lupus anticoagulant (LA)
Often more than one test needed for confirmation
False positive serologic tests for syphilis may indicate APS or SLE

*Maternal Issues*
Arterial and venous thrombosis
Thrombocytopenia
Preeclampsia
Multiple SABs

*Fetal issues*
IUGR
Placental insufficiency
Iatrogenic preterm birth
Fetal death

*Treatment*
Low-dose aspirin
Heparin
Fetal monitoring initiated at 24 wks
Coumadin postpartum

## Systemic Lupus Erythematosus (SLE)
Immune system overstimulation resulting in inflammation and tissue damage; usually 2nd–3rd decade of life
Prevalence 1/700 women (Sacks et al., 2002)
African-American women 1/245 (Sacks et al., 2002)

*Maternal Issues*
Symptoms mimic preeclampsia
Thrombocytopenia
Proteinuria
Renal insufficiency

*Fetal Issues*
SAB
PROM
Heart block
Cardiac defects
Growth restriction
IUFD

*Treatment*
NSAIDs
Antimalarials
Steroids
Immunosuppressants if maternal condition is worsening

**Rheumatoid Arthritis (RA)**

A

Chronic inflammatory, autoimmune disease characterized by bilateral joint involvement; predominantly affects women of childbearing age

*Maternal Issues*

Usually in remission during pregnancy

Effect on pregnancy mild

Preexisting anemia may enhance physiologic anemia

If pelvic deformity, vaginal birth may be difficult

Severe flare up by 2 mos postpartum common

*Fetal Issues*

RA factor does not cross placenta

*Treatment*

Physical therapy

NSAIDs

**Idiopathic Thrombocytopenia (ITP)**

Most common in women

Mean onset 2nd to 3rd decade of life

Not substantially influenced by pregnancy

Dx of exclusion (must R/o HELLP-ITP usually has normal RBC count)

*Maternal Issues*

Increased risk for hemorrhage (especially postpartum)

Method for delivery controversial, partially determined by fetal platelet count

*Fetal Issues*

Fetal thrombocytopenia

Need for early fetal surveillance

*Treatment*

Dependent on severity of disease

Supportive

Immune globulin

Platelets

Steroids

Splenectomy

**SOURCES**

Burrow, G., Duffy, T., & Copel, J. (2004). *Medical complications during pregnancy* (6th ed.). Philadelphia: Elsevier Saunders.

Creasy, R. K., & Resnik, R. (2004). *Maternal-fetal medicine* (5th ed.). Philadelphia: Saunders.

Centers for Disease Control and Prevention. (2002). Trends in deaths from systemic lupus erythematosus—United States, 1979–1998. *Morbidity and Mortality Weekly Report, 51*(RR-17). Retrieved November 24, 2008, from http://www.cdc.gov/mmwr/preview/mmwrhtml/mm5117a3. htm

Sacks, J. J., Helmick, C. G., Langmaid, G., & Sniezek, J. E. (2002). Trends in deaths from systemic lupus erythematosus—United States, 1979–1998. Retrieved May 27, 2008, from http://www.cdc. gov/mmwr/preview/mmwrhtml/mm5117a3.htm

## BACTERIAL VAGINOSIS

### Definition
Lactobacillus of vagina replaced w/ anaerobic bacteria such as *Prevotella* sp.,
*Mobiluncus, G. vaginalis, Mycoplasma hominis*

### Risk Factors
Multiple sex partners
New sex partners
Douching
Lack of lactobacilli

### Signs and Symptoms
Increase in vaginal discharge
Change in vaginal odor
Change in vaginal discharge color
50% asymptomatic

### Diagnosis (3 out of 4 Criteria Required)
Homogeneous white discharge smoothly coating vaginal walls
Clue cells: irregular cell boarders with bacteria coating the membrane
pH > 4.5; test w/ nitrazine paper
Fishy odor before and/or after addition of 10% KOH

### Increased Risk in Pregnancy
PROM/PPROM
PTL
PTD
Intra-amniotic infection
Postpartum endometritis

### Treatment
*See* Table B-1.

### Follow-Up
Not necessary if symptoms resolve
Multiple infections per year, refer for consult
Pregnant pts should be retested 1 month after tx

### Patient Education
No alcohol for 24 h after last dose of metronidazole
D/C douching
Change soaps and laundry detergent to odorless/colorless sensitive skin brands
Use condoms to possibly prevent recurrent BV in sensitive pts
Counsel that creams weaken latex of condoms, so abstinence during tx period is
preferred

### SOURCES
Centers for Disease Control and Prevention. (2006). Sexually transmitted diseases treatment
guidelines, 2006. *Morbidity and Mortality Weekly Report, 55*(RR-11), 50–52.
Epocrates, I. (2008). *Epocrates online.* Retrieved August 1, 2008, from http://www.epocrates.com
Hale, T. W. (2008). *Medications and mothers' milk* (13th ed.). Amarillo, TX: Hale Publishing.

TABLE B-1 Bacterial Vaginosis Treatment

| Medication Information | Dosing | Contraindications/Cautions | Side Effects | Pt Education |
|---|---|---|---|---|
| Metronidazol (Flagyl) | 250 mg PO TID × 7 d | Hypersensitivity to drug/class | Seizures | Do not drink EtOH |
| | or | Not to be used in high doses in first trimester of pregnancy | Neutropenia | |
| | 500 mg PO BID × 7 d | Blood dyscrasia | Peripheral neuropathy | |
| Preg B | | Impaired liver function | N/V | |
| Lact L2 | | CNS disorder | Dyspepsia | |
| | | | Diarrhea | |
| | | | Metallic taste | |
| | | | Dry mouth | |
| | | | Rash | |
| | | | HA | |
| | | | Dizziness | |
| Metronidazol gel 0.75% | 1 applicator (5 g) PV BID × 5 d | Hypersensitivity to drug/class/parabens | Candidiasis | Avoid intercourse during tx |
| | | Seizure disorder | HA | Avoid other vaginal |
| | | CNS disorder | Vaginal uritis | product use during tx |
| Preg B | | Peripheral neuropathy | Abdominal pain | |
| Lact L2 | | Alcohol use | Nausea | |
| | | Impaired liver function | Dysmenorrhea | |

/ continues

**TABLE B-1**   Bacterial Vaginosis Treatment (continued)

| Medication Information | Dosing | Contraindications/Cautions | Side Effects | Pt Education |
|---|---|---|---|---|
| Clindamycin cream 2%<br><br>Preg B<br>Lact L2 | 1 applicator (5 g) PV qhs × 3–7d | Hypersensitivity to drug/class<br>Inflammatory bowel<br>Colitis<br>Systemic absorption possible | Pseudomembranous colitis<br>Vulvovaginal irritation<br>Candidiasis<br>Abdominal cramps<br>N/V<br>Diarrhea<br>HA<br>Rash | May weaken condoms |
| Clindamycin<br><br>Preg B<br>Lact L2 | 300 mg PO BID × 7 d | Hypersensitivity to drug/class<br>Ulcerative colitis<br>Impaired liver function<br>Impaired renal function | C. difficile-associated diarrhea<br>Pseudomembranous colitis<br>Thrombocytopenia<br>Anaphylaxis<br>Stevens-Johnson syndrome<br>Granulocytopenia<br>Esophagitis<br>N/V<br>Diarrhea<br>Rash<br>Jaundice<br>Hypotension | |

/ continues

TABLE B-1  Bacterial Vaginosis Treatment (continued)

| Medication Information | Dosing | Contraindications/Cautions | Side Effects | Pt Education |
|---|---|---|---|---|
| Clindesse<br><br>Preg B<br>Lact L2 | One dose, PV | Hypersensitivity to drug/class<br>Inflammatory bowel disease<br>Colitis<br>Systemic absorption possible | Pseudomembranous colitis<br>Vulvovaginal irritation/pain<br>Abdominal cramps<br>N/V<br>Diarrhea<br>HA<br>Rash | May weaken condoms |

Sources: Adapted from Center for Disease Control and Prevention. (2006). Sexually transmitted diseases treatment guidelines, 2006. Morbidity and Mortality Weekly Report, 55(RR-11). Epocrates, I. (2008). Epocrates online. Retrieved August 1, 2008, from http://www.epocrates.com. Hale, T. W. (2008). Medications and mothers' milk (13th ed.). Amarillo, TX: Hale Publishing. Thompson Healthcare Inc. (2007). MICROMEDEX: Healthcare series. Retrieved May 1, 2008, from http://www.micromedex.com

## BILIRUBIN: JAUNDICE

### Statistics
Affects 60% of full term infants and 80% of preterm infants

### Definition
RBCs break down every 70–90 d in a newborn and form bilirubin
Liver and the bacteria in the GI system break down the bilirubin, which is then excreted
Infants have slow hepatic breakdown and a sterile GI system
Bilirubin gets absorbed by the skin and stains it yellow (jaundice)

### Physiologic Jaundice
Appears after the first 24 h of life w/out signs of illness

### Pathologic Jaundice
Appears w/in the first 24 h of life along w/ other signs of illness

### Risk Factors
Family Hx of CF or blood disorders
Maternal Dx of diabetes
Rh and isoimmune antibody incompatibility
Birth trauma such as cephalohematoma, poor feeding pattern
Decreased output of urine and stool
Temperature instability

### Signs and Symptoms
Cephalocaudal yellowing of the skin
Lethargy
Light-colored stool
Dark urine
Bruising
Petechiae
Temperature instability
Poor feeding
Excessive weight loss
RUQ tenderness

### Diagnosis
Transcutaneous bilirubinometry (TCB) > 19 should have serum levels drawn
Serum levels of total, direct (conjugated), and indirect (unconjugated) bilirubin, CBC w/ differential, platelet count, and albumin
Sometimes blood cultures, urinalysis, and peripheral smear to r/o infection and hemolysis

### Differential Diagnosis
Breastmilk jaundice (not physiologic) = elevated indirect bilirubin w/ normal reticulocyte count and neg Coombs' test
ABO/Rh incompatibility (not RBC abnormalities) = elevated indirect bilirubin and increased reticulocyte count
Hepatitis
Metabolic or obstructive disorders
Sepsis = elevated indirect and direct, neg Coombs' test, normal reticulocyte count
Darker skinned infants tend to have a lower bilirubin level than white infants

### Treatment
Increase intake—adequate intake produces 6 urine saturated diapers and 3 stools each day
Phototherapy
Blue light breaks down bilirubin allowing for urinary and fecal excretion
Bili lights should be 15–20 cm above infant
All skin exposed except genitals and eyes
Temperature should remain stable
Bilirubin levels should fall 1–2 mg/dl every 4–6 h

*See* Figure B-1.
   Phenobarbital—Increases liver excretion of bilirubin
   Transfusion

**Facts**

   Jaundice in breastfed infants can last more than 2–3 wks
   Jaundice in formula-fed infants usually lasts 2 wks
   F/U should occur within 48–120 h

**B**

**SOURCES**

American Academy of Pediatrics: Subcommittee on Hyperbilirubinemia. (2004). Management of hyperbilirubinemia in the newborn infant 35 or more weeks of gestation. *Pediatrics, 114*(1), 297–316.

Cohen, S. M. (2006). Jaundice in the full-term newborn. *Pediatric Nursing, 32*(3), 202–208.

**FIGURE B-1**   Guidelines for Phototherapy In Hospitalized Infants of 35 Weeks or More Gestation.

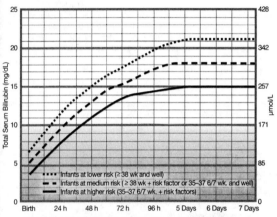

• Use total bilirubin. Do not subtract direct reacting or conjugated bilirubin.
• Risk factors = isoimmune hemolytic disease, G6PD deficiency, asphyxia, significant lethargy, temperature instability, sepsis, acidosis, or albumin > 3.0 g/dL (if measured)
• For well infants 35–37 6/7 wk can adjust TSB levels for intervention around the medium risk line. It is an option to intervene at lower TSB levels for infants closer to 35 wks and at higher TSB levels for those closer to 37 6/7 wk.
• It is an option to provide conventional phototherapy in hospital or at home at TSB levels 2–3 mg/dL (35–50 mmd/L) below those shown but home phototherapy should not be used in any infant with risk factors.

*Source:* Reprinted with permission from American Academy of Pediatrics: Subcommittee on Hyperbilirubinemia. (2004). Management of hyperbilirubinemia in the newborn infant 35 or more weeks of gestation. *Pediatrics, 114*(1), 297–316.

# BIOPHYSICAL PROFILE

**TABLE B-2**  Biophysical Profile Variables

| Biophysical Variable | Normal (score = 2) | Abnormal (score = 0) |
|---|---|---|
| Fetal breathing movements | One or more episode of ≥ 20 second duration in 30 minutes | Absent or no episode of ≥ 20 seconds in 30 minutes |
| Gross body movements | Two or more discrete body/limb movements in 30 minutes (episodes of active continuous movement considered as single movement) | Less than two episodes of body/limb movements in 30 minutes |
| Fetal tone | One or more episode of active extension with return to flexion of fetal limb(s) or trunk (opening and closing of hand considered normal tone) | Slow extension with return to partial flexion, movement of limb in full extension, absent fetal movement, or partially open fetal hand |
| Reactive fetal heart rate | Two or more episodes of acceleration of ≥ 15 bpm and of > 15 seconds associated with fetal movement in 20 minutes | One or no episode of acceleration of fetal heart rate or acceleration of < 15 bpm in 20 minutes |
| Qualitative amniotic fluid volume | One or more pockets of fluid measuring ≤ 2 cm in vertical axis | Either no pockets or largest pocket < 2 cm in vertical axis |

*Source:* Reprinted with permission from Manning, F. (1999). Fetal biophysical profile. *Obstetrics and Gynecology Clinics of North America, 26*(4), 557–577.

## Indications

Maternal IDDM
Post dates (> 42 wks)
Oligohydramnios
Preeclampsia
Nonreactive NST
Positive contraction stress test
Multiple pregnancy
Known or suspected IUGR
Reasoning: "99.946% of fetuses that have a normal BPP score remain healthy for the 7 days following the test" (Frye, 1997, p. 1030)

## Amniotic Fluid Index (AFI)

Normal 5–23 cm at term
5–8 cm is considered borderline oligohydramnios by some practitioners
Standards vary from institution to institution
Maternal abdomen visually divided into four quadrants
Vertical depth of largest clear pocket of amniotic fluid measured in each quadrant
Measurements are totaled to get the AFI

## Management

*See* Table B-3.

### SOURCES

Frye, A. (1997). *Understanding diagnostic tests in the childbearing years* (6th ed.). Portland, OR: Labrys Press.
Manning, F. (1999). Fetal biophysical profile. *Obstetrics and Gynecology Clinics of North America, 26*(4), 557–577.

**B**

**TABLE B-3**  Biophysical Profile Management

| Result | Interpretation | Percent Risk of Asphyxia (umbilical venous blood pH < 7.25) | Risk of Fetal Death (per 1000/week) | Recommended Management |
|---|---|---|---|---|
| 10/10 | Nonasphyxiated | 0 | 0.565 | Conservative management |
| 8/10 (normal AFV) | Nonasphyxiated | 0 | 0.565 | Conservative management |
| 8/8 (NST not done) | Nonasphyxiated | 0 | 0.565 | Conservative management |
| 8/10 (decreased AFV) | Chronic compensated asphyxia | 5–10 (estimate) | 20–30 | If mature (≥ 37 weeks), deliver; serial testing (twice weekly) in the immature fetus |
| 6/10 (normal AFV) | Acute asphyxia possible | 0 | 50 | If mature (≥ 37 weeks), deliver; repeat test in 24 hours in immature fetus; if ≤ 6/10, deliver |
| 6/10 (decreased AFV) | Chronic asphyxia with possible acute asphyxia | > 10 | > 50 | Factor in gestational age; if ≥ 32 weeks, deliver; if < 32 weeks, test daily |
| 4/10 (normal AFV) | Acute asphyxia likely | 36 | 115 | Factor in gestational age; if ≥ 32 weeks, deliver; if ≤ 32 weeks, test daily |
| 4/10 (decreased AFV) | Chronic asphyxia with acute asphyxia likely | > 36 | > 115 | If ≥ 26 weeks, deliver |
| 2/10 (normal AFV) | Acute asphyxia nearly certain | 73 | 220 | If ≥ 26 weeks, deliver |
| 0/10 | Gross severe asphyxia | 100 | 550 | If ≥ 26 weeks, deliver |

AFV = Amniotic fluid volume; NST = nonstress test.

Source: Reprinted with permission from Manning, F. (1999). Fetal biophysical profile. *Obstetrics and Gynecology Clinics of North America, 26*(4), 557–577.

## BIRTH MECHANISMS

### LOA—Left Occiput Anterior

1. Flexion—Chin tucks to chest of baby; head is felt on maternal right
2. Descent—Sagittal suture passes through the pelvis throughout the process
3. Engagement—The biparietal diameter passes through the brim of the pelvis via posterior acyncliticism as the head turns from LOA to LOT and then back to LOA
4. Internal rotation—Head rotates 45° from LOA to OA
5. Extension—The neck of the baby extends, rocking the occiput under the pubic bone
6. Restitution—Once the head is born, the neck turns to align w/ the body by turning 45° from OA back to LOA
7. External rotation—As the body internally rotates to descend, the head turns another 45° from LOA to LOT position

### LOT—Left Occiput Transverse

1. Flexion—Chin tucks to chest of baby; vertex presentation w/ the sagittal suture parallel to the ischial spines and biparietal diameter aligned w/ widest aspects of pelvis
2. Descent—Sagittal suture passes just above or just behind the symphysis
3. Engagement—The biparietal diameter passes through the antioposterior diameter
4. Internal rotation—Head rotates from LOT to OA through a 90° turn
5. Extension—The neck of the baby extends, rocking the occiput under the pubic bone
6. Restitution—Once the head is born, the neck turns to align w/ the body by turning 45° from OA back to LOA
7. External rotation—As the body internally rotates to descend, the head turns another 45° from LOA to LOT position

### ROP—Right Occiput Posterior

1. Occiput posterior, head partially flexed
2. Descent to engagement, flexion increased
3. Internal rotation from ROP to OP, neck twists leaving shoulders at oblique, allows head to maintain flexion w/ the sacral curve
4. Birth of head, face up, as spine flexes and extends, chest descends obliquely
5. Head restitutes from OP to ROP
6. Chest internally rotates to AP, head follows rotating externally from ROP to ROT, shoulders are born

### Compound Presentation

1. After Dx attempt to move the compounding part
2. Try different positions for the mother:
   - Standing w/ one foot supported up on a surface
   - Kneeling on one knee w/ other leg at 90° angle
   - Moving the pelvis
   - Pelvic dangle
3. Try manual reduction of the compounding part by touching the presenting part; may cause it to withdraw
   - Apply counterpressure on mother where pain is felt (usually where compound is located) encouraging body part to move
   - Replace the small part manually by reducing the body part between contractions and easing away the pressure as the contraction builds
4. If not reducible, anticipate slow descent and rapid movement of the compound part away from the head after birth
5. Support compounding part as it emerges and surrounding vaginal tissue during birth to prevent lacerations

#### SOURCE

Frye, A. (2004). *Holistic midwifery: A comprehensive textbook for midwives in homebirth practice.* Portland, OR: Labrys Press.

Varney, H. Kriebs, J. M., & Gegor, C. L. (2004). *Varney's midwifery* (4th ed.). Sudbury, MA: Jones and Bartlett.

# BISHOP'S SCORE

Document: indication, EFW, lung maturity, FHR

**TABLE B-4**  Bishop's Score

| Score | Dilation (cm) | Effacement (%) | Fetal station | Cervical consistency | Cervical position |
|-------|---------------|----------------|---------------|----------------------|-------------------|
| 0 | Closed | 0–30 | −3 | Firm | Posterior |
| 1 | 1–2 | 40–50 | −2 | Medium | Midposition |
| 2 | 3–4 | 60–70 | −1/0 | Soft | Anterior |
| 3 | 5–6 | 80 | +1/+2 | — | — |

Source: Varney, H., Kriebs, J. M., & Gegor, C. L. (2004). *Varney's midwifery* (4th ed.). Sudbury, MA: Jones and Bartlett.

### Score

  0–5: unfavorable

  6: favorable

  4–7: <1% failure rate

### Variations

  +1 for preeclampsia

  +1 for each prior vaginal delivery

  −1 for postdates, nulliparity, preterm or prolonged PROM

#### SOURCES

Varney, H., Kriebs, J. M., & Gegor, C. L. (2004). *Varney's midwifery* (4th ed.). Sudbury, MA: Jones and Bartlett.

Xenakis, E. M., Piper, J. M., Conway, D. L., & Langer, O. (1997). Induction of labor in the nineties: Conquering the unfavorable cervix. *Obstetrics and Gynecology, 90*(2), 235–239.

## BLEEDING

Amenorrhea—Absence of menses for 6 mos or for 3 cycles
  Primary—Delayed puberty
  Secondary—Absence of bleeding for 6 mos once regular cycles have been
    established
Dysmenorrhea—Painful bleeding
  Primary—Intrinsic/early onset physiologic reasons
  Secondary—Late onset
Intermenstrual bleeding (breakthrough)—Bleeding or spotting between menses
  often combined w/ lighter than normal flow
Menorrhagia—Prolonged (> 7 d) or excessive (> 80 ml) bleeding
Menometrorrhagia—Prolonged irregular bleeding
Metrorrhagia—Frequent irregular bleeding of different amounts
Oligomenorrhea—Cycle length > 35 d
Polymenorrhage—Short interval bleeding (< 21 d)

**SOURCE**

Schuiling, K. D., & Likis, F. E. (2006). *Women's gynecologic health.* Sudbury, MA: Jones and Bartlett.

# BLEEDING: ABNORMAL UTERINE BLEEDING

## Causes of Bleeding

*Intermittent Spotting*
Low estrogen withdrawal bleeding
Not enough estrogen in oral contraceptives
Unfavorable estrogen and progesterone ratio
Fibroids
Polyps
Endometrial/cervical cancer
High androgen level (as in PCOS)

*Amenorrhea*
Pregnancy
High estrogen
Excess body wt (resulting in higher estrogen levels)
Athletic lifestyle
High-stress lifestyle
Anorexia
Hyperthyroidism
High androgen (as in PCOS)

*Menorrhagia*
Coagulopathy
Hypothyroidism
Fibroids/polyps
Infection
Endometrial hyperplasia

*Postcoital Bleeding*
Infections
Fibroids/polyps
Endometrial/cervical cancer

*Variable Bleeding Pattern*
Trauma
Foreign body/IUD
Medication
Substance abuse
Cigarettes

## Differential Diagnosis

*Systemic Disease*
Coagulopathies
von Willibrand's
Leukemia
Prothrombin deficiency
Endocrinopathy
Diabetes
Hypo/hyperthyroidism
Adrenal disorder
PCOS
Liver disease
Renal disease

*Autoimmune Diseases*

*Reproductive Tract Diseases/Disorders*
Pregnancy complications
Ectopic pregnancy
Trophoblastic Disease
Cervical/endometrial cancer

    Granulosa/theca cell tumor
    Infections
    Endometrial abnormalities
    Fibroids
    Polyps
    Hyperplasia
    Trauma
    Foreign bodies
    IUD
    Anatomical abnormalities

*Iatrogenic (Medication)*
    OCP
    Steroids
    Tranquilizers
    TCAs
    SSRIs
    Anticoagulants

*Lifestyle*
    Drugs—nicotine, THC, marijuana
    High stress level
    Nutrition—obesity, malnutrition, anorexia
    Exercise excess

## Labs

*General—Done w/ All DUB*
    Labs should be done as an adjunct to bimanual/speculum exam
    CBC
    Basil body temperature chart
    Serum/urine HCG
    TSH
    Pap smear
    GC/CT
    Wet mount
    Endocrine studies
    Prolactin (< 100 ng/ml to r/o pituitary tumor)
    FSH/LH (FSH > 40 mIU/ml suggests premature ovarian failure)

*Adrenal Causes (PCOS)*
    Adrenal studies
    Testosterone level
    DHEAS
    Abdominal CT scan
    Hormone-secreting tumor
    MRI/CT scan
    Cortisol levels

*Structural Abnormalities*
    U/S

*Cervical/Uterine Pathology*
    Colposcopy
    Endometrial biopsy
    FSH/LH
    Prolactin
    TSH
    Progesterone

*Coagulation (von Willenbrand's, Leukemia)*
    von Willebrand's: Ristocetin cofactor
    PTT, PT, and APTT

## Treatment

*Acute Bleeding Treatment*
IV fluids
CEE (note risk of thromboembolitic event) 25 mg IV q 4–6 h PRN
CEE 2.5–5 mg PO 4 times daily × 2–3d then add medroxyprogesterone acetate 10
  mg for 10–14 d while continuing the estrogen
COCs BID–TID then taper down

**B**

*Long Term*
Hormonal contraceptives (Depo, OCPs, patch, ring, Mirena IUD)
"Holiday"—If on long-term contraception like Seasonale, consider occasional break
  hormones
NSAIDs
Oral micronized progesterone 300 mg for 10 d of each cycle
Lupron
Hysterectomy
D&C

*Endometrial Ablation*
Laser/resectoscopic, nonresectoscopic (e.g., cryotherapy, heated free fluid,
  microwaves, radiofrequency energy [novasure], thermal balloon)
Pt can expect decreased menstrual flow, but not necessarily amenorrhea

### SOURCES

American College of Nurse-Midwives. (2002). Abnormal and dysfunctional uterine bleeding: Clinical
  bulletin no. 6. *Journal of Midwifery & Women's Health, 47*(3), 207–213.
American College of Obstetricians and Gynecologists. (2007). Endometrial ablation. ACOG practice
  bulletin no. 81. *Obstetrics and Gynecology, 109*, 1233–1248.
Schuiling, K. D., & Likis, F. E. (2006). *Women's gynecologic health.* Sudbury, MA: Jones and Bartlett.
Speroff, L., & Fritz, M. A. (2005). *Clinical gynecology, endocrinology, infertility* (7th ed.). Philadelphia:
  Lippincott Williams & Wilkins.

## BLEEDING: PREGNANCY

**TABLE B-5**   Bleeding During Pregnancy

| Causes of first and second trimester bleeding | Associated Pain | Concern/Treatment |
|---|---|---|
| Implantation bleed | Painless | None |
| Ectopic | Painful as size increases | Dangerous, needs tx, MD referral |
| Spontaneous abortion threatened | Cramping | Follow-up |
| Incomplete | Cramping | Management options |
| Complete | No pain | Routine follow-up |
| Inevitable | Cramping | Management options |
| Septic | Painful | Needs tx and antibiotics |
| Cervical incompetence | May be painful | May need cerclage |
| Cervical polyp | Painless | None |
| Hydatiform mole | Painless | Needs removal and follow-up |
| **Third trimester bleeding** | | |
| Labor | | |
| Term | Painful | Labor management |
| Preterm | Painful | Preterm assessment |
| Mucous plug | Painless | None |
| **Throughout pregnancy** | | |
| Cervicitis | Painless | Treat if caused by sexually transmitted disease or infection |
| Placenta abruption or partial abruption | Painful | Full evaluation needed |
| Placenta previa | Painless | Pelvic rest, cesarean birth, close monitoring of bleeding |

Rhogam: If a woman is Rh negative she may need rhogam for bleeding during pregnancy or abortion.

*Source:* Varney, H., Kriebs, J. M., & Gegor, C. L. (2004). *Varney's midwifery* (4th ed.). Sudbury, MA: Jones and Bartlett.

# BLOOD: HEMOGLOBIN ELECTROPHORESIS

**TABLE B-6** Hemoglobin Electrophoresis Results and Diagnosis

| | HbA | HbA₂ | HbF | Other Hbs | Phenotype | Patient Care |
|---|---|---|---|---|---|---|
| Normal | > 95% | 1.5–3% | < 2% | None | | |
| Sickle cell trait (HbAS) | 60–70% | | | 30–40% Hb S; If S is reduced, consider α thal trait | Increased incidence of UTIs; risk of sickling crisis when anoxic | Monitor for UTIs; Inform woman that she carries the sickle cell trait; genetic counseling |
| Sickle cell anemia (HbSS) | Absent | Normal | 0–20% | 80–90% HbS | Can be fatal in childhood; reduced fertility; sickling crisis; frequent infections | MD consult and collaborative mngmt; increased risk of IUFD; monitor for sickling crisis/UTIs |
| Sickle HbC disease | Absent | Absent | Absent | 60% HbC; 40% HbS | Hemolytic anemia with mostly normal Hb levels; enlarged spleen; increased risk of sickling crisis in pregnancy | Often undiagnosed until pregnancy; MD consult and collaborative mngmt |
| Beta thalassemia trait (Minor) | Normal | Elevated | Normal to elevated | | Mild anemia; low MCV, MCH; normal MCHC; microcytic, hypochromic; abnormal iron panel | Genetic consult Note: β-thalassemia major causes severe anemia, splenomegaly, bone deformities, iron toxicity, usually fatal in childhood |
| Alpha thalassemia trait | Normal | Normal | Normal | 5–30% HbH; Hb Bart's; any β chain abnormality (β thal, HbC, HbE, HbJ Bangkok, Hb); Hb Constant spring | Mild anemia, microcytic, hypochromic | Will not respond to iron therapy |

*Sources:* Adapted from Desai, S. P. (2004). *Clinician's guide to laboratory medicine: A practical approach* (3rd ed.). Hudson, OH: LexiComp. Frye, A. (1997). *Understanding diagnostic tests in the childbearing years* (6th ed.). Portland, OR: Labrys Press.

B

## BLOOD: THROMBOPHILIAS

### Hereditary Causes of Increased Risk
Protein S deficiency
Antithrombin III deficiency
Plasminogen deficiency
Fibrinogen deficiency
Activated protein C resistance
High homocysteine levels
Mutation in factor II (prothrombin gene mutation)
Factor V Leiden mutation

### Nonhereditary Causes of Increased Risk
Pregnancy
Malignancy
Chronic infection
Diabetes
Trauma
Smoking
Obesity
Bed rest or immobility
OCPs

### Diagnosis
PT, PTT, INR
Coagulation panel
Consider any tests to determine genetic or immunological component (i.e., ANA, LA)

### Treatment
Aspirin or low dose aspirin (if pregnant may stop at 36 wks)
Heparin
Low-molecular weight heparin (Lovenox)
Coumadin (not safe in pregnancy)
All clotting factors (except V, XI, XIII) increase in pregnancy, therefore pregnancy increases the risk of thrombosis
DVTs occur in 0.4 per 1000 pregnancies and are 7 to 10 x more common in pregnancy (highest risk is postpartum)

**SOURCES**
Gabbe, S. G., Niebyl, J. R., & Simpson, J. L., (Eds.). (2002). *Obstetrics: Normal and problem pregnancies* (4th ed.). New York: Churchill Livingstone.
Kaaja, R. J., & Greer, I. A. (2005). Manifestations of chronic disease during pregnancy. *Journal of the American Medical Association, 294*(21), 2751–2757.

# BODY MASS INDEX (BMI)

**TABLE B-7**  BMI Categories

| Category | IOM | NHBLI and *Healthy People 2010* |
|---|---|---|
| Under | < 19.8 | < 18.5 |
| Normal | 19.8 to 26 | 18.5 to 24.9 |
| Over | 26.1 to 29 | 25 to 29.9 |
| Obese Class I | > 29 | 30–34.9 |
| Obese Class II | | 35–39.9 |
| Extreme Obesity | | > 40 |

*Sources:* Adapted from Centers for Disease Control and Prevention. (2007). *Body mass index: BMI for adults.* Retrieved August 29, 2008, from http://www.cdc.gov/nccdphp/dnpa/bmi/adult_BMI/about_adult_BMI.htm. Institute of Medicine Committee on Nutritional Status During Pregnancy and Lactation. (1990). *Nutrition during pregnancy: Part 1 weight gain, part 2 nutrient supplements.* Washington, DC: National Academy Press.

$$BMI = Weight\ (lbs) \times 703\ /\ Height\ (ins)^2$$

**TABLE B-8**  Recommended Weight Gain During Pregnancy

| Weight | Prepregnancy BMI | Total Weight Gain (lb) |
|---|---|---|
| Underweight | < 19.8 | 28–40 |
| Normal weight | 19.8–26.0 | 25–35 |
| Overweight | > 26.0–29.0 | 15–25 |
| Obese | > 29 | At least 15 |

*Source:* Reprinted from Centers for Disease Control and Prevention. (2005). *Pediatric and pregnancy nutrition surveillance system health indicators.* Retrieved May 29, 2008, from http://www.cdc.gov/pednss/what_is/pnss_health_indicators.htm#Maternal%20Health%20Indicators

Excessive wt gain in pregnancy: > 1.5 kg/mo
Inadequate wt gain in pregnancy: < 0.25 kg/wk or < 1 kg/mo
1 kg = 2.2 lb

**SOURCES**
Centers for Disease Control and Prevention. (2007). *Body mass index: BMI for adults.* Retrieved August 26, 2008, from http://www.cdc.gov/nccdphp/dnpa/bmi/adult_BMI/about_adult_BMI.htm
Institute of Medicine Committee on Nutritional Status During Pregnancy and Lactation. (1990). *Nutrition during pregnancy: Part 1 weight gain, part 2 nutrient supplements* (1st ed.). Washington, DC: National Academy Press.
Salazar, S. S. (2006). Assessment and management of the obese adult female: A clinical update for providers. *Journal of Midwifery & Women's Health, 51*(3), 202.

## BMI TABLE

**TABLE B-9  BMI Table**

| BMI | Normal | | | | | | Overweight | | | | | Obese | | | | | | | | | | Extreme Obesity | | | | | | | | | | | | | | |
|---|---|---|---|---|---|---|---|---|---|---|---|---|---|---|---|---|---|---|---|---|---|---|---|---|---|---|---|---|---|---|---|---|---|---|---|---|
| | 19 | 20 | 21 | 22 | 23 | 24 | 25 | 26 | 27 | 28 | 29 | 30 | 31 | 32 | 33 | 34 | 35 | 36 | 37 | 38 | 39 | 40 | 41 | 42 | 43 | 44 | 45 | 46 | 47 | 48 | 49 | 50 | 51 | 52 | 53 | 54 |
| **Height (inches)** | | | | | | | | | | | | **Body Weight (pounds)** | | | | | | | | | | | | | | | | | | | | | | | | |
| 58 | 91 | 96 | 100 | 105 | 110 | 115 | 119 | 124 | 129 | 134 | 138 | 143 | 148 | 153 | 158 | 162 | 167 | 172 | 177 | 181 | 186 | 191 | 196 | 201 | 205 | 210 | 215 | 220 | 224 | 229 | 234 | 239 | 244 | 248 | 253 | 258 |
| 59 | 94 | 99 | 104 | 109 | 114 | 119 | 124 | 128 | 133 | 138 | 143 | 148 | 153 | 158 | 163 | 168 | 173 | 178 | 183 | 188 | 193 | 198 | 203 | 208 | 212 | 217 | 222 | 227 | 232 | 237 | 242 | 247 | 252 | 257 | 262 | 267 |
| 60 | 97 | 102 | 107 | 112 | 118 | 123 | 128 | 133 | 138 | 143 | 148 | 153 | 158 | 163 | 168 | 174 | 179 | 184 | 189 | 194 | 199 | 204 | 209 | 215 | 220 | 225 | 230 | 235 | 240 | 245 | 250 | 255 | 261 | 266 | 271 | 276 |
| 61 | 100 | 106 | 111 | 116 | 122 | 127 | 132 | 137 | 143 | 148 | 153 | 158 | 164 | 169 | 174 | 180 | 185 | 190 | 195 | 201 | 206 | 211 | 217 | 222 | 227 | 232 | 238 | 243 | 248 | 254 | 259 | 264 | 269 | 275 | 280 | 285 |
| 62 | 104 | 109 | 115 | 120 | 126 | 131 | 136 | 142 | 147 | 153 | 158 | 164 | 169 | 175 | 180 | 186 | 191 | 196 | 202 | 207 | 213 | 218 | 224 | 229 | 235 | 240 | 246 | 251 | 256 | 262 | 267 | 273 | 278 | 284 | 289 | 295 |
| 63 | 107 | 113 | 118 | 124 | 130 | 135 | 141 | 146 | 152 | 158 | 163 | 169 | 175 | 180 | 186 | 191 | 197 | 203 | 208 | 214 | 220 | 225 | 231 | 237 | 242 | 248 | 254 | 259 | 265 | 270 | 278 | 282 | 287 | 293 | 299 | 304 |
| 64 | 110 | 116 | 122 | 128 | 134 | 140 | 145 | 151 | 157 | 163 | 169 | 174 | 180 | 186 | 192 | 197 | 204 | 209 | 215 | 221 | 227 | 232 | 238 | 244 | 250 | 256 | 262 | 267 | 273 | 279 | 285 | 291 | 296 | 302 | 308 | 314 |
| 65 | 114 | 120 | 126 | 132 | 138 | 144 | 150 | 156 | 162 | 168 | 174 | 180 | 186 | 192 | 198 | 204 | 210 | 216 | 222 | 228 | 234 | 240 | 246 | 252 | 258 | 264 | 270 | 276 | 282 | 288 | 294 | 300 | 306 | 312 | 318 | 324 |
| 66 | 118 | 124 | 130 | 136 | 142 | 148 | 155 | 161 | 167 | 173 | 179 | 186 | 192 | 198 | 204 | 210 | 216 | 223 | 229 | 235 | 241 | 247 | 253 | 260 | 266 | 272 | 278 | 284 | 291 | 297 | 303 | 309 | 315 | 322 | 328 | 334 |
| 67 | 121 | 127 | 134 | 140 | 146 | 153 | 159 | 166 | 172 | 178 | 185 | 191 | 198 | 204 | 211 | 217 | 223 | 230 | 236 | 242 | 249 | 255 | 261 | 268 | 274 | 280 | 287 | 293 | 299 | 306 | 312 | 319 | 325 | 331 | 338 | 344 |
| 68 | 125 | 131 | 138 | 144 | 151 | 158 | 164 | 171 | 177 | 184 | 190 | 197 | 203 | 210 | 216 | 223 | 230 | 236 | 243 | 249 | 256 | 262 | 269 | 276 | 282 | 289 | 295 | 302 | 308 | 315 | 322 | 328 | 335 | 341 | 348 | 354 |
| 69 | 128 | 135 | 142 | 149 | 155 | 162 | 169 | 176 | 182 | 189 | 196 | 203 | 209 | 216 | 223 | 230 | 236 | 243 | 250 | 257 | 263 | 270 | 277 | 284 | 291 | 297 | 304 | 311 | 318 | 324 | 331 | 338 | 345 | 351 | 358 | 365 |
| 70 | 132 | 139 | 146 | 153 | 160 | 167 | 174 | 181 | 188 | 195 | 202 | 209 | 216 | 222 | 229 | 236 | 243 | 250 | 257 | 264 | 271 | 278 | 285 | 292 | 299 | 306 | 313 | 320 | 327 | 334 | 341 | 348 | 355 | 362 | 369 | 376 |
| 71 | 136 | 143 | 150 | 157 | 165 | 172 | 179 | 186 | 193 | 200 | 208 | 215 | 222 | 229 | 236 | 243 | 250 | 257 | 265 | 272 | 279 | 286 | 293 | 301 | 308 | 315 | 322 | 329 | 338 | 343 | 351 | 358 | 365 | 372 | 379 | 386 |
| 72 | 140 | 147 | 154 | 162 | 169 | 177 | 184 | 191 | 199 | 206 | 213 | 221 | 228 | 235 | 242 | 250 | 258 | 265 | 272 | 279 | 287 | 294 | 302 | 309 | 316 | 324 | 331 | 338 | 346 | 353 | 361 | 368 | 375 | 383 | 390 | 397 |
| 73 | 144 | 151 | 159 | 166 | 174 | 182 | 189 | 197 | 204 | 212 | 219 | 227 | 235 | 242 | 250 | 257 | 265 | 272 | 280 | 288 | 295 | 302 | 310 | 318 | 325 | 333 | 340 | 348 | 355 | 363 | 371 | 378 | 386 | 393 | 401 | 408 |
| 74 | 148 | 155 | 163 | 171 | 179 | 186 | 194 | 202 | 210 | 218 | 225 | 233 | 241 | 249 | 256 | 264 | 272 | 280 | 287 | 295 | 303 | 311 | 319 | 326 | 334 | 342 | 350 | 358 | 365 | 373 | 381 | 389 | 396 | 404 | 412 | 420 |
| 75 | 152 | 160 | 168 | 176 | 184 | 192 | 200 | 208 | 216 | 224 | 232 | 240 | 248 | 256 | 264 | 272 | 279 | 287 | 295 | 303 | 311 | 319 | 327 | 335 | 343 | 351 | 359 | 367 | 375 | 383 | 391 | 399 | 407 | 415 | 423 | 431 |
| 76 | 156 | 164 | 172 | 180 | 189 | 197 | 205 | 213 | 221 | 230 | 238 | 246 | 254 | 263 | 271 | 279 | 287 | 295 | 304 | 312 | 320 | 328 | 336 | 344 | 353 | 361 | 369 | 377 | 385 | 394 | 402 | 410 | 418 | 426 | 435 | 443 |

*Source:* Reprinted from National Heart, Lung, and Blood Institute. (2008). Body mass index table. Retrieved May 10, 2008, from http://www.nhlbi.nih.gov/guidelines/obesity/bmi_tbl.pdf

# BREASTS

## Breast Problems (Descending Order of Frequency)

Breast pain—Most commonly a cyst or fibroadinoma, tx w/ analgesics as well as decrease in caffeine and sodium intake

Mass or asymmetric thickening

Fibroadenoma—Dx by U/S and fine needle aspiration, should be excised if noncystic

Cyst—Dx by U/S or fine-needle aspiration

Fibrocystic mass or vague nodularity—Re-evaluate bimonthly during mid-menstrual cycle, if noncyclical and persists after 3 mos then further F/U is needed

Carcinoma—Immediate referral to surgeon

Occult mammographic abnormality

**TABLE B-10**    BI-RADS System

| Rating | Results |
|--------|---------|
| 0 | Assessment is incomplete, additional imaging evaluation needed |
| 1 | Negative findings |
| 2 | Benign finding |
| 3 | Probably benign finding; short follow-up suggested |
| 4 | Suspicious abnormality; biopsy should be considered |
| 5 | Highly suggestive of malignancy; appropriate action should be taken |

*Source:* Adapted from Eberi, M., Fox, C., Edge, S., Carter, C., & Mahoney, M. (2006). BI-RADS classification for management of abnormal mammograms. *Journal of the American Board of Family Medicine, 19*(2), 161–164.

Category 4 and 5 = immediate referral to surgeon

Category 3 = 2% chance of cancer, complete F/U as directed but reassure pt

Nipple discharge—Milky, green, grey, or black discharge that is unilateral or bilateral and is expressed from multiple ducts requires further investigation

Spontaneous bloody discharge during 3rd trimester is not suspicious of cancer, F/U w/ mammogram postpartum

If accompanied by a mass immediate referral to breast surgeon

Cytologic studies of discharge is rarely helpful

Skin or nipple changes—Breakdown of skin in areola or nipple is suggestive of cancer (Paget's disease)

## Diagnosis

"Triple diagnosis" technique of breast mass diagnosis has been used to improve diagnostic accuracy

Uses the combination of results:

CBE

Mammography

Biopsy

## Absolute Indications for Referral to a Surgeon

A persistent mass at the optimal phase of the menstrual cycle

A mass in a postmenopausal woman

A mass that does not completely disappear after aspiration

A cyst that is grossly bloody

A rapidly reaccumulating cyst (w/in 4–6 wks)

Atypia or malignancy on biopsy

An insufficient specimen on biopsy, unless repeated

Any single component of triple diagnosis that is inconsistent w/ benign disease

**Mass Classification: Aberrations of Normal Development and Involution (ANDI) of the Breasts**

TABLE B-11   Aberrations of Normal Developments and Involutions of the Breasts (ANDI)

| Stage (peak age in yrs) | Normal process | Aberration | | Disease state |
|---|---|---|---|---|
| | | Underlying condition | Clinical presentation | |
| Early reproductive period (15–25) | Lobule formation Stroma formation | Fibroadenoma Juvenile hypertrophy | Discrete lump Excessive breast development | Giant fibroadenoma Multiple fibroadenoma |
| Mature reproductive period (25–40) | Cyclical hormonal effects on glandular tissue and stroma | Exaggerated cyclical effects | Cyclical mastalgia and nodularity generalized or discrete | |
| Involution (35–55) | Lobular involution (including microcysts, apocrine change fibrosis, adenosis Ductal involution (including periductal round cell infiltrates) Epithelial turnover | Macrocysts Sclerosing lesions Duct dilatation Periductal fibrosis Mild epithelial hyperplasia | Discrete lumps X-Ray abnormalities Nipple discharge Nipple retraction Histological report | Periductal mastitis with bacterial infection and abscess formation Epithelial hyperplasia with atypia |

Source: Reprinted with permission from Hughes, L. E. (1991). Classification of benign breast disorders: The ANDI classification based on physiological processes within the normal breast. *British Medical Bulletin, 47*(2), 251–257.

**Commonly Used Lifestyle Modifications to Decrease Fibrocystic Breasts**

Decrease caffeine and sodium intake

Increase water intake

Often related to menstrual cycle, note cyclical changes

Vitamin E and primrose oil supplements

**SOURCES**

Cady, B., Stelle, G. D., Morrow, M., Gardner, B., Smith, B., Lee, N., et al. (1998). Evaluation of common breast problems: Guidance for primary care providers. *CA: A Cancer Journal for Clinicians, 48*(1), 49–63.

Eberi, M., Fox, C., Edge, S., Carter, C., & Mahoney, M. (2006). BI-RADS classification for management of abnormal mammograms. *Journal of the American Board of Family Medicine, 19*(2), 161–164.

Hughes, L. E. (1991). Classification of benign breast disorders: The ANDI classification based on physiological processes within the normal breast. *British Medical Bulletin, 47*(2), 251–257.

Schuiling, K. D., & Likis, F. E. (2006). *Women's gynecologic health.* Sudbury, MA: Jones and Bartlett.

# BREAST: CANCER

**B**

### Statistics
Second leading cancer cause of death in women
Screening contributed to the 23.5% decline in mortality between 1990 and 2000
Overall risk in a lifetime (80 years) = 12.5 (1 in 8)

### Screening Methods

TABLE B-12   Probability of Breast Cancer

| Age | Probability of breast cancer in 1 year (1 in X) |
|-----|-------------------------------------------------|
| 20  | 2044 |
| 30  | 249 |
| 40  | 67 |
| 50  | 36 |
| 60  | 29 |
| 70  | 24 |

*Source:* Adapted from National Cancer Institute. (2008). *Breast cancer risk assessment tool.*
Retrieved February 23, 2008, from http://www.cancer.gov/bcrisktool

Breast self-exam (BSE):
  Cochrane review concludes that BSE only increases the number of biopsies
    performed, and it does not increase early detection
  USPSTF concludes insufficient evidence for or against BSE as screening
  ACS concludes that self-exams are optional
Clinical breast exams (CBE):
  5% of cancers are detected solely by CBE (54% sensitivity, 94% specificity)
  Lack of standardization accounts for a 29% variance in sensitivity and 33%
    variance in specificity
  Suspicious mass = solitary, discrete, firm or hard, fixed or mobile, unilateral,
    non-tender but possibley sensitive
Mammography:
  USPSTF meta-analysis concludes screening w/ mammography should occur
    every 1–2 yr for women over age 40, sensitivity is 60–90%
  Digital and computer-aided detection are increasing these statistics
U/S, MRI, PET, and scintimammography: Not recommended for any women as a
  screening tool

### Factors That Increase Risk
Genetic mutations (BRACA)
Two or more first-degree relatives w/ cancer at an early age
Personal hx of breast cancer
Age > 65
Nodular densities on mammogram
Atypical hyperplasia
High-dose ionizing radiation to chest
Ovaries not surgically removed age < 40
High socioeconomic status
Urban residence
Early menarche (< 12)
Late menopause (> 55)
No term pregnancies or late age of pregnancy (> 30)
No breastfeeding

**Diagnostic Tests**

TABLE B-13   Diagnostic Tests for Breast Symptoms

| | |
|---|---|
| **Diagnostic mammography** | A radiologic procedure performed in women with breast problems detected either by screening mammography or CBE |
| **Breast ultrasound** | A radiologic procedure involving the use of sonic energy to distinguish a cyst from a solid mass, and in experienced settings to differentiate solid masses into benign and suspicious categories |
| **Image-guided biopsy** | A radiologic procedure using mammographic stereotactic images or images by ultrasound to localize an abnormality in order to perform a fine-needle aspiration biopsy or core biopsy |
| **Needle localization/biopsy** | A combined radiological-surgical procedure in which an occult mammographic abnormality is localized with a wire, dye, or both prior to excisional biopsy |
| **Fine-needle aspiration** | An office procedure in which a small (22G) needle is inserted into a mass to distinguish whether it is cystic or solid |
| **Fine-needle aspiration biopsy** | An office procedure in which a small (22G) needle is inserted into a solid mass to obtain a cytologic diagnosis |
| **Core needle biopsy** | An office procedure in which a large-bore needle is inserted into a solid mass to obtain histological sampling |
| **Punch biopsy** | An office procedure using a special device to biopsy a portion of skin for histological diagnosis of a skin lesion |
| **Incisional biopsy** | An operative procedure that removes a portion of a large mass for histological examination |
| **Excisional biopsy** | An operative procedure that removes an entire mass or mammographic abnormality for histological examination |

Source: Schuiling, K. D., & Likis, F. E. (2006). *Women's gynecologic health.* Sudbury, MA: Jones and Bartlett.

**SOURCES**

American College of Obstetricians and Gynecologists. (2003). Breast cancer screening. In *2006 compendium of selected publications* (p. 386). Washington, DC: Author.

Centers for Disease Control and Prevention. (2007). *Breast cancer.* Retrieved March 5, 2008, from http://www.cancer.gov/cancertopics/types/breast

Knutson, D., & Steiner, E. (2007). Screening for breast cancer: Current recommendations and future directions. *American Family Physician, 75*(11), 1660–1666.

National Cancer Institute. (2008). *Breast cancer.* Retrieved March 3, 2008, from http://www.cancer.gov/cancertopics/types/breast

National Cancer Institute. (2008). *Breast cancer risk assessment tool.* Retrieved February 23, 2008, from www.cancer.gov/bcrisktool

Schuiling, K. D., & Likis, F. E. (2006). *Women's gynecologic health.* Sudbury, MA: Jones and Bartlett.

# BREASTFEEDING

## Nutritional Benefits
The right amount and types of protein
Iron more bioavailable in breastmilk than formula
More easily digested and absorbed than formula
Nonpeptide hormones, prostaglandins, vitamins, minerals, and antibodies in breastmilk are specifically adapted from the mother's environment and lifestyle, which the baby will be introduced into

## Developmental Benefits
Nutritional content changes over time to meet the baby's needs
Offers immune system support and protects an infant from disease
Stimulates growth, development, and maturation of the gut, immune system, and neuroendocrine system
Shown to have antiviral activity (i.e., against HSV)
Evidence to suggest that it may increase brain development and IQ
Indirectly reduce the risk of becoming overweight by facilitating self-regulation of energy intake or by activating regulatory systems that maintain energy balance
Protects against various illnesses, infections, and allergic reactions, including GI disease, LRIs, URIs, ear infections, and asthma
May also protect against UTIs and infant botulism
May also protect against IDDM, celiac disease, childhood cancer, and IBS

## Maternal Benefits
Increases rate of uterine contraction after childbirth, resulting in a reduced risk of postpartum blood loss
Reduced risk of breast cancer, particularly premenopausal breast cancer
Reduced risk of ovarian cancer
Possible reduced risk of spinal and hip fractures after menopause
Amenorrhea and decreased fertility that generally accompany lactation can contribute to effective family planning efforts during breastfeeding

## Contraindications
Mothers who use street drugs or alcohol
Infants w/ galactosemia
Mothers w/ HIV
Mothers w/ active TB
Mothers taking medications deemed unsafe for breastfeeding
Mothers undergoing chemotherapy

## Increasing Milk Supply
Express/pump milk after feedings

*Herbal Supplements*
Fenugreek: 1–3 capsules TID (will make mother's body fluids smell like maple syrup)
Blessed thistle 3 capsules TID
Can be taken together, both are effective galactologues

*Medications to increase prolactin level*
Domperidone
Reglan

## Decreasing Milk Supply
If weaning, do so gradually, eliminating feedings over at least 1 wk to avoid engorgement
If deciding not to start breastfeeding: wear a supportive bra, avoid any nipple stimulation
To decrease engorgement, apply fresh chilled cabbage leaves to breasts for 20 min

### Assessing Baby's Intake

Count wet diapers and bowel movements
1–2 wet diapers per day in first 3–4 d
6+ wet diapers per day after day 4
3–4 BMs the size of a quarter or larger per day after day 4

### Breastmilk Storage

Store in glass or plastic
Freshly pumped milk can be kept 2–8 d in refrigerator
Thawed milk can be stored for 24 h in refrigerator
Freshly pumped milk is safe to keep up to 10 h at room temperature
Milk will keep for 3–4 mos in a refrigerator freezer; 6 mos deep freezer

**SOURCES**

American College of Obstetricians and Gynecologists. (2000). Breastfeeding: Maternal and infant aspects practice. In *2006 compendium of selected publications* (p. 274). Washington, DC: Author.

Kent, J. C. (2007). How breastfeeding works [Abstract]. *Journal of Midwifery & Women's Health, 52*(6) 564–570.

Mohrbacher, N., Stock, J., & La Leche League International. (2003). *The breastfeeding answer book* (3rd ed.). Schaumburg, IL: La Leche League International.

# BREASTFEEDING: ENGORGEMENT

B

### How to Avoid
Unrestricted nursing for first wk
Minimum of 11–12 feeding in 24 h

### Risk Factors
Sleepy baby
Poor latch and position
Ineffective suck
H/o engorgement
Supplementation
Pumping

### Etiology
Breast becomes congested w/ milk
Circulation within the breast slows, causing swelling

### Signs and Symptoms
Bilaterally taut, shiny skin
Warmth
Tender breasts
Occasionally accompanied by low-grade fever (< 38.4°C)

### Treatment
Resolves within 24–48 h w/ active management of breastfeeding
Immediately before feeding, warm breast for 5–10 min w/ compresses/shower
Gently massage breast to express milk, which will soften nipple and areola
Encourage frequent feedings (may require waking baby every 2 h)
Finish first breast before going to second (if baby refuses 2nd breast, then offer
     that breast 1st at next feeding)
Use a breast pump to completely drain breast after the baby has nursed
Apply cold compresses between feedings to reduce swelling; can apply cold,
     chilled cabbage leaves for 20 min, but use caution as this can significantly
     decrease the milk supply
Wear a well-fitting bra (not too tight or pinching; avoid underwire)
Usually all engorgement/fullness will resolve in 7–10 d as breast and baby adjust
     supply/demand

### Complications
Slow wt gain for baby
Sore nipples
Increased risk of mastitis
Decreased milk supply

### Reverse Pressure Softening
Steady, gentle pressure inward toward the chest wall is exerted for a full 60 sec
     or longer (2–3 min, repeat if needed), focusing on the areola where it joins the
     base of the nipple.

#### SOURCE
Mohrbacher, N., Stock, J., & La Leche League International. (2003). The breastfeeding answer book
(3rd ed.). Schaumburg, IL: La Leche League International.

## BREASTFEEDING: IMPLANTS/REDUCTION

### Implants

Place of insertion

Scar under breast or near armpit → implant behind milk duct

Scar around areolae → nerves and milk duct damaged

Silicone in breast milk is not an issue (baby's GI system will excrete silicone w/o problem)

Adequate milk supply is largest concern, secondary to compression of milk ducts by implant

### Reduction

How were breasts reduced?

Liposuction → only removed fat, milk ducts and nerves spared

Breast tissue removed → decreased number of milk ducts and nerves

Areola surgically relocated → all milk ducts and nerves damaged; loss of pathway to the nipple

Pt will not know until she tries to breastfeed if there will be enough milk

Typically breastmilk supply increases w/ each successive pregnancy

### SOURCE

Mohrbacher, N., Stock, J., & La Leche League International. (2003). *The breastfeeding answer book* (3rd ed.). Schaumburg, IL: La Leche League International.

# BREASTFEEDING: MASTITIS

**B**

## Risk Factors
Poor latch
Cracked nipples
Ineffective suck
Sustained pressure on breast (typically from ill-fitting or underwire bras)
Stress
Fatigue
Weakened immune system
Irregular feeding pattern
Pacifier use by infant
Supplementation
Nipple shield
High saturated fat and salt diet
Excessive upper arm exercise
Sudden weaning
Postpartum depression

## Signs and Symptoms
General malaise
Headache
Painful/swollen/inflamed/reddened/hard area of the breast
Chills
Fever (39.5–40.0°C)

## Signs and Symptoms of an Abscess
Purulent nipple discharge
Remittent fever w/ chills
Breast swollen generally with an extremely painful palpable breast mass w/
  reddish/bluish tinge

## Nonpharmacological Treatment
Supportive, nonconstricting bra
Careful hand washing and breast care
Warm compresses
Massaging the breast while nursing
Pumping if unable to nurse
Increased fluid intake
Rest
Stress reduction

## Organisms
*S. aureus*, gram negative *Streptococci*, *Candida* (increase suspicion if mother was
  treated w/ intrapartum antibiotics)
\*\*There is no reason to stop breastfeeding due to mastitis!

*See* Table B-14.

**SOURCES**
Betzold, C. M. (2007). An update on the recognition and management of lactational breast
inflammation [Abstract]. *Journal of Midwifery & Women's Health, 52*(6) 595–605.
Mohrbacher, N., Stock, J., & La Leche League International. (2003). *The breastfeeding answer book*
(3rd ed.). Schaumburg, IL: La Leche League International.

TABLE B-14  Breastfeeding Problems and Suggested Treatment

| Breast issue | Antibiotics (Lact Category) | Antifungal | Supportive Therapy |
|---|---|---|---|
| Plugged duct/ cracked nipples/ nipple or duct infections | Mupirocin 2% ointment (15 g) applied to nipples after each nursing/pumping; culture area if no improvement (L1) | If recurrent or h/o recent antibiotic use, Rx fluconazole (Diflucan) 200–400 mg × 1, then 100–200 mg QD × 2–3 wks  *If fungal infection is suspected, mother and infant need to be treated concurrently | Lecithin 1200 mg TID to QID to prevent recurrences  Increase dietary lactobacilli  Dr. Newman's APNO instead of mupirocin, apply after feeding  Sterilize things that come into contact with breast or baby's mouth (bras, breast pads, breast pump parts, pacifiers, etc.) |
| Mastitis | Dicloxacillin 500 mg PO QID × 10–14 d (L2)  Cephalexin (Keflex) 500 mg PO Q 12 h × 10 d (L1)  Erythromycin 250 mg QID × 10 d (L2, L3 in early postnatal period d/t risk of pyloric stenosis)  All are breastfeeding compatible | Intense nipple pain during latch that dissipates with continued feeding, followed by burning breast pain after is indicative of likely yeast infection, treat as above | Topical treatments as stated above when indicated. If recurrent consider longer antibiotic tx |

Sources: Adapted from Mohrbacher, N., Stock, J., & La Leche League International. (2003). The breastfeeding answer book (3rd ed.). Schaumburg, IL: La Leche League International. Betzold, C. M. (2007). An update on the recognition and management of lactational breast inflammation [Abstract]. Journal of Midwifery & Women's Health, 52(6) 595–605.

**ALL PURPOSE NIPPLE OINTMENT**
Mupirocin 2% ointment: 15 g
Betamethasone 0.1% ointment: 15 g
Add miconazole powder to a final concentration of 2%
Do not substitute cream for ointments
Total volume is approximately 30 g
Clotrimazole powder can be substituted to a final concentration of 2% if miconazole is unavailable
Apply the ointment sparingly after each feeding.
No need to wash off the ointment prior to feedings

# BREECH

Incidence: 3–4% of singleton pregnancies

**Positions**

Complete—One or both knees are flexed with the buttocks in the pelvis

Incomplete—One or both hips are not flexed and one or both feet or knees lies below the buttocks

Footling—Incomplete presentation because one or both feet are below the buttocks

Frank—Hips are flexed but both knees are not flexed, one or both feet are up near the head

**Diagnosis**

1. Leopold's defines a hard, round, ballotable fetal head occupying the fundus, and the intertrochanteric diameter of the pelvis at the pelvic inlet
2. Vaginal exam discovers muscular resistance with the anus, meconium extracted, a fetal foot, or genitalia
3. U/S should confirm position

**Complications**

Perinatal morbidity and mortality due to delivery complications

LBW due to PTD and/or growth restriction

Prolapsed cord

Placenta previa

Fetal, neonatal, and infant anomalies

Uterine anomalies and/or tumors

**External Cephalic Version**

Successful 35–85% of the time, average 60%

Indicated for > 36 wks because of possibility of immediate delivery

*Factors Increasing Success*

Increased parity

Type of breech presentation

Amniotic fluid level

Unengaged fetus

Uterine relaxation

*Factors Decreasing Success*

Low amniotic fluid level

Maternal obesity

Anterior placenta

Cervical dilation

Fetal engagement

Anterior or posterior positioning of fetal spine

Difficulty palpating fetal head

Uterine tension

*Technique*

Secure facility equipped to perform an emergency C/S

Real-time U/S confirms position, AFI, placental position, and cardiac movement

Obtain reactive NST

Administer terbutaline 2.5 mg PO or 0.25 mg SC, or another tocolytic agent

Each hand grasps a fetal pole

Buttocks are elevated and displaced laterally

Head is directed toward the pelvis in a "forward roll"

If forward roll is unsuccessful a backward flip is attempted

*Stop* if excessive discomfort, persistent abnormal FHR pattern, multiple failed attempts

Confirm fetal status by repeat NST

*Complications*

Abruption

Uterine rupture

Amniotic fluid embolism
Fetomaternal hemorrhage
Isoimmunization
PTL
Fetal distress
Fetal demise

## Suggestions for Patient-Initiated Breech Version

Visualization of baby turning

Breech tilt—Begin at 32–35 wks TID; at baby's most active time, lie on an ironing board or other flat surface that can be securely tilted from a height of 12–18 inches with head towards the floor; flex knees, but keep feet flat

Moxibustion—Refer to naturopath or similar practitioner

Acupuncture—Usually involves the stimulation of the "moving down" point on the outer aspect of the little toes just adjacent to the corner of the toenail; can stimulate point with clothespins placed parallel to the foot and pinching the pressure point for at least 30 min QD

Webster's breech technique—Chiropractic referral

Knee-chest position for 15 min q 2 h for 1 wk or until turned

## Birth

Most breech presentations at term are delivered by C/S; however, the chance of the midwife being presented with a breech presentation requiring immediate delivery necessitates that all midwives understand the maneuvers for breech delivery

Preparations for a breech birth

Determine type of breech presentation

Ensure complete cervical dilation

Empty maternal bladder

Assess effectiveness of maternal pushing effort

Alert staff regarding possible need for full-scale newborn resuscitation

Place pt in lithotomy position, allowing for adequate room below maternal pelvis necessary for delivery

MD backup notified with a STAT request for his/her presence at the delivery

## Birth Mechanisms

Hands-off approach is best

Descent will occur throughout the delivery, if descent arrests r/o CPD/ hydrocephalus, then perform Pinard maneuver

1. Starting from RSA the buttocks will rotate to RST

2. Birth of the buttocks is by lateral flexion. Generally, the posterior hip is born first, and the anterior hip is impinged beneath the symphysis pubis, which allows the posterior hip to pivot along the curve of Carus.

3. The legs and feet are born spontaneously. If a frank breech is presented, then use Pinard maneuver.

4. Buttocks then externally rotate from RST to RSA and shoulders engage. Continue hands-off approach, but make a request for a warm towel during this stage.

5. When the baby's body emerges to the level of the umbilicus, (1) gently use a finger to pull down a loop of umbilical cord, (2) place the warm towel around the hips and legs, below the umbilicus to allow for a better grip on the baby lower body.

6. Exert downward and outward traction on the baby's body to facilitate the internal rotation of the shoulders; the sacrum will externally rotate to RST. *Important:* Grasp the baby's hips w/ thumbs on the sacroiliac region and fingers on the iliac crests, avoiding any pressure on the abdomen. Continue traction until the anterior shoulder and axilla are visible at the introitus.

7. The shoulders are born by lateral flexion. During this stage, grasp the baby's feet and exert upward traction, drawing the baby's abdomen toward the mother's inner thigh. *Caution:* Do not let the baby's back turn upward! The delivery of the arms may occur spontaneously, or may be gently delivered by inserting two fingers into the vagina, locating the elbow of the posterior arm, and gently

splinting and sweeping the arm across the baby's chest and out of the vagina. Now the anterior shoulder is delivered by exerting downward traction, but use caution to assess for arm position as the extremity may need to be delivered first (see above).

8. Once the body is delivered, the head is now engaged in either the transverse or oblique diameter. Have an assistant apply suprapubic pressure to the maintain head flexion. This pressure should continue until the head is born.

9. Now grasp the hips as before and gently ensure that the head settles in an occiput anterior position.

10. Instruct that suprapubic pressure continue to ensure head flexion and perform the Mauriceau-Smellie-Veit maneuver.

11. Successful delivery is now achieved, but be prepared for neonatal resuscitation.

### SOURCES

Cunningham, G., Leveno, K. J., Bloom, S. L., Hauth, J. C., Gilstrap, L. C., & Wenstrom, K. D. (2005). *Williams obstetrics* (22nd ed.). New York: McGraw-Hill Professional.

Frye, A. (2004). *Holistic midwifery: A comprehensive textbook for midwives in homebirth practice.* Portland, OR: Labrys Press.

Varney, H., Kriebs, J. M., & Gegor, C. L. (2004). *Varney's midwifery* (4th ed.). Sudbury, MA: Jones and Bartlett.

**B**

## CALCIUM AND VITAMIN D

TABLE C-1  Foods Rich in Vitamin D

| Selected Foods | Vitamin D Content (IUs/serving) |
|---|---|
| Cod liver oil, 1 Tbsp | 1360 |
| Salmon, cooked, 3.5 oz | 360 |
| Mackerel, cooked, 3.5 oz | 345 |
| Tuna fish, canned in oil, 3 oz | 200 |
| Milk, vitamin D fortified | 98 |
| Cereal, fortified | 40 |
| Egg, whole (vitamin D in yolk) | 20 |
| Liver, beef, 3.5 oz | 15 |
| Cheese, Swiss, 1 oz | 12 |

Source: Adapted from Office of Dietary Supplements National Institutes of Health. (2008). Dietary supplement fact sheet: Vitamin D. Retrieved June 29, 2008, from http://ods.od.nih.gov/factsheets/vitamind.asp

TABLE C-2  Food Rich in Calcium

| Selected Foods | Calcium Content (mg) |
|---|---|
| Milk, nonfat, 8 fl oz | 302 |
| Milk, reduced fat (2%), 8 fl oz | 297 |
| Milk, whole, 8 fl oz | 291 |
| Milk, lactose reduced, 8 fl oz | 285–302 |
| Yogurt, plain, low fat, 8 oz | 415 |
| Yogurt, fruit, low fat, 8 oz | 245–384 |
| Orange juice w/ calcium, 6 fl oz | 200–260 |
| Cheddar cheese, 1 oz | 204 |
| Mozzarella, part skim, 1½ oz | 275 |
| Cottage cheese, low fat, 1 cup | 138 |
| Cheese, cream, regular, 1 Tbsp | 12 |
| Ricotta, part skim, 4 oz | 335 |
| Turnip greens, boiled, ½ cup | 99 |
| Broccoli, cooked from raw, 1 cup | 136 |
| Broccoli, cooked from frozen, 1 cup | 100 |
| Soybeans, cooked, 1 cup | 131 |
| Collards, cooked, 1 cup | 357 |
| Kale, cooked, 1 cup | 94 |
| Salmon, pink/canned, w/ bones, 3 oz | 181 |
| Cereal, calcium fortified, 1 cup | 100–1000 |
| Almonds, 1 oz | 75 |

Source: Adapted from Office of Dietary Supplements National Institutes of Health. (2005). Dietary supplement fact sheet: Calcium. Retrieved June 29, 2008, from http://ods.od.nih.gov/factsheets/calcium.asp

TABLE C-3    Vitamin D and Calcium Requirements by Age

| Age | RDA Calcium | RDA Vitamin D |
|-----|-------------|---------------|
| Birth to 6 months | 210 mg | |
| 7 months to 12 months | 270 mg | |
| 1 to 3 years | 500 mg | |
| 4 to 8 years | 800 mg | 5 mcg (200 IU) |
| 9 to 18 years | 1300 mg | |
| 19 to 50 years | 1000 mg | |
| 51 to 70 years | 1200 mg | 10 mcg (400 IU) |
| 71+ years | 1200 mg | 15 mcg (600 IU) |
| For Pregnancy and lactation increase to 1300–1500 mg/d | | |

*Source:* Adapted from Office of Dietary Supplements National Institutes of Health. (2005). *Dietary supplement fact sheet: Calcium.* Retrieved June 29, 2008, from http://ods.od.nih.gov/factsheets/calcium.asp

**C**

**Supplements**

Calcium carbonate

Calcium phosphate

Calcium citrate

Base choice on tolerance, convenience, cost, availability

Consider purity, absorbability (best taken several times /d in divided doses), and calcium interactions w/ other medications/foods

Often combined w/ vitamin D supplements, which can increase absorption

**SOURCES**

National Institute of Health Osteoporosis and Related Bone Diseases—National Resource Center. (2005). *Calcium supplements: What to look for* [Patient Handout]. Bethesda, MD: National Institute of Health.

Office of Dietary Supplements National Institutes of Health. (2005). *Dietary supplement fact sheet: Calcium.* Retrieved June 29, 2008, from http://ods.od.nih.gov/factsheets/calcium.asp

Office of Dietary Supplements National Institutes of Health. (2008). *Dietary supplement fact sheet: Vitamin D.* Retrieved June 29, 2008, from http://ods.od.nih.gov/factsheets/vitamind.asp

## CANDIDIASIS

### Cause
C. albicans most common

### Signs and Symptoms
Pruritus
Vaginal soreness
Dysparunia
External dysuria
Abnormal vaginal discharge

### Diagnosis
Thick curdy vaginal discharge
Vulvar edema
Fissures
Excoriations
Wet mount w/ pseudohyphae
Positive culture results
Normal vaginal pH

### Complicated Cases
Recurrent infection (> 4 per yr)
Non-albicans candidiasis (test on Sabouraud's medium)
Other condition (diabetes, immunosuppression, pregnancy)

### Treatment
Butoconazole 2% cream 5 g PV × 1 or QD × 3 d
Clotrimazole 1% cream 5 g PV × 7–14 d
Miconazole 1200 mg PV once
Nystatin 100,000 units PV × 14 d
Terconizole 0.4% cream 5 g PV × 7 d
Fluconazole 150 mg PO once (not during pregnancy)
Fluconazole 100 mg PO daily × 5 d (not during pregnancy)

*Pregnant*
Topical antifungal cream for 7 d
All of the above antifungal creams are Preg Cat C

*Non-albicans Candidiasis*
Longer duration of therapy 7–14 d
600 mg boric acid in a gelatin capsule vaginally QD × 14 d

### Patient Education
Cotton underwear
Avoid long periods in wet swim suits
No tight pants
Creams are oil based and may weaken latex condoms and diaphragms
No soaps w/ color or odor
Sensitive skin laundry detergent

**SOURCE**
Centers for Disease Control and Prevention. (2006). Sexually transmitted diseases treatment guidelines, 2006. *Morbidity and Mortality Weekly Report, 55*(RR-11), 54–56.

# CARDIOVASCULAR HEALTH ASSESSMENT

### Cholesterol

1. Measure lipoprotein levels after fasting 9–12 h (never do on a pregnant woman as level will be artificially elevated as the fetus mobilizes cholesterol for development)

TABLE C-4  Classifications of LDL, Total, and HDL Cholesterol (mg/dl) According to the ATP III

| LDL Cholesterol—Primary Target of Therapy | |
| --- | --- |
| < 100 | Optimal |
| 100–129 | Near optimal/above optimal |
| 130–159 | Borderline high |
| 160–189 | High |
| ≥ 190 | Very high |
| **Total Cholesterol** | |
| < 200 | Desirable |
| 200–239 | Borderline high |
| ≥ 240 | High |
| **HDL Cholesterol** | |
| < 40 | Low |
| ≥ 60 | High |

Source: Reprinted from National Institutes of Health: National Heart, Lung, and Blood Institute. (2001). ATP III guidelines at-a-glance quick desk reference. Retrieved April 2, 2008, from http://www.nhlbi.nih.gov/guidelines/cholesterol/atglance.pdf

2. Assess risk factors noting s/sx of CAD
Increased risk if:
   - Smoke
   - HTN (or BP > 140/90)
   - Low HDL
   - Family hx of CHD < 55 yr old (men) or < 65 yr old (women)
   - Age > 45 yr old (men) or > 55 yr old (women)
3. If 2+ risk factors, do Framingham Risk Assessment
4. Create target LDL levels and start therapeutic lifestyle changes
   - Saturated fat < 7% of total calories/d
   - Cholesterol < 200 mg/d
   - Increase fiber to 10–25 g/d
   - Increase plant sterols to 2 g/d
   - Decrease wt
   - Increase physical activity
5. Add medication: HMG-CoA reductase inhibitors (statins), bile acid sequestrants, nicotonic acid (niacin), fibric acids

If no improvement assess for metabolic syndrome and treat accordingly

*Cholesterol Drug Therapy*

▶ HMG-CoA Reductase Inhibitors (Statins)
Medications: Atorvastatin, Fluvastatin, Lovastatin Pravastatin, Simvastatin, Rosuvastatin
Expected lipid changes:
LDL ↓ 18–55%,
HDL ↑ 5–15%,
TG ↓ 7–30%
Side effects:
Myopathy,
↑ LFTs
Contraindications: active or chronic liver disease, elevated LFTs, pregnancy, breastfeeding, concurrent administration of drugs that inhibit or are processed

through cytochrome p450 pathway (cyclosporine, azole antifungals, protease inhibitors, macrolide antibiotics, grapefruit juice > 1 quart QD)

▶ Bile Acid Sequestrants

Medications: Cholestyramine, Colestipol, Colesevelam

Expected lipid changes:

LDL ↓ 15–30%,

HDL ↑ 3–5%,

TG—no change

Side effects:

GI distress

Constipation

↓ Absorption of other medications

Contraindication:

TG > 400, due to no effect on TG levels

▶ Nicotinic Acid (Niacin)

Medications: Available OTC

Lipid changes:

LDL ↓ 5–25%

HDL ↑ 15–35%

TG ↓ 20–50%

Side effects:

Flushing

Hyperglycemia

Hyperuricemia

Gout

Upper GI distress

Liver toxicity

Contraindications:

Chronic liver disease

Severe gout

▶ Fibric Acids

Medications: Fenofibrate, Gemfibrozil

Lipid changes:

LDL ↓ 5–20%

LDL ↑ in pts w/ high TG,

HDL ↑ 10–20%,

TG ↓ 20–50%

Side effects:

Dyspepsia

Gallstones

Myopathy

Contraindication: Severe renal or liver disease

## Framingham Risk Assessment

See Table C-5.

## Hypertension

Dx = 2 elevated BPs on 2 separate occasions

See Table C-6.

See Figure C-1.

Lifestyle modifications × 3 mo then repeat BP

Refer to primary care or cardiologist for drug management

See Table C-7.

## Metabolic Syndrome

Insulin resistance, hyperandrogenemia, and obesity

TABLE C-5 Framingham Risk Assessment for Women

## Framingham Point Scores

| Age | Points |
|---|---|
| 20-34 | -7 |
| 35-39 | -3 |
| 40-44 | 0 |
| 45-49 | 3 |
| 50-54 | 6 |
| 55-59 | 8 |
| 60-64 | 10 |
| 65-69 | 12 |
| 70-74 | 14 |
| 75-79 | 16 |

| Total Cholesterol | Points | | | | |
|---|---|---|---|---|---|
| | Age 20-39 | Age 40-49 | Age 50-59 | Age 60-69 | Age 70-79 |
| <160 | 0 | 0 | 0 | 0 | 0 |
| 160-199 | 4 | 3 | 2 | 1 | 1 |
| 200-239 | 8 | 6 | 4 | 2 | 1 |
| 240-279 | 11 | 8 | 5 | 3 | 2 |
| ≥ 280 | 13 | 10 | 7 | 4 | 2 |

| | Points | | | | |
|---|---|---|---|---|---|
| | Age 20-39 | Age 40-49 | Age 50-59 | Age 60-69 | Age 70-79 |
| Nonsmoker | 0 | 0 | 0 | 0 | 0 |
| Smoker | 9 | 7 | 4 | 2 | 1 |

| Systolic BP (mm Hg) | If Untreated | If Treated |
|---|---|---|
| < 120 | 0 | 0 |
| 120-129 | 1 | 3 |
| 130-139 | 2 | 4 |
| 140-159 | 3 | 5 |
| ≥ 160 | 4 | 6 |

| HDL (mg/dl) | Points |
|---|---|
| ≥ 60 | -1 |
| 50-59 | 0 |
| 40-49 | 1 |
| < 40 | 2 |

| Point Total | 10-Year Risk % |
|---|---|
| < 9 | < 1 |
| 9 | 1 |
| 10 | 1 |
| 11 | 1 |
| 12 | 1 |
| 13 | 2 |
| 14 | 2 |
| 15 | 3 |
| 16 | 4 |
| 17 | 5 |
| 18 | 6 |
| 19 | 8 |
| 20 | 11 |
| 21 | 14 |
| 22 | 17 |
| 23 | 22 |
| 24 | 27 |
| ≥ 25 | ≥ 30 |

10-Year Risk _____ %

C

Source: Reprinted from National Institutes of Health: National Heart, Lung, and Blood Institute. (2001). ATP III guidelines at-a-glance quick desk reference. Retrieved April 2, 2008, from http://www.nhlbi.nih.gov/guidelines/cholesterol/atglance.pdf

Increased risk for cerebrovascular disease, elevated cholesterol, triglycerides, LDL, and C-peptides but lower HDL and apolipoprotein A-1

*Diagnosis (need at least 3 out of 5)*
Abdominal obesity > 35 in
Trigylcerides > 150 mg/dl
HDL-C < 50 mg/dl
BP > 130/85
Fasting glucose 110–126 mg/dl
2 h GTT 140–199 mg/dl

**SOURCES**

National Institutes of Health: National Heart, Lung, and Blood Institute. (2003). *Seventh report of the joint national committee on prevention, detection, evaluation, and treatment of high blood pressure (JNC 7)*. Retrieved April 4, 2008, from http://www.nhlbi.nih.gov/guidelines/hypertension/phycard.pdf

Schuiling, K. D., & Likis, F. E. (2006). *Women's gynecologic health*. Sudbury, MA: Jones and Bartlett.

U.S. Department of Health and Human Services. (2001). *ATP III guidelines at-a-glance quick desk reference*. Retrieved April 23, 2008, from http://www.nhlbi.nih.gov/guidelines/cholesterol/atglance.pdf

TABLE C-6   Classifications of Blood Pressure

| Category | SBP mm Hg | | DBP mm Hg |
|---|---|---|---|
| Normal | < 120 | and | < 80 |
| Prehypertension | 120–139 | or | 80–89 |
| Hypertension, Stage 1 | 140–159 | or | 90–99 |
| Hypertension, Stage 2 | ≥ 160 | or | ≥ 100 |

SBP = systolic blood pressure; DBP = diastolic blood pressure.

*Source:* Reprinted from National Heart, Lung, and Blood Institute. (2003). *Seventh report of the joint national committee on prevention, detection, evaluation, and treatment of high blood pressure (JNC 7)*. Retrieved April 4, 2008, from http://www.nhlbi.nih.gov/guidelines/hypertension/phycard.pdf

TABLE C-7   Lifestyle Modification Recommendations

| Modification | Recommendation | Avg. SBP Reduction Range† |
|---|---|---|
| Weight reduction | Maintain normal body weight (body mass index 18.5–24.9 kg/m²). | 5–20 mm Hg/10 kg |
| DASH eating plan | Adopt a diet rich in fruits, vegetables, and low-fat dairy products with reduced content of saturated and total fat. | 8–14 mm Hg |
| Dietary sodium reduction | Reduce dietary sodium intake to ≤ 100 mmol per day (2.4 g sodium or 6 g sodium chloride). | 2–8 mm Hg |
| Aerobic physical activity | Regular aerobic physical activity (e.g., brisk walking) at least 30 minutes per day, most days of the week. | 4–9 mm Hg |
| Moderation of alcohol consumption | Men: limit to ≤ 2 drinks* per day. Women and lighter weight persons: limit to ≤ 1 drink* per day. | 2–4 mm Hg |

*1 drink = 1/2 oz or 15 ml ethanol (e.g., 12 oz beer, 5 oz wine, 1.5 oz 80-proof whiskey).

† Effects are dose and time dependent.

*Source:* Reprinted from National Heart, Lung, and Blood Institute. (2003). *Seventh report of the joint national committee on prevention, detection, evaluation, and treatment of high blood pressure (JNC 7)*. Retrieved April 4, 2008, from http://www.nhlbi.nih.gov/guidelines/hypertension/phycard.pdf

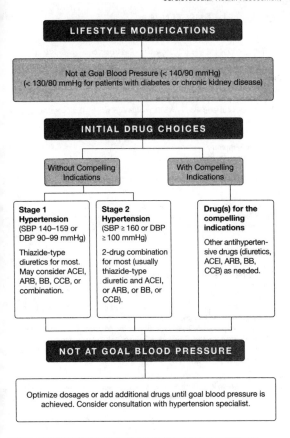

FIGURE C-1 Algorithm for Treatment of Hypertension. *Source:* Reprinted from National Heart, Lung, and Blood Institute. (2003). *Seventh report of the joint national committee on prevention, detection, evaluation, and treatment of high blood pressure (JNC 7).* Retrieved April 4, 2008, from http://www.nhlbi.nih.gov/guidelines/hypertension/phycard.pdf

## CERVICAL INCOMPETENCE

### Definition

Painless cervical changes that occur in the 2nd trimester and can result in pregnancy loss

### Contributing Factors

Cervical abnormality—congenitally short cervix, distal Mullerian duct abnormality (high in bicornuate uteruses), exposure in utero to DES

Trauma: cervical laceration w/ NSVD, postcervical surgery (e.g., cone biopsy and/or mechanical dilation of the cervix)

Over distended uterus d/t multiple gestation

### Signs and Symptoms

Vaginal fullness/pressure

Contractions

Increased vaginal discharge (often brown or red tinged)

### Diagnosis

Visualization and digital exam of the cervix

TVU/S for cervical length: progressive shortening of endocervical canal to < 20 mm or funneling of fetal membranes into endocervical canal indicative of incompetence

### Treatment

Pelvic rest

TVU/S surveillance of cervical changes

Bed rest

Prophylactic cerclage

Preventing dilation w/ a suture through the cervix placed by a surgeon at 12–15 wk gestation and removed at 37–38 wk or w/ preterm labor

Risks of this procedure include infection, trauma to cervix, PTD, PROM, PPROM

Evidence suggests that TVU/S surveillance q 2 wk to assess for cervical shortening (< 25 mm) before cerclage placement can decrease the number of unnecessary cerclages

**SOURCE**

Cunningham, G., Leveno, K. J., Bloom, S. L., Hauth, J. C., Gilstrap, L. C., & Wenstrom, K. D. (2005). *Williams obstetrics* (22nd ed.). New York: McGraw-Hill.

# CERVICAL LIP

Do you really need to intervene?

**Definition**

Dilation > 8–9 cm
Cervix absent everywhere except anteriorly/posteriorly/laterally

**Risk Factors**

Posterior babies
Posterior os during most of labor
Long labor
Lack of position change during labor
Presenting part low and ctx strong
Bearing down before complete dilation

**Management**

Change to hands and knees position
Rock side to side on back
Alternate between left and right lateral sides q 2 ctx
Breath through urge to push
If epidural in place and woman not able to move:
    McRoberts: hold knees up and back (hyperflexion of knees onto abdomen)
    Trendelenburg: head lower than pelvis
    Manual reduction: push it back during a ctx (can be very painful)

**EDEMATOUS ANTERIOR LIP**

Remove baby's head pressure w/ position change (knee–chest position)
Apply ice to cervix (put ice in a glove and hold it on the lip through 2 ctx)
Apply arnica gel directly to cervix

**SOURCE**

Frye, A. (2004). Holistic midwifery: A comprehensive textbook for midwives in homebirth practice. Portland, OR: Labrys Press.

## CERVICITIS

### Definition
Inflammation of the cervix
Present in 30–45% of pts in STI clinics
GC/CT only account for 50% of the cases

### Signs and Symptoms
Cervical ectopy (extension of columnar epithelium onto the visible ectocervix)
Friable cervix
Mucopurulent or yellow discharge
Abundance of WBCs on microscopic examination
Polymorphonuclear leukocytes on gram stain examination
Caused by: gonorrhea, chlamydia, *Mycoplasm genitalium*, *Mycoplasm hominis*,
    *Uralasma uralytium*, BV, HSV, cytomegalovirus, *Tricamonas vaginalis*, adenovirus
Can lead to endometritis, PID, and adverse outcomes in pregnancy and newborns
Cervicitis increases the risk of contracting and transmitting HIV

### Treatment
Empiric tx for CT of pt and her partner
Empiric GC tx not generally suggested
Chronic cervicitis w/o STI can be tx w/ ablation

**SOURCES**
Lusk, M. J., & Konecny, P. (2008). Cervicitis: A review. *Current Opinions in Infectious Diseases, 21*, 49–55.
Nazeer, S. (2007). *Unaided visual inspection of the cervix "clinical downstaging" picture atlas.* Retrieved April 15, 2008, from http://www.gfmer.ch/Books/Cervical_cancer_modules/Unaided_visual_inspection_atlas.htm

# CHLAMYDIA

### Definition
*C. trachmoatis* (gram neg, small, obligate intracellular parasite) present on cervix
  or in urethra

### Screening
Annually < 25 yr old
Risk factors > 25 yr old

### Signs and Symptoms
Mostly asymptomatic
Cervicitis

### Sequelae
PID
Ectopic pregnancy
Infertility
Cervicitis
Endometritis
Salpingitis
Perinatal retinitis

### Diagnosis
Urine collection and dip
Endocervical/vaginal/rectum specimen

### Treatment
Anyone (all tx are Preg Cat B):
  Azithromycin 1 g PO × 1
  Erythromycin base 500 mg PO QID × 7 d
  Erythromycin ethylsuccinate 800 mg PO QID × 7 d
Not pregnant:
  Doxycycline 100 mg PO BID × 7 d
  Ofloxacin 300 mg PO BID × 7 d
  Levofloxacin 500 mg PO QD × 7 d

### Follow-up
No test of cure needed in nonpregnant pts, but encouraged 3–12 mo post tx
Test of cure 3 wk after tx in pregnant women
Partners should be tested and treated
It is appropriate for same provider to treat pt's partner at the same time

### Patient Education
Abstain from sex during tx and for 7 d after tx completed by both partners
Transmission risks
Partner notification
Prevention

### Newborn
Prophylactic antibiotics not recommended
Culture conjunctiva
Assess for pneumonia characterized by repetitive staccato cough, no fever, no
  wheezing
Nasopharynx cultures
If positive, treat w/ erythromycin ethyl succinate 50 mg/kg/d PO QID × 14 d
Do test of cure (often needs 2 rounds of tx)

### SOURCE
Centers for Disease Control and Prevention. (2006). Sexually transmitted diseases treatment
guidelines, 2006. *Morbidity and Mortality Weekly Report, 55*(RR-11), 38–42.

## CHOLESTASIS OF PREGNANCY

### Definition
Normal bile flow from the gallbladder is obstructed

### Statistics
2.4% singleton pregnancies
20.9% twin pregnancies
70% of cases occur in 3rd trimester

### Maternal Risk
Postpartum hemorrhage
Development of gallstones postpartum

### Fetal Risks
Fetal distress
PTL
IUFD (9% of cases)

### Signs and Symptoms
Pruritis—especially palmar, solar, abdominal
Dark colored urine
Light colored stools
Fatigue/exhaustion
Loss of appetite
Depression
Jaundice

### Diagnosis
Serum bile acids—10 to 100 fold increase
Alkaline phosphatase—7 to 10 fold increase
Increased AST (65% cases)
Increased ALT (60% cases)

### Differential Diagnosis
Viral hepatitis
Gallbladder disease

### Treatment
Deliver as soon as lungs are mature (*See also* Fetal Lung Assessment)
Pruritis usually does not respond to antihistamines
Reduction in bile acids w/ cholestyramine and/or aluminum-containing antacids
   may help
Cold baths and ice packs
Ursodeoxycholic acid 15–25 mg/kg/d decreases liver tranaminases, no studies of
   safety in pregnancy
Vitamin K/Mephyton (for maternal and fetal clotting)
Steroids to increase fetal lung maturation (when indicated)
NSTs (2/wk)
Fetal kick counts
Monitor LFTs and bile salts

### Resolution
Maternal symptoms usually resolve w/in 2 d after delivery
Counsel woman regarding increased risk for reoccurrence in subsequent
   pregnancy or while taking OCP

Dandelion root and/or milk thistle to help support liver health

### SOURCE
Burrow, G., Duffy, T., & Copel, J. (2004). *Medical complications during pregnancy* (6th ed.).
   Philadelphia: Elsevier Saunders.

# CHORIOAMNIONITIS

### Definition
Inflammation of chorion and/or amnion
Pathogens: GBS, *E.coli*, *U. urealyticum*, *G. vaginalis*, *B. bivius*

### Statistics
1–2% of all pregnancies, common in PTD
Neonatal mortality 1–2% at term, 10% preterm

### Signs and Symptoms
Maternal fever > 37.8°C; 100% frequency
Maternal tachycardia > 100 bpm; 50–80% frequency
Fetal tachycardia > 160 bpm; 40–70% frequency
Maternal WBCs > 15,000; 70–90% frequency
Foul odor of amniotic fluid; 5–22% frequency
Uterine tenderness; 4–25% frequency

### Diagnosis = Maternal temperature + 2 other s/sx

### Risk Factors
PROM (> 24 h), w/ or w/out prolonged labor
Repeated vaginal exams
Manipulative vaginal or intrauterine procedures

### Complications
Inadequate contractions
Decreased response to pitocin
Labor dystocia
Slowed cervical dilation
Fetal acidosis
Neonatal pneumonia

### Labor Management

| | |
|---|---|
| Deliver w/in 24 hours of dx | VS q 1 h |
| ROM as necessary | Pitocin to expedite delivery |
| FSE | MD consult |
| IV fluids | |

### Increased Risk of

| | |
|---|---|
| Atony | Sepsis |
| Uterine abscess | Seizure |
| Thromboembolism | Low 5-min Apgar |
| Wound infections | |

### Treatment

*Combination Therapy*
Ampicillin 2 g IV load, then 1 g IV Q 4–6 h (Preg Cat B; Lact Cat L1) with
   gentamicin 120 mg load, then 80–100 mg (or 1.5 mg/kg) IV Q 8 h (Preg Cat C,
   but considered safe in intrapartum; Lact Cat L1)

*Single Agent Therapy*
Ampicillin-sulbactam (Unasyn) 3g Q 6 h (Preg Cat B; Lact Cat L1)
Cefuroxime (Ceftin) 1.5 g Q 8 h (Preg Cat B; Lact Cat L2)

*If PCN Allergic*
Clindamycin 900 mg IV Q 8 h (Preg Cat B; Lact Cat L1)
Erythromycin 1 g Q 6 h (Preg Cat B; Lact Cat L2/L3)
Vancomycin 500 mg Q 6 h (Preg Cat C; Lact Cat L1)

*Adjunct Therapy*
Acetaminophen 1000 mg PO or PR, repeated Q 3–4 h (Preg Cat B; Lact Cat L1)

### SOURCES
Cunningham, G., Leveno, K. J., Bloom, S. L., Hauth, J. C., Gilstrap, L. C., & Wenstrom, K. D. (2005).
   *Williams obstetrics* (22nd ed.). New York: McGraw-Hill.
Fahey, J. O. (2008). Clinical management of intra-amniotic infection and chorioamnionitis: A review of
   the literature [Abstract]. *Journal of Midwifery & Women's Health, 53*(3) 227–235.
Newton, E. (2005). Preterm labor, preterm premature rupture of membranes, and chorioamnionitis.
   *Clinics of Perinatology, 32*(3), 571.

## CIRCUMCISION

**Definition**
Removal of the foreskin that covers the tip of the penis

**Reasons to Choose Circumcision**
Penis is easier to clean
Decreased risk of penile cancer
Social reasons ("I want my child to look like his father")
Religious or cultural reasons

**Reasons Not to Circumcise**
It is easy to teach a child to care for his penis
Circumcision is a form of genital mutilation
It can be painful for infants
Risk of infection from the procedure
Circumcision can be done later
Circumcision exposes sensitive parts of the penis

**Care of the Circumcised Penis**
Care will depend on the type of instrument used to do the circumcision (check w/
   the provider)
Generally, a thin layer of petrolatum or A&D ointment is applied to a 2 × 2 dressing
   prior to diapering to prevent wound from sticking to diaper for 2–3 d post
   procedure
Watch for signs of infection

**Care of the Uncircumcised Penis**
Wash the exposed skin surfaces when the genitals are washed
No need to retract the foreskin or clean under it until it naturally retracts

**Academy of Pediatrics Statement**

FIGURE C-2   Summary of Recommendations from American Academy of Pediatrics

Existing scientific evidence demonstrates potential medical benefits of newborn
male circumcision; however, these data are not sufficient to recommend routine
neonatal circumcision. In the case of circumcision, in which there are potential
benefits and risks, yet the procedure is not essential to the child's current well-
being, parents should determine what is in the best interest of the child. To make
an informed choice, parents of all male infants should be given accurate and
unbiased information and be provided the opportunity to discuss this decision.
It is legitimate for parents to take into account cultural, religious, and ethnic
traditions, in addition to the medical factors, when making this decision. Analgesia
is safe and effective in reducing the procedural pain associated with circumcision;
therefore, if a decision for circumcision is made, procedural analgesia should be
provided. If circumcision is performed in the newborn period, it should only be
done on infants who are stable and healthy.

*Source:* Reprinted with permission from Task Force on Circumcision. (1999). Circumcision policy
statement. *Pediatrics, 102*(3), 686.

**SOURCE**
Task Force on Circumcision. (1999). Circumcision policy statement. *Pediatrics, 102*(3), 686.

# CODING

Step 1: Preventative services vs. office visit: Preventative services visits get coded according to the pt age

Step 2: New vs. established pt

Step 3: How many elements of the HPI or Chief Complaint did you cover?

HPI = location, quality, severity, duration, timing, context, modifying factors, associated s/sx

1–3 = Brief

4+ = Extended

3+ inactive/chronic conditions = Extended

Step 4: How many body systems did you review?

ROS includes immunological/allergy, constitutional symptoms, integumentary, psychiatric

1 = Pertinent

2–9 = Extended

10+ = Complete

Step 5: How complex was your decision making?

Straightforward = 5–10 min

Low complexity = 15–30 min

Moderate complexity = 30–45 min

High complexity = > 45 min

Using your responses to Steps 3–5, find the appropriate code on the following charts

NEW pts = the lowest code

Established pts = the middle code

When does time trump all codes?

When 50% of the clinicians face-to-face time is spent on counseling only, then code according to total time spent w/ the pt

**TABLE C-8**   New Patient Coding Chart

| Visit Code | HPI | ROS | Decision Making |
|---|---|---|---|
| 99201 | Brief | Pertinent | Straightforward |
| 99202 | Brief | Extended | Straightforward |
| 99203 | Extended | Extended | Low complexity |
| 99204 | Extended | Complete | Moderate complexity |
| 99205 | Extended | Complete | High complexity |

**TABLE C-9**   Established Patient Coding Chart

| Code | History | ROS | Decision Making |
|---|---|---|---|
| 99211 | Provider not required | | |
| 99212 | Focused | Brief | Straightforward |
| 99213 | Extended | Extended | Low complexity |
| 99214 | Extended | Extended | Moderate complexity |
| 99215 | Extended | Complete | High complexity |

**SOURCE**

International Classification of Diseases 9th Revision Clinical Modification. (2006). In Hart, A. C., Hopkins, C. A., & Ford, B. (Eds.), *ICD-9-CM professional* (6th ed.). Salt Lake City, UT: Ingenix.

## CONSTIPATION

### Definition
Within the last 12 mo, or at least 12 wk (not necessarily consecutive), at least two of the following:
  Straining
  Lumpy or hard stool
  Feeling of incomplete evacuation
  Feeling of anorectal obstruction
  Manual maneuvers to assist defecation or fewer than 3 defecations per wk

### Causes
  Inadequate fluid intake
  Low-fiber diet
  Poor bowel habits
  Age
  Lack of exercise
  Pregnancy
  Illness
  Medications
  Hormonal changes d/t menstrual cycle/menopause

### Assessment
  Detailed diet history
  Detailed bowel history
  Thorough abdominal exam, including bowel sounds (r/o obstruction)
  Rectal exam to assess for masses or obstructions

### Labs
  CBC
  Serum electrolytes
  Calcium
  TSH

### Prevention (and Often Treatment)
  Increase fiber content of diet: fruits, vegetables, whole grains
  Drink plenty of noncaffeinated fluids
  Increase physical activity
  Use the bathroom promptly with urge
  Medications (caution against relying on stimulant laxatives)
  Increase intake of lactobacilli (probiotic)

### Treatment
  *See* Table C-10.
  1st line: bulking agents, lubricants
  2nd line: saline agents, hyperosmotics
  3rd line: stimulants

### HERBAL LAXATIVE SYRUP (NOT FOR PREGNANT/NURSING MOTHERS)
  1 tsp honey
  2 tsp cascara sagrada bark tincture (herbal laxative)
  1 tsp licorice root tincture
  ½ tsp tincture of fennel, ginger, or peppermint
  Warm honey, enough to make it liquid
  Combine w/ remaining ingredients and stir well
  Take 1 tsp

**SOURCES**

Arcangelo, V. P., & Peterson, A. M. (Eds.). (2006). *Pharmacotherapeutics for advanced practice: A practical approach* (2nd ed.). Philadelphia, PA: Lippincott Williams & Wilkins.

Epocrates, I. (2008). *Epocrates online.* Retrieved May 22, 2008, from http://www.epocrates.com

Hackley, B., Kriebs, J. M., & Rousseau, M. E. (2007). *Primary care of women.* Sudbury, MA: Jones and Bartlett.

Hale, T. W. (2008). *Medications and mothers' milk* (13th ed.). Amarillo, TX: Hale.

**TABLE C-10** Constipation Treatment

| Category | Drug | Side Effects | Advantages | Disadvantages | Contraindications |
|---|---|---|---|---|---|
| Bulking agents | Psyllium (Metamucil) 1–2 tsp QD-TID<br>Methylcellulose (Citrucel) 2–6 g/d; 1 heaping tsp mixed in 8 oz water 1–3 ×/d | Flatulence, bloating | No systemic absorption | Must drink plenty of water<br>Can be high in sugar | GI obstruction, undiagnosed abd pain, DM |
| Lubricants and surfactants | Ducosate sodium (Colace) 50–500 mg/d; 100 mg QD-BID<br>Mineral oil 5–45 ml/d<br>Glycerin 1 supp PR PRN | Stomach upset, rectal seepage | No systemic absorption; prevents straining | Use for prevention, except supp<br>BEST for pregnancy | Do not use colace with mineral oil |
| Saline agents | Sodium phosphate enema (Fleet) 118 ml/d<br>Magnesium hydroxide (milk of magnesia) 30–60 ml/d | GI upset, diarrhea | | Electrolyte imbalance | CHF, HTN, edema, CRF, some abx and antifungals |
| Hyperosmotic agents | Sorbitol 15–60 ml<br>Lactulose 15–60 ml (15–30 ml PO QD-BID)<br>Miralax 17 g PO QD | GI upset, diarrhea, gas | | Some are high in sugar | Electrolyte problems, renal insufficiency, DM |
| Stimulants | Senna (Senakot) 2–4 tabs PO QD-BID or 1 supp Qhs<br>Castor oil 15–60 ml PO × 1 | Cramping, diarrhea, gas<br>Rapid onset w/ castor oil | | **Potential laxative abuse Extreme! Not for routine use! NO pregnancy | GI obstruction, abdominal pain, hemorrhoids/anal fissures |

1st line: bulking agents, lubricants
2nd line: saline agents, hyperosmotics
3rd line: stimulants

Sources: Epocrates, 2008; Hale, 2008.

C

## CONTRACEPTION

Percentages of women experiencing an unintended pregnancy during the first year of typical and perfect use of each contraceptive type

**TABLE C-11**  Failure Rates of Contraceptive Methods

| Method | Perfect Use | | Typical Use | |
|---|---|---|---|---|
| | Multip | Primip | Multip | Primip |
| Cervical cap | 26% | 9% | 32% | 16% |
| Combined oral contraceptives | 0.3% | | 8% | |
| Male condom | 2% | | 15% | |
| Female condom | 5% | | 21% | |
| Depo | 0.3% | | 3% | |
| Diaphragm | 6% | | 16% | |
| Mirena | 0.2% | | 0.2% | |
| Paraguard | 0.6% | | 0.8% | |
| Patch/ring | 0.3% | | 8% | |
| Periodic abstinence | 8% | | 25% | |
| Abstinence/delayed sexual intercourse | 0% | | Unknown | |
| Implanon | 0.05% | | 0.05% | |
| Progestin-only contraceptive pills | 0.3% | | 8% | |
| Spermicides | 18% | | 29% | |
| Sponge | 20% | 9% | 32% | 16% |
| Female sterilization | 0.5% | | 0.5% | |
| Male sterilization | 0.1% | | 0.15% | |
| Withdrawal | 4% | | 27% | |
| No method | 85% | | 85% | |
| Fertility awareness | 25% | | Unknown | |

*Source:* Reprinted with permission from Hatcher, R. A. (2007). *Contraceptive technology* (19th ed.). New York, NY: Ardent Media.

**SOURCE**
Hatcher, R. A. (2007). *Contraceptive technology* (19th ed.). New York, NY: Ardent Media.

# CONTRACEPTION: ABSTINENCE

Perfect Use: 0%
Typical Use: Unknown

**Mechanism of Action**
No sperm in or near the vagina

**Candidates**
Everyone

**C**

**Types**
Primary abstinence—waiting until marriage
Return to abstinence—no sex until marriage w/ new partner
Abstinence for a while—until OCPs take effect, for STD results, postpartum
Abstinence right now—tonight or today because we don't have a condom

**Advantages**
Increased self-esteem/confidence
Increased communication and negotiation skills
Reduced risk of STIs
Incorporates religious and cultural values
Reduced risk of cervical cancer
Learning alternative ways of pleasing self and partner

**Disadvantages**
Frustration
Fear of rejection by partner
Requires commitment and self-control
Risk of being unprepared for unplanned intercourse

**SOURCE**
Hatcher, R. A. (2007). *Contraceptive technology* (19th ed.). New York, NY: Ardent Media.

# CONTRACEPTION: COMBINED ORAL CONTRACEPTIVE PILLS (COCs)

Perfect use: 0.3
Typical use: 8%

## Progestin MOA

Thicken cervical mucus to prevent sperm penetration into upper genital tract
Block LH surge inhibiting ovulation
Inhibit capacitation of sperm
Slow tubal motility delaying sperm transport
Disrupt transport of fertilized ovum
Induce endometrial atrophy

## Estrogen MOA

Decrease FSH release, which may help suppress LH surge
May induce localized edema in endometrial lining, reducing probability of implantation

## WHO 3/4

Breastfeeding < 6 mo postpartum
Postpartum < 21 d
Age > 35 yr and smoking any amount of cigarettes
Multiple cardiac risk factors (thromboembolic disorder, hx of current DVT or pulmonary embolism, CVA, or CAD)
Multiple risk factors for arterial CVD (valvular heart disease, uncontrolled HTN, diabetes w/ vascular involvement)
H/As w/ focal aura
Migraines w/o aura > 35 yr old
Major surgery w/ prolonged immobilization (d/c COCs 1 mo prior to surgery)
Acute/chronic hepatocellular disease w/ abnormal liver function
Hepatic adenomas or hepatic carcinomas
Anticonvulsant therapy
Hx of cancer
Known hyperlipidemia
Nephropathy
Gallbladder disease
Active hepatitis

## Advantages

Highly effective
Safer for health than pregnancy
Easily reversible
Decreased risk of ectopic pregnancy
Decreased dysmenorrhea
Decreased menstrual flow
Less PMDD symptoms
Decreased anovulatory bleeding
Cessation of mittelschmerz
Decreased ovarian cysts
Decreased menstrual migraines

## Disadvantages

Daily administration
Need for storage and ready access
Expense and access
No protection against STIs
Increased risk for MI (not true for pills w/ 20 mcg EE)
Increased risk for stroke in high-risk women
Increased risk for venous thromboembolism
Hormone induced HTN
Increased risk of HIV/chlamydia infection

Increased incidence of cervical dysplasia and carcinoma
Increased risk for gall bladder disease, cholestatic jaundice, or hepatic neoplasms
Increased breast cancer risk (weak evidence)

**Patient Education**

3–6 mo BP check after initiation
Call if miss 2 periods or s/sx of pregnancy
Instructions for missed pills
STI protection
Severe mood swings or depression
Jaundice
Breast lump
Fainting attack
Seizure or difficulty speaking
BP above 160/95
Server allergic skin rash
Prolonged immobilization (d/c COCs 1 mo prior to surgery)
Review ACHES: **A**bdominal pain, **C**hest pain. **H**/As, **E**ye/vision problems, **S**evere leg/arm pain

**General COC Info**

Broad spectrum antibiotics do not decrease the effectiveness of any COCs
Heavier women do not need higher dosages
COCs do not cause weight changes (gain or loss)

**TABLE C-12**   Common OCP Problems

| Too Much Estrogen | Too Little Estrogen |
|---|---|
| Heavy bleeding | Bleeding (spotting) early in cycle |
| Cystic breast | Too-light bleeding |
| Breast enlargement | Bleeding throughout the cycle |
| Dysmenorrhea | Amenorrhea |
| Bloating | |
| Premenstrual edema, H/A, irritability | |
| GI | |
| Cervical extrophy | |

| Too Much Progestin | Too Little Progestin |
|---|---|
| Increased appetite | Bleeding fewer days |
| Candidiasis | Bleeding (spotting) late in cycle |
| Depression | Heavy bleeding |
| Fatigue | Delayed-withdrawal bleeding |
| Cervicitis | Bloating |
| | Dysmenorrhea |
| | Premenstrual edema, H/A, irritability |
| | GI |

Source: Reprinted with permission from Hatcher, R. A. (2004). *Contraceptive technology* (18th ed.). New York, NY: Ardent Media.

**Types of COCs**

Monophasic COC: Good to manage breakthrough bleeding and for those that are sensitive to hormone fluctuations
Biphasic and triphasic COC: Good if experiencing progestin-related side effects, goal is to mimic normal menstrual cycle w/out ovulation, change in hormones takes place Q 7–10 d, no proven difference in efficacy, less net estrogen per cycle than monophasic

**SOURCES**

Dickey, R. P. (2005). *Managing contraceptive pill patients* (12th ed.). Dallas, TX: EMIS Medical.
Hatcher, R. A. (2007). *Contraceptive technology* (19th ed.). New York, NY: Ardent Media.
World Health Organization. (2004). *Medical eligibility criteria for contraceptive use.* Geneva, Switzerland: WHO Library Cataloguing-in-Publication Data.

## CONTRACEPTION: COMBINED ORAL CONTRACEPTIVE PILL INSTRUCTIONS FOR PATIENTS

When starting pills for the first time, or restarting pills:
1. Start taking pills on the day decided upon by you and your healthcare provider.
2. You must use another birth control method, such as condoms, for the entire first 7 days of taking the pills.
3. Please do NOT stop taking the pills even if you have irregular vaginal bleeding, breast tenderness, or nausea.

If you miss 1 "active" pill:
1. Take it as soon as you remember. Take the next pill at your regular time. If you forget 1 pill for an entire day then you will take 2 pills the following day.
2. If the missed pill is during the first week of your first pack, you should take emergency contraception (EC).
3. You do not need to use a backup birth control method if you have sex.

If you miss 2 "active" pills in a row within week 1 or 2 in your pack:
1. Take 2 pills on the day you remember and 2 pills the next day.
2. Then take 1 pill a day until you finish the pack.
3. You could become pregnant if you have sex within 7 days after your missed pills. Please use another method of birth control in addition to the pills, such as condoms, for all 7 days.

If you miss 2 "active" pills in a row in week 3:
1. If you are a Sunday starter: Keep taking 1 pill every day until Sunday. On Sunday, throw away the rest of the pack and start a new pack of pills on that Sunday.
2. If you are a day 1 starter: throw out the rest of the pills in that pack and start a new pack that day.
3. You may not have your period this month but that is expected. However, if you miss your period for 2 months in a row, call your healthcare provider because you might be pregnant.
4. You could become pregnant if you have sex in the first 7 days after your 2 missed pills. You must use another birth control method in addition to the pills, such as condoms, for a full 7 days.

If you miss 3 or more "active" pills in a row during any of the 3 weeks:
1. If you are a Sunday starter: keep taking 1 pill every day until Sunday. On Sunday, throw out the rest of that pack and start a new pack of pills that Sunday.
2. If you are a day 1 starter: throw out the rest of that pill pack and start a new pack that same day.
3. You may not have your period this month but that is expected. However, if you do not get your period the second month, please call your healthcare provider because you might be pregnant.
4. You could become pregnant if you have sex in the 7 days after your missed pills. You must use another birth control method, such as condoms, for a full 7 days.

If you forget any of the 7 "reminder/sugar" pills in week 4:
1. Throw away the pills you missed.
2. Keep taking one pill each day until the pack is empty.
3. You do not need a back up method.

If you are still not sure what to do about the pills you have missed:
1. Use another birth control method, such as condoms, every time you have sex.
2. Keep taking 1 "active" pill each day until you can reach your healthcare provider.

**SOURCES**

Hatcher, R. A. (2007). *Contraceptive technology* (19th ed.). New York, NY: Ardent Media.
Dickey, R. P. (2005). *Managing contraceptive pill patients* (12th ed.). Dallas, TX: EMIS.

# CONTRACEPTION: CONDOMS

Male: Perfect 2%, Typical 15%
Female: Perfect 5%, Typical 21%

## Mechanism of Action

Physical barrier between penile glans and shaft and vagina
Blocks semen and other sexually transmitted infections
Available in latex and nonlatex, many colors, flavors, sizes, and thicknesses

**WHO 3/4**

Latex allergy

## Candidates

Anyone at risk for STIs or pregnancy

## Advantages

No hormones
Protects against STIs
Cheap
Readily available
May help men maintain erection longer
Added sexual pleasure w/ the process of condom placement
Male involvement in fertility control
Sex is less messy
Easily transportable

## Disadvantages

Interrupts love making
Requires discipline for perfect use
May cause men to lose erection
Blunting of sensation
Decrease natural lubrication
Requires prompt withdrawal after ejaculation
Latex allergy
Requires communication and cooperation

## Patient Education

No petroleum products (no baby oil, edible oils, massage oils, petroleum jelly,
   suntan lotions, vaginal infection creams, body lotion, or rubbing alcohol)
Keep them handy, but do not overheat
Check expiration date
Teach correct placement
Encourage having EC on hand in case condom breaks or slips off

## Five Steps to Use a Condom

1. New condom for every sex act
2. Before any genital contact, place condom on tip of erect penis and roll sides
   down shaft
3. Unroll condom all the way to the base of the penis
4. Immediately after ejaculation hold the condom and withdraw the penis
5. Throw away used condom safely

**SOURCES**

Hatcher, R. A. (2007). *Contraceptive technology* (19th ed.). New York, NY Ardent Media.
World Health Organization. (2004). *Medical eligibility criteria for contraceptive use.* Geneva,
   Switzerland: WHO Library Cataloguing-in-Publication Data.

## CONTRACEPTION: DIAPHRAGM, CERVICAL CAP, SPONGE

Diaphragm: perfect 6%, typical 16%
Cervical Cap: perfect 26% (multip), 9% (nullip); typical 32% (multip), 16% (nullip)
Sponge: perfect 20% (multip), 9% (nullip); typical 32% (multip), 16% (nullip)

### Mechanism of Action

Physical barrier between egg and sperm
Spermicide kills any sperm that get past the barrier

### WHO 3/4

HIV pos
Hx of toxic shock
Latex or spermicide allergy
Obese pts harder to fit
Increased risk of UTI
Cervical lesions
Abnormalities in vaginal anatomy
Inability to perform correct technique
Full-term delivery w/in the past 6 wk
Recent spontaneous or therapeutic Ab

### Advantages

No hormones
Better spontaneity than condoms
Reusable
Some available OTC

### Disadvantages

Toxic shock syndrome
UTI
Pelvic pressure
Vaginal irritation/infection
Allergy
No STI protection
Insertion and removal difficulty
Messy
Must touch genitals
*See* Table C-13.

### Patient Education

Placement and use of spermicide
No STI protection
Less effective in parous women
Cleaning technique:
    Store in clean, cool, dark, convenient location
    Wash all parts w/ mild soap
    Do not use talcum powder
    Do not use oil-based products for lubrication or cleaning, it can deteriorate the
        rubber

### Fitting a Diaphragm

Measure length of vaginal vault between index/middle finger and palm (distance
    between posterior fornix and pubic bone)
Compare length measured on hand w/ lengths of fitting diaphragms
Insert fitting diaphragm and check rim for secure fit behind pubic bone
Choose largest diaphragm that comfortably fits behind pt's pubic bone, should be
    minimally felt by pt
Encourage pt to practice removing and inserting diaphragm during fitting
Clean fitting diaphragms in autoclave or w/ bleach and alcohol

TABLE C-13  Comparison of Barrier Methods

| | Diaphragm | Male/Female Condom | Lea's Shield/ FemCap | Sponge | Spermicide |
|---|---|---|---|---|---|
| Waiting time between insertion and sex (min and max) | 0 min<br>18 hrs max | 0<br>No max stated | 0<br>No max stated | 0<br>24 hrs max | 0–15 min<br>0–15 hrs max |
| Waiting time between sex and removal (min and max) | 6 hrs min<br>24 hrs max | No min or max—with female condom remove before standing to decrease messiness | 6 hrs (min FemCap)<br>8 hrs (min Lea's Shield)<br>48 hrs max both | 6 hrs (min)<br>30 hrs (max) | None |
| Reusable | Yes | No | Yes | No | No |
| Available without Rx | No | Yes | No | Yes | Yes |
| OK for multiple acts of sex after insertion | Yes | No | Yes | Yes | No |

Source: Reprinted with permission from Hatcher, R. A. (2007). Contraceptive technology (19th ed.). New York, NY: Ardent Media.

C

**SOURCES**

Hatcher, R. A. (2007). Contraceptive technology (19th ed.). New York, NY: Ardent Media.
World Health Organization. (2004). Medical eligibility criteria for contraceptive use. Geneva, Switzerland: WHO Library Cataloguing-in-Publication Data.

## CONTRACEPTION: DMPA—DEPO-PROVERA

Perfect use: 0.3%
Typical use: 3%
Dosage: 150 mg/ml IM or 104 mg/ 0.65 ml SC

**Mechanism of Action**

No ovulation d/t suppression in the GnRH therefore suppressing LH and FSH surge
Cervical mucus thickened creating physical plug
Thin atrophic endometrium not receptive to implantation

**Candidates**

No desire for pregnancy soon
Convenient
Easily hidden
Seizure disorders
Sickle cell disease

**WHO 3/4**

Migraine w/focal symptoms
Seizure medications
Breastfeeding < 6 wk
Multiple cardiovascular risk factors
BP > 160/100
Vascular disease
Current DVT/PE
Hx of ischemic disease
Stroke
Unexplained vaginal bleeding
Nephropathy
Vascular disease
Active hepatitis
Hx of cancer
Severe cirrhosis
Liver tumors
Caution:
    Desires pregnancy soon
    Osteoporosis

**Advantages**

8–10 mo until returned fertility
Easy to remember
Does not interfere w/ breastfeeding
No estrogen
Reduced risk of ectopic pregnancy
Absence of menses
Decreased menstrual symptoms
Minimal drug interactions
Decreases seizure threshold
Decreases sickle cell crises events
Decreases endometriosis symptoms
Decreases risk of PID

**Disadvantages**

Wt gain—average of 9 lb in the first year, higher baseline BMI means more likely
    to gain wt
Depression—WHO category 2 for known hx of depression
Bone density decrease temporarily—loss greatest in first 2 yr then rate of loss
    slows. Women > 21 yr old recovered all density w/in 30 mo of discontinuation.
    No need to d/c before menopause because loss of estrogen-sensitive bone
    density has already occurred and can not be recovered
Not possible to d/c immediately

Return visits required Q 11–13 wk
Lipid changes (decrease in HDL, increase in LDL)
Allergic reactions
H/As
Decreased libido
Breast discomfort
Irregular bleeding
Menstrual changes

C

## Warning Signs and Symptoms of Adverse Reaction
Very painful H/As
Heavy bleeding
Severe depression
Severe lower abdominal pain
Prolonged pain at injections site

## Patient Education
Return every 11–13 wk for injection
Irregular bleeding
S/sx of warning signs
Long-term side effects
Calcium
NSAIDs w/ monthly bleeding

**SOURCES**
Hatcher, R. A. (2007). *Contraceptive technology* (19th ed.). New York, NY: Ardent Media.
World Health Organization. (2004). *Medical eligibility criteria for contraceptive use.* Geneva,
Switzerland: WHO Library Cataloguing-in-Publication Data.

## CONTRACEPTION: EMERGENCY CONTRACEPTION

59–94% effective
More effective the sooner it is taken
Can be taken up to 120 hours after unprotected sex

### Mechanism of Action

Inhibits or delays ovulation
Possibly alters endometrium lining
Increases cervical mucus
Alters the corpus luteum

### Indications

No other contraceptive was used
Condom broke, fell off, or leaked
Diaphragm or cervical cap was inserted incorrectly or came out too early
Missed birth control pills
LAM > 6 mo
Late (more than 7 d) for DMPA injection
2 or more d late to insert ring or reapply patch
Withdrawal did not get timed correctly
IUD was partially or completely expelled 7 d or less from act
Break in abstinence

### Contraindications

Pregnancy
Hypersensitivity to medication components
Undiagnosed abnormal genital bleeding

### Side Effects

N/V (worse w/ EE containing pills)
Menstrual changes
IUD insertion side effects
1–6% of drug level ends up in breast milk

### Plan B

OTC > 18 yr old
Approx $40–$50
Directions: Take 1 pill now and 2nd pill 12 hours later, or take both pills now
Each pill contains 750 mcg levonorgestrel
Yutzby

TABLE C-14   Yutzby Method of Emergency Contraception

| | |
|---|---|
| Alesse | 5 pink tablets, then again in 12 h |
| Levlen | 4 pink tablets, repeat in 12 h |
| Lo-Ovral | 4 white tablets, repeat in 12 h |
| Nordette | 4 light orange tablets, repeat in 12 h |
| Tri-Levlen | 4 yellow tablets, repeat in 12 h |
| Triphasil | 4 yellow tablets, repeat in 12 h |
| Ovral | 2 white tablets, repeat in 12 h |
| Seasonale | 4 pink pills repeat in 12 hours |
| Plan B | 1 tablet, repeat in 12 h (levonorgestrel alone) |

*Source:* Reprinted with permission from Hatcher, R. A. (2007). *Contraceptive technology* (19th ed.).
New York, NY: Ardent Media.

### IUD

Paraguard 0.1% failure rate if inserted w/in 7 d of unprotected sex

### SOURCES

Hatcher, R. A. (2007). *Contraceptive technology* (19th ed.). New York, NY: Ardent Media.
World Health Organization. (2004). *Medical eligibility criteria for contraceptive use.* Geneva,
    Switzerland: WHO Library Cataloguing-in-Publication Data.

# CONTRACEPTION: IMPLANON

0.05% risk of unintended pregnancy in perfect and typical use
Provider must be trained by Organon before prescribing and inserting or removing
Single rod (4 cm long, 2 mm wide) implanted under the skin between the bicep and
the tricep of the nondominant arm that slowly releases 68 mg etonogestrel over
a 3-year period

**C**

## Mechanism of Action

High progestin level prevents ovulation by decreasing GnRH, which suppresses the
LH and FSH
Thin atrophic endometrium not receptive to implantation
Thicker cervical mucus creating a physical plug in cervix

## WHO 3/4

Pregnancy
Current DVT or pulmonary embolus
Unexplained vaginal bleeding
Liver disease active hepatitis, cirrhosis
Breast cancer or hx of disease in past 5 yr
Allergy to products in Implanon

## Advantages

Very effective
Easy to use
No estrogen
Discrete
No adverse effects on acne
Relief for dysmenorrhea and endometriosis symptoms
Few side effects
Easily reversible

## Disadvantages

Abnormal uterine bleeding (same average number of days bleeding over 3-year
period but dates and amount unpredictable)
Insertion complications
Possible weight gain < 5.5 lb over 3 yr
Possible adverse effects
No STI protection
Risk of thromboembolic conditions

## General Risks

Insertion failure
Removal difficulties
Pain, swelling, itching, bruising, infection at insertion site
Scarring
Device malfunction
Interactions w/ other medicines
Thrombosis

## Side Effects

Irregular menstrual bleeding
H/A
Emotional lability
Abdominal pain
Nausea
Loss of libido
Vaginal dryness

## Patient Education

Need backup for 7 d after insertion
Pt must check her arm to make sure she can feel device
Management of irregular bleeding

**SOURCES**

Hatcher, R. A. (2007). *Contraceptive technology* (19th ed.). New York, NY: Ardent Media.
Organon USA. (2007). Implanon. Retrieved August 30, 2008, from http://www.implanon-usa.com

# CONTRACEPTION: LACTATIONAL AMENORRHEA METHOD

98% effective for 6 mo if:
>  Exclusive breastfeeding at least 8 times per 24 h (~ q 3 h)
>  Pumping cannot be substituted for actual breast suckling
>  No postpartum menses (menses = any bleeding after 56 d postpartum)

## Mechanism of Action

Exclusive breastfeeding during the postpartum period extends the depression of ovarian function

Infant suckling and the production of prolactin disturbs the pulsatile release of GnRH, which therefore disrupts the normal pattern of LH release

W/out the normal pulsatile release of LH the ovary is not stimulated to produce a follicle

## Statistics

60% of women ovulate before their first postpartum period
Possibility of ovulation before first menses increases w/ time
1–3 mo postpartum 33–45% ovulate before menses
4–12 mo postpartum 64–71% ovulate before menses
> 12 mo postpartum 87–100% ovulate before menses

## Advantages

Breastmilk is good for the baby
Natural period of infertility for child spacing

## Disadvantages

Not as effective as some other methods of birth control
Only effective for a 6-month period

**SOURCE**
Hatcher, R. A. (2007). *Contraceptive technology* (19th ed.). New York, NY: Ardent Media.

# CONTRACEPTION: MIRENA IUD

Perfect use: 0.1%
Typical use: 0.1%

## Mechanism of Action

Thin atropic endometrium impenetrable to implantation
Decreased ovulation
Increase in cervical mucus
Increase in foreign body mediators, which decrease implantation
Inhabitation of sperm mobility and survival

## WHO 3/4

Cancer
Pregnancy
Immediately postpartum, post septic abortion
Abnormal uterine cavity (fibroids,
    cavity < 6 or > 10 cm)
Current DVT or pulmonary embolism
Migraine w/ aura
Unexplained vaginal bleeding
Trophoblastic disease
Cervical or endometrial cancer

PID
Current infection
Current STI
Increased risk of infection
AIDS
Known pelvic tuberculosis
Severe cirrhosis
Liver tumors and
    malignancies

## Candidates

Hx of mennorhagia
Monogamous relationship
Quick return of fertility desired
Convenient
HIV pos
Heart problems (HTN)
Diabetes
Smokers
Obese pts
Postabortion

## Advantages

Shorter/lighter monthly periods (90% decrease in menstrual blood loss)
Highly effective
Protects against endometrial cancer
Long-term cost effective
Good for menopause
Convenient
Long-lasting

## Disadvantages

Irregular bleeding
Risk of perforation
Cramping and pain during placement
Risk of expulsion (2–10%)
Difficulty locating strings
Complications if pt becomes pregnant
Risk of upper genital tract infection
Actinomyces-like organisms on Pap smear

## Patient Education

RTC 6 wk to check placement
Bleeding changes
Check strings Q month
PAINS: **P**eriod late, **A**bdominal pain, **I**nfections, **N**ot feeling well, **S**trings missing

S/sx of infection
STI protection stressed

### SOURCES

Hatcher, R. A. (2007). *Contraceptive technology* (19th ed.). New York, NY: Ardent Media.
World Health Organization. (2004). *Medical eligibility criteria for contraceptive use.* Geneva,
    Switzerland: WHO Library Cataloguing-in-Publication Data.

## CONTRACEPTION: NATURAL FAMILY PLANNING

### Mechanism of Action

Determine most fertile time each month and plan sexual activity around that time for pregnancy facilitation or prevention

Requires determination of the "fertile window," which can be done in a number of ways

### Calendar

Record the length of 6 to 12 cycles and determine the longest and shortest cycles

First fertile day = shortest cycle minus 18

Last fertile day = longest cycle minus 11

First fertile day until the last fertile day is the "fertile window"

### Standard Days Method

For women whose cycles are 26–32 d

Fertile window is days 8–19 of menstrual cycle

Cycle beads can be used to help keep track of fertile window (www.cyclebeads.com)

### Postovulation Method

Calculate average cycle length

Average length minus 14 = predicted day of ovulation

Abstinence or barrier method used for first half of cycle and until 4 d after predicted day of ovulation

This method uses the longest period of abstinence

### Signs and Symptoms of Ovulation

Basal body temperature (BBT):

BBT rises at time of ovulation and remains elevated for the rest of the cycle

Difficult to use alone because when temperature rises you have already ovulated

Usually combined w/ the Billings method

Billings method:

Assessment of cervical mucus to determine fertile window

Looking for an increase in clear, stretchy, slippery cervical secretions associated w/ ovulation

The fertile time lasts from the day ovulatory secretions are observed until 4 d after they are last observed

Two-day method:

Simplified version of Billings

Check daily for cervical secretions

Considered fertile if cervical secretions are present that day or were present the day before

Symptothermal:

Observing multiple indicators

Cervical mucus can indicate beginning of fertile window and BBT temp rise can signal the end

Others:

Cervical position

Mittelschmertz

Home ovulation tests

**RESOURCES**

Billings ovulation method: www.billingsmethod.com

Institute for natural family planning: www.marquette.edu/nursing/nfp/index.html

Institute for reproductive Health: www.irh.org

Taking charge of your fertility: www.tcoyf.com

Fertility Friend: www.fertilityfriend.com

**SOURCES**

Hatcher, R. A. (2007). *Contraceptive technology* (19th ed.). New York, NY: Ardent Media.

Schuiling, K. D., & Likis, F. E. (2006). *Women's gynecologic health*. Sudbury, MA: Jones and Bartlett.

# CONTRACEPTION: ORTHO EVRA PATCH

Perfect use: 0.3%
Typical use: 8%

**Progestin MOA**

Thicken cervical mucus to prevent sperm penetration into upper genital tract
Block LH surge inhibiting ovulation
Inhibit capacitation of sperm
Slow tubal motility delaying sperm transport
Disrupt transport of fertilized ovum
Induce endometrial atrophy

**Estrogen MOA**

Decrease FSH release, which may help suppress LH surge
May induce localized edema in endometrial lining reducing probability of implantation

**WHO 3/4**

Wt > 198 lb effectiveness reduced
Breastfeeding < 6 mo postpartum
Postpartum < 21 d
Age > 35 y and smoking any amount of cigarettes
Multiple cardiac risk factors
Thromboembolic disorder
Hx or current DVT/PE
Cerebrovascular or CAD
Multiple risk factors for CHD or CAD
Valvular heart disease
Uncontrolled HTN
Diabetes w/ vascular involvement
H/As w/ focal aura

Migraines w/o aura > 35 yr old
Prolonged immobilization (d/c COCs 1 mo prior to surgery)
Acute/chronic hepatocellular disease w/ abnormal liver function
Hepatic adenomas or hepatic carcinomas
Anticonvulsant therapy
Hx of cancer
Known hyperlipidemia
Nephropathy
Gallbladder disease
Active hepatitis

**Advantages**

Only change weekly
Effective up to 9 d per patch even though changed every 7 d
Adheres well
Visual reassurance of birth control
No wt gain
Rapidly reversible
Nonlatex

**Disadvantages**

Change weekly
Local skin irritation
Difficult to conceal
H/As
Nausea
Sticky residue around patch
No STI protection

**Patient Education**

BP check 3–6 mo after initiation
Weekly patch change schedule
What to do if it falls off
Patch placement: abdomen, buttocks, upper torso (not breasts), or lateral aspect of upper arm
STI protection
Severe mood swings or depression
Jaundice

Breast lump
Fainting attack
Seizure or difficulty speaking
BP above 160/95
Server allergic skin rash
Immobilization
ACHES: **A**bdominal pain, **C**hest pain, **H**/As, **E**ye problems, **S**evere leg pain

**SOURCES**

Hatcher, R. A. (2007). *Contraceptive technology* (19th ed.). New York, NY: Ardent Media.
World Health Organization. (2004). *Medical eligibility criteria for contraceptive use.* Geneva, Switzerland: WHO Library Cataloguing-in-Publication Data.

## CONTRACEPTION: PARAGUARD IUD

Perfect use: 0.6%
Typical use: 0.8%

### Mechanism of Action
Copper impairs sperm function
IUD obstructs implantation
Strings increase cervical mucus
Not an abortifacient

### WHO 3/4
Puerperal sepsis
Immediately post septic Ab
Unexplained vaginal bleeding
Trophoblastic disease
Cervical, endometrial, ovarian cancer
Fibroids causing uterine distortion
Abnormal uterine shape
PID, current STI
Increased risk of STI
AIDS
Known pelvic tuberculosis

### Advantages
No hormones
Regular monthly cycles
Cost effective due to long-term use (12 yr per device)

### Disadvantages
Uncomfortable to place
Increased bleeding and cramping
No STI protection
Risk of infection, uterine perforation, expulsion

### Patient Education
NSAIDs w/ monthly bleeding/cramping
Check for strings Q mo
6 wk f/u
Period changes
S/sx of infection
PAINS: Period late, Abdominal pain, Infections, Not feeling well, Strings missing

**SOURCES**
Hatcher, R. A. (2007). *Contraceptive technology* (19th ed.). New York, NY: Ardent Media.
World Health Organization. (2004). *Medical eligibility criteria for contraceptive use.* Geneva,
    Switzerland: WHO Library Cataloguing-in-Publication Data.

# CONTRACEPTION: POSTPARTUM

## If Breastfeeding

*Immediately*
> LAM—for 6 mo only (*see corresponding page*)
> Condoms (male or female)
> Sperimicides
> Female/male sterilization
> Abstinence

*At 6 weeks postpartum*
> Progestin only methods preferred: POPs, Implanon, DMPA, Mirena IUD
> Other barrier methods (diaphragms and cervical caps)
> Paraguard IUD

*At 6 months postpartum*
> COCs if lactation is well established, however generally not recommended if breastfeeding

## If Not Breastfeeding

*Immediately*
> Condoms (male or female)
> Spermicides
> Female/male sterilization
> Progestin-only methods: POPs, DMPA, Implanon
> Female/male sterilization

*At 3 Weeks Postpartum*
> COCs

*At 6 Weeks Postpartum*
> Diaphragm
> Cervical cap
> Sponge
> Mirena IUD
> Paraguard IUD

## Postabortion (1st Trimester)

*Immediately*
> All methods

## Postabortion (2nd Trimester)

*Immediately*
> Condoms (male or female)
> Sperimicides
> Progestin-only—POPs, DMPA, Implanon, Mirena IUD
> Paraguard IUD
> Sterilization
> COC

*At 6 Weeks Post 2nd Trimester Abortion*
> Diaphragm
> Cervical cap
> Sponge

Note: Insertion of IUD postabortion is best done 10 minutes after procedure or within 48 h of the procedure; if not done in that time frame, it is best to wait until the next menstrual cycle

### SOURCES
Hatcher, R. A. (2007). *Contraceptive technology* (19th ed.). New York, NY: Ardent Media.
World Health Organization. (2004). *Medical eligibility criteria for contraceptive use*. Geneva, Switzerland: WHO Library Cataloguing-in-Publication Data.

C

## CONTRACEPTION: PROGESTIN-ONLY PILLS

Perfect use = 0.3%
Typical use = 8%

**Mechanism of Action**

No ovulation because GnRH inhibited
Cervical mucus thickened
Thin atrophic endometrium
Reduced activity of cilia in fallopian tubes decreases transport of sperm and egg

**WHO 3/4**

Anticonvulsant therapy
Breastfeeding < 6 wk
Multiple cardiovascular risk factors
BP > 160/100
Vascular disease
Current DVT or pulmonary embolism
Development of ischemic disease
Stroke
Migraine w/ aura

Unexplained vaginal bleeding
Nephropathy
Vascular disease
Active hepatitis
Hx of cancer w/in the last 5 yr
Severe cirrhosis
Liver tumors
Active hepatitis
Current breast cancer

**Candidates**

Desire quick return to fertility
Mennorrhagia
PMS
Menstrual migraines
Cramps
Older women
Endometriosis
Pt w/ estrogen contraindications
Anticonvulsant
Smokers age > 35 yr old
Breastfeeding

**Advantages**

No estrogen
Does not interfere w/ breastfeeding
Fewer contraindications w/ other health concerns
Easily reversible

**Disadvantages**

Vulnerable efficacy (need for obsessive regularity)
Extremely low-dose contraceptive (certain drugs decrease effectiveness of POPs)
Lack of protection against STI
Menstrual cycle disturbances
Wt gain
Breast tenderness
Depression
Decreased libido
Less ovarian suppression than COCs for hx of ovarian cysts
Limited availability

**Patient Education**

BP check 3–6 mo after initiation
Expect irregular bleeding and breast tenderness
Report H/A and mood changes
Decreased libido
Must take at EXACT same time every day
Missed pill precautions
No STI protection

**SOURCES**

Hatcher, R. A. (2007). *Contraceptive technology* (19th ed.). New York, NY: Ardent Media.
World Health Organization. (2004). *Medical eligibility criteria for contraceptive use.* Geneva, Switzerland: WHO Library Cataloguing-in-Publication Data.

# CONTRACEPTION: SPERMICIDE

Films, gels, applicators, w/ caps/diaphragms/sponge
Typical use: 29%
Perfect use: 15%

**Mechanism of Action**

Barrier to sperm reaching cervical os
Detergent disrupts sperm motility

C

**Advantages**

Heightened lubrication
Ease of application
Nonhormonal
Either partner can apply
Widely available
Inexpensive

**Disadvantages**

May require time to dissolve
Must be comfortable inserting applicator into vagina
Messy during sex
Possible vaginal and urethral irritation
Tastes unpleasant
High failure rate due to need for reapplication between sex acts
Toxic shock syndrome
Allergic reaction

**Instructions**

Wash and dry hands
Insert as close to the cervix as possible
Do not wash out vagina for 6 h after insertion
Reapply for every penetrative act
Store in cool, dry place
Have Plan B on hand

**SOURCE**
Hatcher, R. A. (2007). *Contraceptive technology* (19th ed.). New York, NY: Ardent Media.

## CONTRACEPTION: STERILIZATION

### Female
Perfect use: 0.5%
Typical use: 0.5%

*Types*
Salpingestomy (full/partial)
Silastic bands
Bipolar cautery
Spring clip application
Filshie clip
Essure—tubal blockage w/ spring fiber
  Advantages
    No surgery
    OK for obese women
    Done in office
  Disadvantages
    Hysterosalpingogram must be done at 3 mo to confirm blockage
    Cannot be done immediately postpartum
    Expulsion possible
    Perforation possible
    Not reversible

*Mechanism of Action*
Interrupt path of egg

*Advantages*
Decreased worry of pregnancy
Decrease risk of ovarian cancer
Permanent
Highly effecting
Nonhormonal

*Disadvantages*
Regret
Requires surgery
Failure occurs
Not considered reversible

*Discussion Points*
Other methods available
Vasectomy vs. tubal
Absolute no desire for more children
Details about surgery (informed consent)
Regret discussion
Obtain informed consent (partner does not have to consent in most states/
  countries)

### Male
Perfect use: 0.10%
Typical use: 0.15%

*Mechanism of Action*
Interrupts vas deferens preventing passage of sperm into seminal fluid

*Advantages*
No interference w/ sexual function
Highly effective
Cost effective
Simple and safe outpatient procedure

*Disadvantages*
Regret
Backup method needed until no motility
  left (approx. 20 ejaculations)
Does not decrease STIs
Postoperative discomfort
Development of antisperm antibodies
  (health risks unclear)

**SOURCE**
Hatcher, R. A. (2007). *Contraceptive technology* (19th ed.). New York, NY: Ardent Media.

# CONTRACEPTION: VAGINAL RING

Perfect use: 0.3%
Typical use: 8%

**Progestin MOA**

Thicken cervical mucus to prevent sperm penetration into upper genital tract
Block LH surge inhibiting ovulation
Inhibit capacitation of sperm
Slow tubal motility delaying sperm transport
Disrupt transport of fertilized ovum
Induce endometrial atrophy

**Estrogen MOA**

Decrease FSH release, which may help suppress LH surge
May induce localized edema in endometrial lining reducing probability of
   implantation

**WHO 3/4**

Breastfeeding < 6 mo postpartum
Postpartum < 21 d
Age > 35 y and smoking any amount of cigarettes
Multiple cardiac risk factors
Thromboembolic disorder
Hx or current DVT or pulmonary embolism
Cerebrovascular or CAD
Multiple risk factors for arterial cardiovascular disease
Valvular heart disease
Uncontrolled HTN
Diabetes w/ vascular involvement
H/As w/ focal aura
Migraines w/o aura > 35 y old
Major surgery w/ prolonged immobilization (d/c 1 mo prior to surgery)
Acute/chronic hepatocellular disease w/ abnormal liver function
Hepatic adenomas or hepatic carcinomas
Anticonvulsant therapy
Hx of cancer
Known hyperlipidemia
Nephropathy
Gallbladder disease
Active hepatitis

**Advantages**

Only change q 3 wk
Local hormone effect
Hormones effective up to 3 d after removal date
Rapidly reversible
No wt gain
No adverse effects to vaginal and cervical epithelium
OK to use w/ tampons
Can be removed up to 3 h per 24 h period w/o decreasing effectiveness
No effect on bone density

**Disadvantages**

Needs to be kept refrigerated if kept longer than 3 mo
Must be comfortable w/ genitalia to insert and remove
Sex partner may notice it
May fall out
May change vaginal discharge
No STI protection
Toxic shock syndrome
H/As
Breast tenderness

### Patient Education

BP check 3–6 mo after initiation
Monthly change schedule
How to clean it
How long it can be out during sex
How to place it correctly
STI protection
Severe mood swings or depression
Jaundice
Breast lump
Fainting attack
Seizure or difficulty speaking
BP above 160/95
Server allergic skin rash
Immobilization
ACHES: **A**bdominal pain, **C**hest pain, **H**/As, **E**ye problems, **S**evere leg pain

**SOURCES**

Hatcher, R. A. (2007). *Contraceptive technology* (19th ed.). New York, NY: Ardent Media.

World Health Organization. (2004). *Medical eligibility criteria for contraceptive use.* Geneva, Switzerland: WHO Library Cataloguing-in-Publication Data.

# CORD PROLAPSE

## Definition
Frank: cord falls through the cervix
Occult: cord along the presenting part but not through the cervix

## Risk Factors
Abnormal presentation
Small fetus
Multiple gestation
Long umbilical cord
Polyhydramnios
SROM or AROM w/ unengaged head

## Assessment
Any time there is ROM the FHR or fetal movement should be assessed to evaluate
  fetal status

## Treatment
Call backup for stat C/S
Move woman into a position in which the presenting part of the fetus is not
  pressing on the cord
  Knees to chest
  Reverse Trendelenberg
  Any position in which her bottom is higher than her head
Explain to the woman what is happening and what you need her to do to protect
  her baby
Manually hold presenting part up and away from the cord w/out putting any
  pressure on the cord
Put hand into the vagina and spread fingers to support fetal head or buttocks in an
  effort to move it away from the cord (avoid the fontanels)
Do not remove hand
Give oxygen
Monitor FHR
Consider stopping contractions
Prepare the woman for C/S

**SOURCE**
Varney, H., Kriebs, J. M., & Gegor, C. L. (2004). *Varney's midwifery* (4th ed.). Sudbury, MA: Jones and
  Bartlett.

C

## COOMBS

### Direct Coombs

Done on baby

Direct antiagglutination test to detect antibodies attached to erythrocytes

If baby is negative Coombs then Rh neg mom gets Rhogam

### Indirect Coombs

Assesses increasing anti-Rh antibodies in maternal blood

Positive with fetal–maternal transplacental hemorrhage

Occurs 75% of the time

Rhogam given at 28 wk protects against sensitization to fetomaternal bleeds during the 3rd trimester

Rhogam is effective for 12 wk

Given up to 28 d after birth, common practice to give Rhogam prior to discharge from hospital

Rh neg women must be given Rhogam because sensitization to D antibodies can cause hemolytic disease of the newborn (erythroblastosis fetalis) in subsequent pregnancies

**SOURCE**

Varney, H., Kriebs, J. M., & Gegor, C. L. (2004). *Varney's midwifery* (4th ed.). Sudbury, MA: Jones and Bartlett.

# DATING A PREGNANCY

## Information to Gather for Accurate Dating
Last menstrual period
Date of positive pregnancy test
Possible date(s) of conception
Uterine size
Contraception hx

## Signs and Symptoms of Pregnancy

*Presumptive*
Maternal observations
Basal body temp
Amenorrhea
Breast changes (milk can be expressed by the 12th wk)
Urinary frequency
Fatigue (primarily 1st trimester)
N/V (not usually beyond 1st trimester)
Bowel changes
Engorgement
Skin changes (linea nigra, cholasma, striae) occur by the 5–6 mo of pregnancy
Wt changes
Appetite changes
Olfactory changes
Emotional changes
Quickening

*Probable (Noted on Exam)*
Positive pregnancy tests
Uterine enlargement
Abdominal landmarks
Chadwicks: violet vagina caused by increased blood flow by 6 wk
Goodell's: globular fundus, uterus gets larger and rounder by 6 wk
Hegar's: softening of isthmus at 6–8 wk

*Positive (Directly Linked to Fetus)*
FHTs (by 6 wk on U/S and 10–12 wk doppler)
Leopold's maneuver for fetal position
U/S
Fetal movement
Cervical exam revealing presenting part

## Indications for U/S Dating
Unknown LMP
Unknown conception date
Hx of irregular periods
Contraception irregularities
Size/dates discrepancy

## Size > Dates
Inaccurate dating
Different examiners
Full bladder
Multiple gestations
Fibroids
Ovarian cysts
Fetal/chromosomal anomaly
Polyhydramnios
Macrosomia
Gestational diabetes
Breech presentation
Placenta previa
Excessive maternal weight gain

### Size < Dates

Inaccurate dates
Different examiners
IUGR
Missed Ab
Ectopic pregnancy
Fetal anomaly
Placental pathology
Fetal death
Fetal infection
Transverse or oblique lie
Poor maternal wt gain
Oligohydramnios

### Naegele's rule: LMP - 3 mo + 7 d + 1 yr = EDD

### U/S dates = LMP dates if the measurement is obtained between:

6–10 wk then dating is accurate +/– 3 d

10–14 wk then +/– 5 d

14–20 wk then +— 7 d

**If the U/S date is not within these time frames then the EDD should be changed to the U/S date**

### UTERINE SIZE (FOR COMPARISONS)

6 wk = orange
10 wk = large grapefruit
16 wk = halfway to umbilicus
20 wk at umbilicus

**SOURCES**

Lockwood C. L., Lemons, J. A. (Eds.). (2007). *Guidelines for perinatal care* (6th ed.). Elk Grove Village, IL: American Academy of Pediatrics, American College of Obstetricians and Gynecologists.

Varney, H., Kriebs, J. M., & Gegor, C. L. (2004). *Varney's midwifery* (4th ed.). Sudbury, MA: Jones and Bartlett.

# DEPRESSION/ANXIETY

## Depression
Estimated rate of 17% of adults
Women at twice the risk of men

TABLE D-1   Mnemonic Tool for Depression Screening

| Mnemonic | Question |
|---|---|
| **S**leep | Has there been a change in your sleep pattern? |
| **I**nterest | Have you lost pleasure in your usual activities? |
| **G**uilt | Do you feel worthless, do you have inappropriate guilt? |
| **E**nergy | Are you feeling more fatigued or do you tire easily? |
| **C**oncentration | Are you having difficulty concentrating? |
| **A**ppetite | Has there been a change in your appetite? |
| **P**sychomotor agitation | Do you feel restless, agitated, or is it difficult to remain on task? |
| **S**uicide | Have you felt that life is not worth living? Have you considered suicide? |

*Source:* Reprinted with permission from Sanders, L. (2006). Assessing and managing women with depression: A midwifery perspective. *Journal of Midwifery & Women's Health, 51*(3).

*Effects on Pregnancy*
PTD
LBW
Fetal growth restriction
Postnatal complications

## Anxiety
Estimated rate of 18.1% of adults
Women at twice the risk of men
Panic disorder
Obsessive compulsive disorder
Generalized anxiety disorder
Post-traumatic stress disorder
Social anxiety
Phobias

*Signs and Symptoms*
Panic reaction occurs spontaneously to situations that usually do not cause anxiety

*Effects on pregnancy*
Spontaneous Ab
PTD
Delivery complications

## Postpartum Depression

*Signs and Symptoms*
Dysphoric mood
Loss of interest in usually pleasurable activities
Difficulty concentrating or making decisions
Psychomotor agitation/retardation
Fatigue or changes in appetite/sleep
Recurrent thoughts of death/suicide
Feelings or worthlessness/guilt, especially failure at motherhood
Excessive anxiety over child's health
See Table D-2.

## Pharmacology
See Table D-3.

TABLE D-2  Depression/Postpartum Depression Screening Tools

| Screening Tool Information | Available From |
| --- | --- |
| Beck Depression Inventory (BDHI*), $70.00, 21 questions | http://pearsonassess.com/HAIWEB/Cultures/en-us/Productdetail.htm?Pid=015-8018-370&Mode=summary |
| Zung Self-Rating Depression Scale, Free, 20 questions | http://www.counselingpros.com/zung-scale.pdf |
| Patient Health Questionnaire,† Free, 9 questions | http://www.phqscreeners.com |
| Hamilton Depression Scale, Free, 23 questions | http://healthnet.umassmed.edu/mhealth/HAMD.pdf |
| Edinburgh Postnatal Depression Scale, Free, 10 questions | http://health.utah.gov/rhp/pdf/EPDS.pdf |
| Postpartum Depression Screening Scale, $152.00, 7 questions short form | http://www.psychtest.com/curr01/CATLG012.HTM |

*Coefficient alpha = .92.
†Sensitivity/specificity 88%.

*Source:* Reprinted with permission from Sanders, L. (2006). Assessing and managing women with depression: A midwifery perspective. *Journal of Midwifery & Women's Health, 51*(3).

**SOURCES**

American College of Obstetricians and Gynecologists. (2007). Use of psychiatric medications during pregnancy and lactation. *ACOG 2008 compendium of selected publications volume II: Practice bulletins* (pp. 978–997). Washington, DC: American College of Obstetricians and Gynecologists.

Epocrates, I. (2008). *Epocrates online.* Retrieved May 22, 2008, from http://www.epocrates.com

Hale, T. W. (2008). *Medications and mothers' milk* (13th ed.). Amarillo, TX: Hale Publishing.

Sanders, L. (2006). Assessing and managing women with depression: A midwifery perspective. *Journal of Midwifery & Women's Health, 51*(3).

Thompson Healthcare Inc. (2007). *MICROMEDEX: Healthcare series.* Retrieved May 24, 2008, from http://www.micromedex.com

TABLE D-3 Pharmacology Treatment for Depression (continued)

| Category | Medication Information | Dose | Contraindications/ Caution | Side Effects | Peak in Mother's Plasma |
|---|---|---|---|---|---|
| Selective serotonin-reuptake inhibitors | Sertraline (Zoloft) Preg C Lact L2 | 50–200 mg/d | Hypersensitivity to drug/class MAOI use within 14 d Disulfiram use Impaired liver function Volume depletion Diuretic use Seizure disorder Mania Caution in pregnancy > 20 wk gestation Alcohol use | Suicidality Depression Serotonin syndrome Withdrawal Mania Seizures Hyponatremia SIADH Bleeding Glaucoma Anaphylaxis Hypoglycemia Neonatal pulmonary hypertension (> 20 wk gestation) Neonatal serotonin syndrome (3rd trimester) Neonatal withdrawal (3rd trimester) Nausea HA insomnia | 7–8 h |

/ continues

**TABLE D-3** Pharmacology Treatment for Depression (continued)

| Category | Medication Information | Dose | Contraindications/ Caution | Side Effects | Peak in Mother's Plasma |
|---|---|---|---|---|---|
| Selective serotonin-reuptake inhibitors (continued) | Paroxetine (Paxil) Preg Cat C Lact L2 | 20–60 mg/d | Hypersensitivity to drug/class MAOI use within 14 d Impaired liver function Volume depletion Diuretic use Seizure disorder Impaired renal function Glaucoma Mania Suicidality Alcohol Bleeding risk | Suicidality Depression Serotonin syndrome Withdrawal Mania Seizures Hyponatremia SIADH Bleeding Glaucoma Extrapyramidal Hypoglycemia Teratogenicity (1st trimester) Neonatal pulmonary hypertension (> 20 wk gestation) Neonatal serotonin syndrome (3rd trimester) Neonatal withdrawal (3rd trimester) Nausea H/A | 4 h |

/ continues

TABLE D-3 Pharmacology Treatment for Depression (continued)

| Category | Medication Information | Dose | Contraindications/ Caution | Side Effects | Peak in Mother's Plasma |
|---|---|---|---|---|---|
| Selective serotonin- reuptake inhibitors (continued) | Citalopram (Celexa)<br><br>Preg Cat C<br>Lact L3 | 20–40 mg/d | Hypersensitivity to drug/class<br>MAOI use within 14 d<br>Impaired liver function<br>Impaired renal function<br>Seizure disorder<br>Mania<br>Volume depletion<br>Diuretic use<br>Pregnancy > 20 wk gestation<br>Alcohol use | Suicidality<br>Depression<br>Serotonin syndrome<br>Withdrawal<br>Mania<br>Seizures<br>Hyponatremia<br>SIADH<br>Abnormal bleeding<br>Neonatal pulmonary hypertension (> 20 wk gestation)<br>Neonatal serotonin syndrome (3rd trimester)<br>Neonatal withdrawal (3rd trimester)<br>Nausea<br>Dry mouth<br>Insomnia | 2–4 h |

/ continues

D

TABLE D-3 Pharmacology Treatment for Depression (continued)

| Category | Medication Information | Dose | Contraindications/ Caution | Side Effects | Peak in Mother's Plasma |
|---|---|---|---|---|---|
| Selective serotonin-reuptake inhibitors (continued) | Fluoxetine (Prozac)<br><br>Preg Cat C<br>Lact L2 in older infants, L3 if used in neonatal period | 20–60 mg/d | Hypersensitivity to drug/class<br>MAOI use within 5 wk<br>Impaired liver function<br>Diabetes<br>Volume depletion<br>Diuretic use<br>Seizure disorder<br>Mania<br>Pregnancy > 20 wk gestation<br>Alcohol use | Depression<br>Suicidality<br>Serotonin syndrome<br>Withdrawal<br>Mania<br>Seizures<br>Hyponatremia<br>SIADH<br>Hypoglycemia<br>Serum sickness<br>Vasculitis<br>Anaphylaxis<br>Rash<br>Erythema multiforme<br>Pulmonary fibrosis<br>Abnormal bleeding<br>Glaucoma<br>Neonatal pulmonary hypertension (> 20 wk gestation)<br>Neonatal serotonin syndrome (3rd trimester)<br>Neonatal withdrawal (3rd trimester)<br>Nausea<br>H/A<br>Insomnia<br>Anxiety | 6 h |

**TABLE D-3** Pharmacology Treatment for Depression (continued)

| Category | Medication Information | Dose | Contraindications/ Caution | Side Effects | Peak in Mother's Plasma |
|---|---|---|---|---|---|
| Tricyclic antidepressants | Nortriptyline

Preg Cat C
Lact L2 | 25–150 mg/d | Hypersensitivity to drug/class
MAOI use within 14 d
Heart problems
GI obstruction
Urinary problems
Glaucoma
Increased intraocular pressure
Seizure disorder
Thyroid disease
Diabetes mellitus
Asthma
Parkinson's disease
Impaired liver function
Schizophrenia
Bipolar disorder
Alcohol abuse
Suicide risk | Hypotension
HTN
Heart problems
Stroke
Seizures
Extrapyramidal symptoms
Ataxia
Tardive dyskinesia
Paralytic ileus
Increased intraocular pressure
Agranulocytosis
Leucopenia
Thrombocytopenia
Hallucinations
Psychosis exacerbation
Mania
Depression
Suicidality
SIADH
Hepatitis
Angioedema
Hyperthermia
Drowsiness
Dry mouth
Dizziness | |

/ continues

D

**TABLE D-3** Pharmacology Treatment for Depression (continued)

| Category | Medication Information | Dose | Contraindications/ Caution | Side Effects | Peak in Mother's Plasma |
|---|---|---|---|---|---|
| Tricyclic antidepressants (continued) | Desipramine (Norpramin)<br><br>Preg Cat C<br>Lact L2 | 25–300 mg/d | Hypersensitivity to drug/class<br>MAOI use within 14 d<br>Cardiovascular disease<br>GI obstruction<br>Urinary problems<br>Glaucoma<br>Increased intraocular pressure<br>Seizure disorder<br>Thyroid disease<br>Diabetes<br>Asthma<br>Parkinson's<br>Impaired liver function<br>Schizophrenia<br>Bipolar<br>Alcohol abuse<br>Suicide risk | Hypotension<br>HTN<br>Syncope<br>Heart problems<br>Stroke<br>Seizures<br>Extrapyramidal symptoms<br>Paralytic ileus<br>Increased intraocular pressure<br>Agranulocytosis<br>Leucopenia<br>Thrombocytopenia<br>Hallucinations<br>Psychosis<br>Mania<br>Suicidality<br>SIADH<br>Hepatitis<br>Angioedema<br>Hyperthermia<br>Drowsiness<br>Dry mouth<br>Dizziness | |

TABLE D-3 Pharmacology Treatment for Depression (continued)

| Category | Medication Information | Dose | Contraindications/Caution | Side Effects | Peak in Mother's Plasma |
|---|---|---|---|---|---|
| Serotonin-noreppinephrine reuptake inhibitors | Venlafaxine (Effexor) Preg Cat C Lact L3 | 75–300 mg/d | Hypersensitivity to drug/class MAOI use within 14 d Impaired liver function Impaired renal function Seizure disorder Mania Suicidal HTN Hypovolemia Dehydration Glaucoma Bleeding risk Hyperthyroidism Heart failure Caution in 3rd trimester | Seizures Suicidality Depression Withdrawal Anaphylaxis Mania HTN Hyponatremia SIADH Serotonin syndrome Extrapyramidal symptoms Bleeding Blood dyscrasias Arrhythmias Skin reaction Glaucoma Pancreatitis Interstitial lung disease Pneumonia Nausea HA Dry mouth Dizziness Insomnia | |

/ continues

TABLE D-3  Pharmacology Treatment for Depression (continued)

| Category | Medication Information | Dose | Contraindications/Caution | Side Effects | Peak in Mother's Plasma |
|---|---|---|---|---|---|
| Other | Bupropion (Wellbutrin) | 300–450mg/d | Hypersensitivity to drug/class | Seizures | 2 h |
| | | | MAOI use within 14 d | Arrhythmias | |
| | | | Seizure disorder | Tachycardia | |
| | Preg Cat B | | Bulimia | Stevens-Johnson syndrome | |
| | Lact L3 | | Anorexia | Erythema multiforme | |
| | | | Withdrawal | Anaphylaxis | |
| | | | Head injury | Hallucinations | |
| | | | Alcohol/drug abuse | Paranoia | |
| | | | Diabetes | Mania | |
| | | | Impaired liver function | Psychosis | |
| | | | Impaired renal function | Suicidality | |
| | | | Recent heart attach | Depression | |
| | | | HTN | Hepatotoxicity | |
| | | | Bipolar | HTN | |
| | | | Suicidal | Migraine | |
| | | | | Dry mouth | |
| | | | | H/A | |
| | | | | Agitation | |
| | | | | Nausea | |
| | | | | Dizziness | |

/ continues

**TABLE D-3** Pharmacology Treatment for Depression (continued)

| Category | Medication Information | Dose | Contraindications/Caution | Side Effects | Peak in Mother's Plasma |
|---|---|---|---|---|---|
| Other | Nefazodone | 100–600 mg/d | Hypersensitivity to drug/class | Hepatotoxicity | |
| | | | MAOI use within 14 d | Hypotension | |
| | Preg Cat C | | Liver disease | Seizures | |
| | Lact L4 | | Elevated liver function tests | Mania | |
| | | | Cardiovascular disease | Depression | |
| | | | Cerebrovascular disease | Suicidality | |
| | | | Hypotension | Bradycardia | |
| | | | Bipolar disorder | Tachycardia | |
| | | | Suicide risk | Arrhythmias | |
| | | | Seizure disorder | Heart block | |
| | | | | Anaphylaxis | |
| | | | | H/A | |
| | | | | Dry mouth | |
| | | | | Nausea | |
| | | | | Dizziness | |

/ continues

TABLE D-3 Pharmacology Treatment for Depression (continued)

| Category | Medication Information | Dose | Contraindications/ Caution | Side Effects | Peak in Mother's Plasma |
|---|---|---|---|---|---|
| Other | Mirtazapine (Remeron)  Preg Cat C Lact L3 | 15 mg PO qhs | Hypersensitivity to drug/class MAO inhibitor use within 14 d Impaired liver function Impaired renal function Bipolar disorder Seizure disorder Cardiovascular disease Cerebrovascular disease Hypotension Dehydration Alcohol | Agranulocytosis Neutropenia Hypotension Suicidality Depression Mania Seizures Torsades de pointes Somnolence Dry mouth Weight gain Hypercholesterolemia Constipation Flu symptoms Abnormal dreams/thinking Confusion | |

/ continues

TABLE D-3  Pharmacology Treatment for Depression (continued)

| Category | Medication Information | Dose | Contraindications/ Caution | Side Effects | Peak in Mother's Plasma |
|---|---|---|---|---|---|
| Benzodiazepines | Alprazolam (Xanax)<br><br>Preg D<br>Lact L3 | | Hypersensitivity to drug/class<br>Glaucoma<br>CNS depression | Syncope<br>Tachycardia<br>Seizures<br>Respiratory depression<br>Coma<br>Dependency<br>Withdrawal<br>Suicidal ideation<br>Mania<br>Drowsiness<br>Insomnia | |
| | Diazepam (Valium)<br><br>Preg Cat D<br>Lact L3, L4 if used chronically | 2–10 mg PO BID–QID | Hypersensitivity to drug/class<br>Myasthenia gravis<br>Impaired respiratory function<br>Coma<br>Shock<br>Sleep apnea<br>Glaucoma | Dependency<br>Withdrawal<br>Respiratory depression<br>Bradycardia<br>Hypotension<br>Cardiovascular collapse<br>Seizure exacerbation<br>Depression<br>Hallucinations<br>Psychosis<br>Neutropenia<br>Blood dyscrasias<br>Fatigue<br>Muscle weakness | |

/ continues

D

TABLE D-3 Pharmacology Treatment for Depression (continued)

| Category | Medication Information | Dose | Contraindications/ Caution | Side Effects | Peak in Mother's Plasma |
|---|---|---|---|---|---|
| Benzodiazepines (continued) | Lorazepam (Ativan)<br><br>Preg Cat D<br>Lact L3 | 0.5–1 mg PO/ IM/IV BID-TID PRN anxiety | Hypersensitivity to drug/class<br>Intra-arterial administration<br>Glaucoma<br>Renal failure<br>Hepatic failure<br>Alcohol intoxication<br>CNS depression<br>Respiratory impairment<br>Psychosis<br>Depression | Dependency<br>Withdrawal<br>Respiratory depression/failure<br>Seizures<br>Depression<br>Suicidality<br>Blood dyscrasias<br>Intra-arterial gangrene<br>Sedation<br>Dizziness<br>Hypoventilation<br>Hypotension | |

# DERMATOLOGY

**D**

## Primary Lesions

Flat: macules—small

Patch: large macule

Elevated: papule < 0.5 cm

Plaque: solid, palpable, raised plateau

Firm: nodules—firmer than a papule, rounded

Tumor: larger than nodule

Blister: vesicle—filled with serous fluid < 0.5 cm

Bullae: serous fluid filled > 0.5 cm

Pustule: filled with pus

Wheal: palpable, hive, red, caused by papillary edema, usually disappears in 1–2 d

## Secondary Lesions

Atrophy: thinning of the skin layers

Crust: surface formed by drying of exudate

Fissure: separation of the skin, generally along cleavage lines

Hyperkeratosis: thickening of the skin

Lichenification: thickening and induration, accentuation of skin lines/markings

Scale: dry flaking of skin

Ulcer: skin problem that is deeper than the top layer of skin and forms a scar when healing

## Shape

Umbilicated (depressed center)

Round

Oval

Pedunculated (on a stalk)

## Skin Cancer

Basal cell: often in areas exposed to sun, unlikely to spread, lesion that does not heal on its own

Squamous cell: scaly plaque, lesion that does not heal on its own

Malignant melanoma: irregular border, multicolored, asymmetrical

## Lesions

Acrochordon (skin tags): soft, round, or oval pedunculated papilloma (polyp), constricted at the base; tend to grow during pregnancy; can be removed by cutting, electrode, or cryosurgery

Candidiasis: *see* Candida

Chancre: often painless ulcer after primary syphilis lesion appears 2 to 6 mo after infection

Condyloma lata: secondary syphylitic lesion, flat-topped nodules or plaques

Condyloma acuminata (genital warts): turn white with acetic acid application

Dermatitis: inflammatory reaction that is characterized by puritis, thickening, dry skin; healing usually takes 2 wk of avoiding triggers, use barrier creams as necessary and topical class I glucocorticoids

Eczema: see dermatitis above, often on the flexor surfaces (elbows and knees)

Folliculitis: infection of the hair follicle, tx w/ doxycycline 100 mg BID × 7 d

Impetigo:

Ulcer often characterized by a honey colored crust

Caused by *S. aureus* and *S. pyogenes*

Very contagious, tx anybody in the family who has it, emphasize handwashing

Tx w/ benzoyl peroxide or hibiclins wash daily plus topical 2% mupirocin ointment TID to involved skin for 7–10 d

Consider swabbing nostrils with Mupirocin ointment BID to prevent reinfection

Recommended that all family members rpt antibacterial wash 2 wk after resolution of the infection to prevent reoccurrence

Lichen sclerosis: ivory white atrophic plaque often in an 8 pattern characterized by puritis, burning, pain, and soreness; tx w/ Clabatozol propianate 0.05% QD × 2 wk PRN

Molescum: viral infection of skin and mucosa, self-limited in duration, spread by contact; tx w/ Imiquimod cream 5% applied 3 × per wk for 1–3 mo

Psoriosis: scaling, flaky, erythematous skin (scalp dandruff); tx w/ topical glucocorticoids, tar; or ketaconazole shampoos

PUPPs: Pruritic Urticarial Papules and Plaques of Pregnancy/Polymorphic Eruption of Pregnancy

Typically occurs in the 3rd trimester primigravidae

Characterized by erythematous papules that combine to form uticarial plaques on abdomen and may spread to other areas of the body (but not usually on the face)

Plaques are extremely puritic, no increased risk of fetal morbidity or mortality

Condition usually resolves by 10 d postpartum

Important to R/o cholestasis as the cause of pruritis

Tx w/ high-potency topical steroids (clobetasol) and antihistamines (Atarax, Benadryl, Zyrtec) or over-the-counter Sarna Lotion

*Topical Steroid Classification*

▶ Group I (Ultra-High Potency)
Betamethasone dipropionate 0.05% (cream, ointment, gel, lotion in augmented vehicle)
Clobetasol propionate 0.05% (cream, emollient cream, scalp application, gel, ointment)
Diflorasone diacetate 0.05% (ointment)

▶ Group II (High Potency)
Desoximetasone 0.25% (cream, ointment)
Fluocinonide 0.05% (cream, ointment, gel)
Mometasone furoate 0.1% (ointment)

▶ Group III (Moderate-High Potency)
Betamethasone valerate 0.1% (ointment)
Fluticasone propionate 0.005% (ointment)
Triamcinolone acetonide 0.1% (ointment)

▶ Group IV (Moderate Potency)
Fluocinolone acetonide 0.025% (ointment)
Hydrocortisone valerate 0.2% (ointment)
Triamcinolone acetonide 0.1% (cream, ointment)

▶ Group V (Moderate-Low Potency)
Betamethasone dipropionate 0.05% (lotion)
Betamethasone valerate 0.1% (cream)
Fluocinolone acetonide 0.025% (cream)
Fluticasone propionate 0.05% (cream)
Hydrocortisone butyrate 0.1% (cream)
Hydrocortisone valerate 0.2% (cream)

▶ Group VI (Low Potency)
Alclometasone dipropionate 0.05% (cream, ointment)
Betamethasone valerate 0.05% (lotion)
Desonide 0.05% (lotion, cream, ointment)
Triamcinolone acetonide 0.1% (cream)

▶ Group VII (Lowest Potency)
Hydrocortisone hydrochloride 0.1% (cream, ointment)
Hydrocortisone hydrochloride 2.5% (cream, lotion, ointment)
Hydrocortisone acetate 1% (cream, lotion, ointment)

**SOURCE**
Wolff, K., Johnson, R. A., & Suurmond, R. (2005). *Fitzpatrick's color atlas & synopsis of clinical dermatology* (5th ed.). Boston, MA: McGraw-Hill Professional.

# DIARRHEA

## Causes
Pathogens
Diet
Antibiotics
Large doses of vitamin C
Change in eating habits
Implementation of high-fiber diet

## Management

**D**

If acute and associated with severe dehydration, check electrolytes, administer IV fluids

Encourage clear fluids of any type that are tolerated (see electrolyte replacement fluid recipe below)

Encourage small meals (BRAT diet: bread/bananas, rice, apple sauce, tea; not shown to cause significant improvement in diarrhea symptoms, but is well tolerated)

If no resolution within 48 h obtain stool sample to assess for ova/parasites and *C. difficile*

## Treatment
See Table D-4.
1st line: Loperamide
2nd line: Antisecretory agents, adsorbents
3rd line: Lomotil

**ELECTROLYTE REPLACEMENT FLUID (SAFE IN PREGNANCY)**
½ tsp salt
1 tsp baking soda
8 tsp sugar
8 oz orange juice
Dilute to 1 liter with clean water

## SOURCES
Arcangelo, V. P., & Peterson, A. M. (Eds.). (2006). *Pharmacotherapeutics for advanced practice: A practical approach* (2nd ed.). Philadelphia, PA: Lippincott Williams & Wilkins.
Epocrates, I. (2008). *Epocrates online.* Retrieved May 22, 2008, from http://www.epocrates.com
Hale, T. W. (2008). *Medications and mothers' milk* (13th ed.). Amarillo, TX: Hale Publishing.
Thompson Healthcare Inc. (2007). *MICROMEDEX: Healthcare series.* Retrieved May 24, 2008, from http://www.micromedex.com

**TABLE D-4**　Diarrhea Treatments

| Category | Medication Information | Dose | Contraindications/Cautions | Side Effects |
|---|---|---|---|---|
| Antimotility agents | Loperamide (Imodium)<br>Preg B<br>Lact L2 | 4–16 mg/d, divided doses | Pt w/ bloody stools, fever, possible parasites | Abd discomfort, constipation, drowsiness, dry mouth |
| | Diphenoxylate (Lomotil)<br>Preg C<br>Lact L3 | 2.5–5 mg QID | Pt w/bloody stools, fever, liver disease | Dry mouth/eyes, urinary retention, blurred vision, drowsiness |
| | Adsorbent | Fiber-Con 1–6 g/d | Impaired drug absorption | Bloating, gas, abdominal cramps |
| Antisecretory Agents | Bismuth subsalicylate (Pepto-Bismol)<br>Preg Cat C 1st trimester, D 2nd and 3rd trimesters<br>Lact L3 | 2 tabs or 30 ml, not to exceed 8 doses in 24 h | Pt w/ aspirin allergy, adolescents, warfarin therapy | Dark stools, darkening of the tongue, tinnitus |
| | Kaopectate<br>Preg Cat C<br>Lact L1 | 2 tabs or 30–120 ml after each loose bowel movement; not to exceed 7 doses in 24 h | May prevent absorption of medications/nutrients, alter timing of medication administration | Constipation, bloating |

Sources: Adapted from Arcangelo & Peterson, 2006; Epocrates, 2008; Hale, 2008; Thompson Healthcare Inc., 2007.

# DRUG CLASSIFICATIONS

## Pregnancy

TABLE D-5   Pregnancy Drug Classifications

| Category | Interpretation |
|----------|----------------|
| A | Adequate, well-controlled studies in pregnant women have not shown an increased risk of fetal abnormalities to the fetus in any trimester of pregnancy. |
| B | Animal studies have revealed no evidence of harm to the fetus; however, there are no adequate and well-controlled studies in pregnant women. *or* Animal studies have shown an adverse effect, but adequate and well-controlled studies in pregnant women have failed to demonstrate a risk to the fetus in any trimester. |
| C | Animal studies have shown an adverse effect, and there are no adequate and well-controlled studies in pregnant women. *or* No animal studies have been conducted, and there are no adequate and well-controlled studies in pregnant women. |
| D | Adequate well-controlled or observational studies in pregnant women have demonstrated a risk to the fetus. However, the benefits of therapy may outweigh the potential risk. For example, the drug may be acceptable if needed in a life-threatening situation or serious disease for which safer drugs cannot be used or are ineffective. |
| X | Adequate well-controlled or observational studies in animals or pregnant women have demonstrated positive evidence of fetal abnormalities or risks. The use of the product is contraindicated in women who are or may become pregnant. |

*Source:* Thompson Healthcare Inc. (2007). *MICROMEDEX: Healthcare series.* Retrieved May 22, 2008, from http://www.micromedex.com

## Lactation

*L1 Safest*

Drug that has been taken by a large number of breastfeeding mothers without any observed increase in adverse effects in the infant. Controlled studies in breastfeeding women fail to demonstrate a risk to the infant, and the possibility of harm to the breastfeeding infant is remote, or the product is not orally bioavailable in an infant.

*L2 Safer*

Drug that has been studied in a limited number of breastfeeding women without an increase in adverse effects in the infant. And/or, the evidence of a demonstrated risk that is likely to follow use of this medication in a breastfeeding woman is remote.

*L3 Moderately Safe*

There are no controlled studies in breastfeeding women; however, the risk of untoward effects to a breastfed infant is possible; or, controlled studies show only minimal nonthreatening adverse effects. Drugs should be given only if the potential benefit justifies the potential risk to the infant. (New medications that have absolutely no published data are automatically categorized in this category, regardless of how safe they may be.)

*L4 Possibly Hazardous*

There is positive evidence of risk to a breastfed infant or to breastmilk production, but the benefits of use in breastfeeding mothers may be acceptable despite the risk to the infant (e.g., if the drug is needed in a life-threatening situation or for a serious disease for which safer drugs cannot be used or are ineffective).

D

*L5 Contraindicated*

Studies in breastfeeding mothers have demonstrated that there is significant and documented risk to the infant based on human experience, or it is a medication that has a high risk of causing significant damage to an infant. The risk of using the drug in breastfeeding women clearly outweighs any possible benefit from breastfeeding. The drug is contraindicated in women who are breastfeeding an infant.

**SOURCES**

Epocrates, I. (2008). *Epocrates online.* Retrieved May 22, 2008, from http://www.epocrates.com

Hale, T. W. (2008). *Medications and mothers' milk* (13th ed.). Amarillo, TX: Hale Publishing.

Thompson Healthcare Inc. (2007). *MICROMEDEX: Healthcare series.* Retrieved May 22, 2008, from http://www.micromedex.com

# ECTOPIC PREGNANCY

### Definition
Pregnancy that occurs in a location other than the uterus

### Risk Factors

| | |
|---|---|
| Tubal surgery | Previous genital tract infections |
| Sterilization | Multiple sexual partners |
| Previous ectopic | Smoking |
| Exposure to DES | Douching |
| Use of IUD | Early age of 1st intercourse |
| Tubal pathology | Advanced maternal age |
| Infertility and associated tx | Endometriosis |

### Signs and Symptoms
Abdominal pain (especially early in pregnancy)
Irregular bleeding
Shock
Usual s/sx of pregnancy
Shoulder or diaphragmatic pain

### Signs and Symptoms of Rupture

| | |
|---|---|
| Tachycardia | Shock |
| BP changes | Shoulder or diaphragmatic pain |
| Bleeding | |

### Differential Diagnosis

| | |
|---|---|
| Endometriosis | Kidney stones |
| Appendicitis | Bowel diseases |

### Diagnosis

| | |
|---|---|
| SAB | CMT |
| UTI | Uterine displacement d/t enlarged adnexal mass |
| Ovarian torsion | Tenderness on abdominal palpation |
| Ovarian cyst | TVU/S |
| Fibroids | Serial serum B-hCG measurements |

### Labs
B-hCG can be detected as early as 8 d after LH surge if pregnancy has occurred
IUP usually visible on TVU/S when B-hCG = 1500–2000 IU/L
B-hCG doubles every 48 h until 41 d in normal pregnancy; B-hCG plateaus
  ~100,000 IU/L
B-hCG rises slower in an ectopic pregnancy
B-hCG > 2000 IU/L and no IUP on U/S is strongly suggestive of ectopic pregnancy
B-hCG > 1500 IU/L plus an adnexal mass and no evidence of IUP suggests ectopic
B-hCG < 1500 IU/L with a neg TVU/S for IUP should be repeated, including TVU/S
  in 48–72 h to follow rising or falling levels

### Natural Course
Spontaneously regresses
Tubal rupture—profound hemorrhage requiring surgical intervention
Tubal abortion—expulsion of the POCs through the fimbria that may lead to severe
  abdominal bleeding requiring surgical intervention or slight bleeding requiring no
  intervention
15% reoccurrence after the first, and 30% following 2 ectopic pregnancies

### Treatment
Methotrexate (85–95% successful tx rate)
*Criteria:*

| | |
|---|---|
| Hemodynamically stable | Pt able to return for F/U care |
| Nonlaparoscopic dx | Unruptured mass < 3.5 cm |
| Pt desires future fertility | No fetal cardiac motion |
| General anesthesia contraindicated | B-hCG < 6–15,000 IU/L |

Immediate surgery

FIGURE E-1   Ectopic Pregnancy Workup Decision-Making Tree

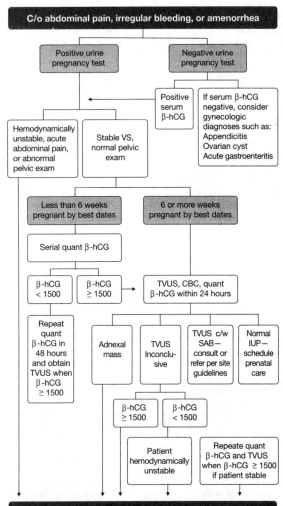

**Follow-Up**
B-HCG
TVU/S

**SOURCES**

American College of Obstetricians and Gynecologists. (1998). Medical management of tubal pregnancy. [Practice bulletin no. 3]. In *2008 compendium of selected publications* (p. 1023). Washington, DC: American College of Obstetricians and Gynecologists.

Kriebs, J. M., & Fahey, J. O. (2006). Ectopic pregnancy. *Journal of Midwifery & Women's Health, 51*, 431.

# ELECTRONIC FETAL MONITORING

Paper: 3 cm/min
Baseline: 110–160 bpm
Variability: fluctuations in baseline FHR > 2 cycles per min (peak to trough);
   irregular in amplitude and frequency
   Absent—undetectable
   Minimal—5 bpm or less
   Moderate—6–25 bpm
   Marked—25 bpm or more

## Acceleration

*Abrupt*
   Acceleration to peak level in < 30 sec
   At least 15 bpm above baseline
   At least 15 sec in duration
   Less than 2 min in duration
   Less than 32 wk, 10 bpm above
      baseline × 10 sec
   Less than 26 wk no accelerations

*Prolonged*
   Lasting > 2 min, but < 10 min
   Tachycardia if > 10 min

**E**

## Deceleration

*Late*
   Gradual decrease > 30 sec to nadir
   Nadir delayed
   After uterine contraction

*Early*
   Gradual decrease > 30 sec to nadir
   Nadir coincides with peak of uterine
      contraction

*Variable*
   Abrupt decrease < 30 sec to nadir
   > 15 bpm and 15 sec in duration
   < 2 min total
   Timing varies with relation to uterine
      contractions

*Prolonged*
   15 bpm or more below baseline
   Lasting > 2 min, but < 10 min
   Bradycardia if > 10 min

Change in baseline—acceleration or deceleration of greater than 10 min in duration
Sinusoidal—no variability, regular amplitude and frequency

### NICHD 2008 Electronic Fetal Monitoring Documentation Guidelines

Category 1: Tracing must include all of the following:
   Baseline 110–160 bpm
   Moderate FHR variability
   Absent late or variable decelerations
   Present or absent early deceleration
   Present or absent accelerations
Category 2: Any tracing that is not characterized by Category 1 or Category 3
Category 3: Tracing must include either
   A. Absent baselines FHR variability and any of the following:
      1. Recurrent late decerations
      2. Recurrent variable decerations
      3. Bradycardia
   B. Sinusoidal pattern

**SOURCES**

Association of Womens Health Obstetrics and Neonatal Nurses. (2003). *Fetal heart monitoring: Principles and practices* (3rd ed.). Dubuque, IA: Kendall/Hunt.

Greulich, B., & Tarrant, B. (2007). The latent phase of labor: Diagnosis and management. *Journal of Midwifery & Women's Health, 52*, 190–198.

Macones, G. A., Hankins, G. D. V., Spong, C. Y., Hauth, J., & Moore, T. (2008). The 2008 National Institute of Child Health and Human Development Workshop report on electronic fetal monitoring: Update on definition, interpretation, and research guidelines. *Obstetrics & Gynecology, 112*(3), 661–666.

## ENDOMETRIAL BIOPSY

**Statistics**
> < 2% of hyperplasias w/o atypia developed into cancer over 10 years
> 23% of hyperplasias w/ atypia became cancerous over a 4 year period

**Indication**
Identification of source of DUB
R/o endometrial cancer and precancerous lesions
Identify cause of postmenopausal bleeding
Evaluate infertility
F/U to endometrial cells on Pap smear
Assess effect of HRT
Assess impact of tamoxifen

**Contraindications**
Pregnancy
Active cervicitis or endometritis
PID
Coagulation disorders
Blood dyscrasias
Heart murmur
Rheumatic heart disease
Fever
Cervical stenosis

**Side Effects**
Cramping
Uterine spasm
Vasovagal reaction
Excessive bleeding
Uterine perforation
Bacteremia
Septicemia
Endocarditis

**Risk Factors for Endometrial Cancer**
Age > 50 yr old
Natural menopause after age 52
PCOS
Obesity > 50 lbs
Infertility
Nulliparity
Unopposed exogenous estrogen
Diabetes
Tamoxifen use

**Patient Education**
Nothing in vagina for 2–3 d post biopsy
Call if fever develops
Call if persistent pain/cramping past 48 h
Call if bleeding heavier than a period in the next 24–48 h

**Procedure**
Administer NSAIDs 1 h before procedure
Perform bimanual exam to document uterine size, shape, and position

FIGURE E-2   Procedure for Endometrial Biopsy Using the Pipelle System

1. Insert vaginal speculum and visualize cervix.
2. Cleanse cervix with antiseptic solution.
3. If the cervix is not in midposition, a tenaculum may be needed to align the uterus and enable the sampler to reach the fundus.
4. If a tenaculum is required, apply 20% benzocaine gel to tenaculum site.
5. Gently introduce the sampling device (piston fully inserted to distal end of the sheath) through the cervical os, endocervical canal, internal os, and lower uterine segment. Proceed slowing and stop at any time resistance is met. Once the lower uterine segment is reached, continue up to the uterine fundus. The fundus of the uterus must be reached for accurate sampling.
6. Document the depth of the uterus.
7. Stabilize the sheath with one hand and draw the piston completely back by using one continuous motion (creating a negative pressure within the lumen).
8. Roll the sheath or turn it one direction between the thumb and forefinger AND at the same time, move the sheath in and out of the fundus and internal os three or four times. (Note: DO NOT bring the sheath outside of the external os or you will lose the negative pressure.)
9. Withdraw the device when the lumen is as full of tissue as possible.
10. Cut the tip off the distal tip with the scissors and discard. Expel the specimen into the formalin bottle by pushing the piston into the sheath thereby discharging the specimen. Label the bottle.
11. If a tenaculum was used, gently remove it at this time.
12. Remove any excess blood from the cervix and vagina.
13. Remove the speculum from the vagina.
14. Allow the woman to recover on the examination table.

*Source:* Reprinted with permission from American College of Nurse-Midwives. (2001). Endometrial biopsy: Clinical bulletin no. 5. *Journal of Midwifery and Women's Health, 46*(5), 321.

## Postprocedure Care

Remain semirecumbent for a few moments
Assist with elevation to avoid vasovagal response
Provide pad for spotting
NSAIDs for persistent pain

## Results and Follow-Up

Inadequate—not enough of a sample to make dx
Benign—no problems
Cystic or adenomatous hyperplasia
Atypical adenomatous hyperplasia
Carcinoma—cancer specialist referral needed

## Hyperplasia Results

Simple hyperplasia—proliferative lesion without any glandular complexity
Complex hyperplasia—proliferative lesion with glandular complexity
Simple hyperplasia with atypia—proliferative lesion with enlarged epithelial cells
Complex with atypia—proliferative lesion with enlarged epithelial cells
F/U for hyperplasia depends on pt's age, menopause status, and biopsy results
Options for F/U include: medroxyprogesterone cyclically, GnRH agonists, COC pills, hysteroscopy, and repeat endometrial biopsy

### SOURCES

American College of Nurse-Midwives. (2001). Endometrial biopsy [Clinical bulletin no. 5]. *Journal of Midwifery & Women's Health, 46*(5), 321.

Montgomery, B. E., Daum, G. S., & Dunton, C. J. (2004). Endometrial hyperplasia: A review. *Obstetrical and Gynecological Survey, 59*(5), 368–378.

Varney, H., Kriebs, J. M., & Gegor, C. L. (2004). *Varney's midwifery* (4th ed.). Sudbury, MA: Jones and Bartlett.

E

# ENDOMETRIOSIS

**Statistics**
- 7–10% of women
- 50% of premenopausal women
- 38% of infertile women
- 71–87% of women with chronic pelvic pain

**Etiological Theories**
- Retrograde menstruation from fallopian tubes during menstruation causes endometrial tissues to adhere in the peritoneal cavity creating endometriomas
- Hematogenous or lymphatogenous transport
- Coelomic metaplasia

**Risk Factors**
- Shorter menstrual cycles
- Long bleeding time
- Early menarche
- Family Hx

**Signs and Symptoms**
- Pelvic pain/dyspareunia—caused by inflammatory cytokines in the peritoneal cavity, bleeding from the endometriomas, and irritation of the nerves of the pelvic floor
- Infertility—endometriomas distort the pelvic anatomy, block the fallopian tubes, and impair transportation of the ovum

**Diagnosis**
- Laparoscopic visualization of at least 2 of the following:
  - Endometrial epithelium
  - Endometrial glands
  - Endometrial stroma
  - Hemosiderin-laden macrophages

**Pertinent History**
- Pelvic pain starting before onset of menses that worsens over time
- Irregular menstrual cycle patterns (usually secondary dysmenorrhea)
- Symptoms associated with menses
- Dyspareunia
- H/o infertility or pregnancy complications

**Physical Exam**
- Abdominal—palpation for tenderness
- Pelvic/rectal exam—noting tenderness, enlargements (blue or red implants/lesions in the posterior fornix), uterine position (often retroverted), mobility of uterus (usually fixed), uterine motion tenderness

**Labs:** U/S, hystosalpingography, MRI, serum marker CA-125 (severe disease only)

**Differential Diagnosis**
- Recurrent painful periods—R/o adenomyosis and physiological dx
- Painful intercourse—R/o psychosexual dysfunction and atrophy
- Painful micturition—R/o cystitis
- Painful defecation during menses—R/o constipation
- Chronic lower abdominal pain—R/o IBS
- Chronic lower back pain—R/o musculoskeletal strain
- Adnexal mass—R/o fibroids, tumors, ovarian cysts
- Infertility—R/o other sources of infertility

**Treatment**
- Decrease the frequency of menstruation with contraception so as to decrease number of endometriomas
- Analgesics
- Surgery to remove endometriomas

Hysterectomy

GnRH agonists inhibit estrogen thereby decreasing endometrial tissue growth

    Lupron—3.75 mg IM Q mo or 11.25 mg Q 3 mo

    Synarel—400–800 mcg/d nasal spray

    Zoladex—3.6 mg SC Q mo

## SOURCES

Farquhar, C. (2007). Endometriosis. *British Medical Journal, 334*(7587), 249–253.

Moghissi, K. S., & Winkel, C. A. (1999). Medical management of endometriosis. In *ACOG 2008 compendium of selected publications* [Volume II: Practice Bulletins], (p. 1036). Washington, DC: American College of Obstetricians and Gynecologists.

Mounsey, A. L., Wilgus, A., & Slawson, D. C. (2006). Diagnosis and management of endometriosis. *American Family Physician, 74*(4).

Schuiling, K. D., & Likis, F. E. (2006). *Women's gynecologic health.* Sudbury, MA: Jones and Bartlett.

Speroff, L., & Fritz, M. A. (2005). *Clinical gynecology, endocrinology, infertility* (7th ed.). Philadelphia: Lippincott Williams & Wilkins.

E

## ENDOMETRITIS

**Statistics:**
0.2–0.9% vaginal delivery
5–30% C/S delivery

**Risk Factors**
Abdominal delivery
Low SES
Prolonged labor
Prolonged ROM
Multiple vaginal exams
Internal monitoring
Preexisting infection

**Pathogen**
Aerobic gram pos cocci (GBS and enterococci)
Aerobic gram neg (E. coli, Klebsiella pneumoniae, Proteus)

**Signs and Symptom**
Fever (37.5–39.5°C) 24 to 48 h after delivery (saw-toothed fever pattern)
Tachycardia
Tachypnea
Lower abdominal pain
Pain with uterine palpation
Foul smelling lochia
Elevated WBCs

**Differential Diagnosis**
Atelectasis
UTI
Pyelonephritis
Appendicitis
Pneumonia

**Labs**
CBC
Urine culture
Blood cultures if immunocompromised or infection is persistent
Chest X-ray to r/o pneumonia

**Treatment**
See Table E-1.

**Prevention and Prophylaxis**
Hand washing
Aseptic technique
Diligent postpartum assessment
Prophylactic antibiotics during C/S decrease incidence by 75% (cephalosporin commonly used)

**SOURCES**

Cunningham, F. G. (2002). Postoperative complications. In L. C. Gilstrap, F. G. Cunningham, & J. P. VanDorsten (Eds.), Operative Obstetrics (2nd ed.). New York: McGraw-Hill.

French, L. M., & Smaill, F. M. (2004). Antibiotic regimens for endometriosis after delivery. Cochrane Database of Systematic Reviews, 4, CD001067.

Gabbe, S. G., Niebyl, J. R., & Simpson, J. L. (Eds.). (2002). Obstetrics: Normal and problem pregnancies (4th ed.). New York: Churchill Livingstone.

Gilbert, D. N., Moellering, R. C., Eliopoulos, G. M., & Sande, M. A. (2007). Table 1: Clinical approach to initial choice in antimicrobial therapy. In The Sanford Guide to Antimicrobial Therapy. Hyde Park, VT: Antimicrobial Therapy.

Tharpe, N. (2008). Postpregnancy genital tract and wound infections. Journal of Midwifery & Women's Health, 53(3). 236–246.

Varney, H., Kriebs, J. M., & Gegor, C. L. (2004). Varney's midwifery (4th ed.). Sudbury, MA: Jones and Bartlett.

TABLE E-1   Selected Antibiotics for Obstetrics Infections

| Infection Type | Pathogens | Sample Regimens Generic (Brand) | Comments |
|---|---|---|---|
| Septic abortion | Bacteroides Group B, A streptococcus Enterobacteria Chlamydia | Cefoxitin (Mefoxin) 2 g IV q 6–8 h, or Ticarcillin/clavulanate (Timentin) 3.1 g IV q 4–6 h, with doxycycline 100 mg q 12 h IV or PO | Consult or refer for evaluaton and treatment Refer for uterine evacuation, prn |
| Endometritis parenteral therapy | Bacteroides Group B, A streptococcus Enterobacteria Chlamydia | Clindamycin (Cleocin) 450–900 mg IV q 8 h, with gentamicin (Garamycin), 1.5 mg/kg IV q 8 h, or Cefoxitin (Mefoxin) 2 g IV q 6–8 h, or Ticarcillin/clavulanate (Timentin) 3.1 g IV q 4–6 h, plus Chlamydia suspected: add doxycycline* (Vibramycin hyclate for injection) 100 mg IV or PO q 12 h | Consult or refer for evaluation and treatment plan |
| Endometritis oral therapy | Chlamydia M. hominis | Ofloxacin (Flozin) 400 mg PO bid, or Doxycycline* (Doryx, Monodox, Vibramycin, and others) 100 mg PO q 12 h, or | Reserved for mild cases in afebrile women |
| Wound infection | S. aureus Group A, B, C strep, enterococci bacteroides | Piperacilin/tazobactam (Zosyn) 4 g q 6 h, or Cefotaxime (Claforan) 2 g q 4–8 h, plus metronidazole (Flagyl IV) 1 g q 12 h | Refer for wound exploration and/or surgical debridement, prn |

E

*Doxycycline not compatible with breastfeeding.

Data from: Cunningham, 2002; French & Smaill, 2004; Gilbert, Moellering, Eliopoulos, & Sande, 2007.

Source: Reprinted with permission from Tharpe, N. (2008). Postpregnancy genital tract and wound infections. Journal of Midwifery & Women's Health, 53(3).

## EPIDURALS

TABLE E-2   Medications Commonly Used for Epidural Analgesia During Labor

| Drug | Usual Dose | Duration (h) |
| --- | --- | --- |
| Morphine | 3–5 mg | 4–12 |
| Meperidine | 25–50 mg | 2–4 |
| Methadone | 5 mg | 6–8 |
| Butorphanol | 2–4 mg | 6–12 |
| Diamorphine | 5 mg | 6–12 |
| Fentanyl | 50–100 mcg | 1–2 |
| Sufentanil | 5–10 mcg | 1–3 |

*Source:* Reprinted with permission from McCool, W. F., Packman, J., & Zwerling, A. (2004). Obstetric anesthesia: Changes and choices. *Journal of Midwifery & Women's Health, 49,* 505.

### Administration

Catheter placement via needle into epidural space at L2 to L5
Covers dermatomes of T10 to T12 and S2 to S4

### Advantages

Quick acting (5–20 min; about 3 ctx)
Can be used for surgical (C/S) anesthesia if necessary, with less risk to mom and baby than general anesthesia
Useful when there is a reason to suppress pushing urge (i.e., cardiac disease)
Provide rest for maternal exhaustion
Useful for women unable to tolerate 2nd-stage due to sexual trauma
If a surgical delivery, women is awake to witness birth

### Midwifery Role

Ensure that pt understands procedure and that she will be confined to the bed for the duration of her labor
Ensure that pt has patent IV, and has received appropriate fluid bolus prior to epidural placement per institution protocols
Position pt for epidural placement either side-lying with knees towards chest, or on the side of the bed; a pillow can be used for pt to curl around
Help pt visualize correct positioning, "Curve your back like a cat"
Ensure that baby is monitored during epidural placement
Watch for fetal bradycardia during/immediately after loading dose

### Side Effects

*Insertion*

Infection
Nerve damage (very rare, d/t placement at L2 to L5)
Respiratory distress secondary to anesthesia administration
Maternal discomfort during placement
Hypotension

*Labor*

Increased need for labor augmentation
Bladder distension (need for catheterization)
Difficulty feeling sensations necessary for pushing
1–2% higher chance of malpresentation and operative delivery (controversial, mixed results from multiple randomized trials)
Longer 2nd stage (better outcomes are seen when fetal descent occurs prior to initiation of pushing; "laboring down")
Increased maternal fever
Itching
N/V

*Postpartum*
   Spinal headache (1 in 100)
   Baby may be slow to breastfeed

**Contraindications**
   Some valvular heart conditions
   Coagulopathy
   Hypovolemia (i.e., hemorrhage)
   Progressive neurologic Dx
   Bacteremia
   Use of heparin
   Skin infection over site
   Increased intracranial pressure
   Patient refusal

**E**

**Caution**
   Hx of spinal surgery or injury
   Pulmonary disease
   Low platelets
   Anesthetic allergies
   BMI > 30

**Possible Immediate Reactions to Placement**
   Mild hypotension
   Fetal distress

**Responses to Reactions**
   Give O$_2$
   IV hydration
   Reposition
   Vassopressor may be necessary for severe or prolonged hypotension (commonly
   managed by anesthesiologist)

**SOURCES**
American College of Obstetricians and Gynecologists. (2002). Obstetric analgesia and anesthesia.
   In *2006 compendium of selected publications* (p. 765). Washington, DC: American College of
   Obstetricians and Gynecologists.
Jacobson, P., & Turner, L. (2008). Management of the second stage of labor in women with epidural
   analgesia. *Journal of Midwifery & Women's Health, 53*(1), 82–85.
McCool, W. F., Packman, J., & Zwerling, A. (2004). Obstetric anesthesia: Changes and choices. *Journal
   of Midwifery & Women's Health, 49,* 505.
Smith, L. J. (2007). Impact of birthing practices on the breastfeeding dyad [Abstract]. *Journal of
   Midwifery & Women's Health, 52*(6) 621–630.
Varney, H., Kriebs, J. M., & Gegor, C. L. (2004). *Varney's midwifery* (4th ed.). Sudbury, MA: Jones and
   Bartlett.

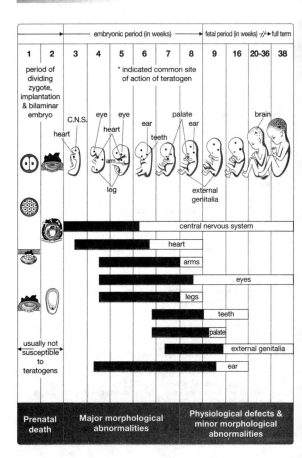

FIGURE F-1 Fetal Development. *Source:* Reprinted from Moore, K. (1982). *The developing human: Clinically oriented embryology.* Philadelphia: WB Saunders.

# FETAL FIBRONECTIN (fFN)

### Definition

"Trophoblastic glue"

Glycoprotein that promotes the adhesion between the decidua and chorion

Present in amniotic fluid

Found in cervicovaginal secretions prior to 20 wk, but is an abnormal finding once the membranes and decidua have completely fused

Levels of fFN found in vaginal secretions increases at 34 wk gestation

### Management

Hx of previous PTD, test Q 2 wk starting at 24 wk

Only useful in gestations between 24–34 wk  6 d

Use to R/O PTL

Membranes must be intact

No cervical manipulation in past 24 h (sex or vaginal exam)

No vaginal bleeding

No intravaginal lubricants or medications

Cervical dilation < 3 cm

Requires a sterile speculum exam

### Procedure

Do this test prior to cervical check

Place fFN swab in posterior fornix of vagina

Lightly rotate the sterile swab across the posterior fornix of the vagina for approximately 10 sec

Keep specimen cold until test can be performed

\*\*If PTL is suspected, fFN testing must be done *prior* to a vaginal exam for results to be accurate

### Results

Negative result = 99.5% will not deliver in the next 7–10 d; 97% will not deliver for at least 14 d

Positive result = 87% will deliver in 7 d (increases risk from 3% to 14%)

TABLE F-1   Interpretations of fFN Results

| fFN ≥ 50 ng/ml | 22–24 wk | 27–28 wk | 31–32 wk |
|---|---|---|---|
| Sensitivity | 18.9 | 21.4 | 41.2 |
| Specificity | 95.1 | 94.5 | 92.5 |
| Positive predictive value | 35.0 | 30.0 | 30.4 |
| Negative predictive value | 89.4 | 91.6 | 95.2 |

*Source:* Adapted from Iams, J. D., Newman, R. B., Thom, E. A., Goldenberg, R. L., Mueller-Heubach, E., Moawad, A., et al. (2002). Frequency of uterine contractions and the risk of spontaneous preterm delivery. *New England Journal of Medicine, 346*(4), 250–255.

### Cervical Length Assessment

A measurement of cervical length increases the PPV of fFN

Requires a TVU/S

Cervical length ≤ 2.5–3.0 cm = increased risk of PTD

Used in conjunction with fFN increases the PPV of both tests

### SOURCES

Cunningham, G., Leveno, K. J., Bloom, S. L., Hauth, J. C., Gilstrap, L. C., & Wenstrom, K. D. (2005). *Williams obstetrics* (22nd ed.). New York: McGraw-Hill Professional.

Gomez, R., Romero, R., Medina, L., Nien, J. K., Chaiworapongsa, T., Carstens, M., et al. (2005). Cervicovaginal fibronectin improves the prediction of preterm delivery based on sonographic cervical length in patients with preterm uterine contractions and intact membranes. *American Journal of Obstetrics and Gynecology, 192*(2), 350–359.

Iams, J. D., Newman, R. B., Thom, E. A., Goldenberg, R. L., Mueller-Heubach, E., Moawad, A., et al. (2002). Frequency of uterine contractions and the risk of spontaneous preterm delivery. *New England Journal of Medicine, 346*(4), 250–255.

Revah, A., Hannah, M., & Sue-A-Quan, A. (1998). Fetal fibronectin as a predictor of preterm birth: An overview. *American Journal of Perinatology, 15*(11), 613–621.

## FETAL LUNG MATURITY ASSESSMENT

Used to determine maturity of fetal lungs in relation to gestational age

Preterm infants are at high risk for RDS, which results from a lack of sufficient alveolar surfactant necessary for adequate lung expansion

Surfactant production increases as the fetal lungs mature

Measurement of lecithin/sphingomyelin ratio (L/S ratio) in amniotic fluid is considered the gold standard of fetal lung maturity, with a ratio of at least 2:1 indicating sufficient fetal lung maturity

May require amniocentesis, but vaginal pool collection is valid in some cases

### When to Assess

Need for delivery prior to term secondary to deteriorating maternal or fetal status

Diabetic pregnancies to be delivered 36–37 wk gestation (DM-complicated pregnancies, whether type I, II, or GDM exhibit a decreased rate of fetal lung maturity)

TABLE F-2    Fetal Lung Maturity Tests

| Test | Technique | Cutoff | Notes |
|------|-----------|--------|-------|
| Lecithin/sphingomyelin ratio (L/S ratio) | Thin-layer chromatography | 2:1 | Blood decreases mature and increases immature result |
| Phosphatidylglycerol (PG) | Thin-layer chromatography | Present | Not affected by blood or meconium, but heavy genital bacterial contamination may yield a false positive mature result |
| Foam stability index | Ethanol dilution | Stable foam ring in 1:1 dilution | Simple test, but skewed by contamination with blood and/or meconium |
| Lamellar body counts | Cell counter | 50,000/mcl uncentrifuged; 30,000/mcl centrifuged | Reliable if no blood contamination, plts increase count, while coagulation decreases count |
| Surfactant/albumin ratio | Fluorescent polarization | ≥ 55 mg/g of albumin | Simple test, not valid with blood and/or meconium contamination |

*Sources:* Adapted from American College of Obstetricians and Gynecologists. (1996). Assessment of fetal lung maturity (Educational Bulletin No. 230). In *2006 compendium of selected publications* (p. 267). Washington, DC: Author. Creasy, R. K., & Resnik, R. (2004). *Maternal-fetal medicine* (5th ed.). Philadelphia: Saunders.

**SOURCES**

American College of Obstetricians and Gynecologists. (1996). Assessment of fetal lung maturity (Educational Bulletin No. 230). In *2006 compendium of selected publications* (p. 267). Washington, DC: Author.

Creasy, R. K., & Resnik, R. (2004). *Maternal-fetal medicine* (5th ed.). Philadelphia: Saunders.

# FEVER: POSTPARTUM

**Puerperal Fever**
Septicemia accompanied by fever, in which the focus of infection is the uterus
The etiologic agent is frequently a streptococcus
Also called childbed fever or puerperal sepsis

**Diagnosis**
Temp ≥ 38°C (100.4°F) on any 2 of the first 10 d postpartum (exclusive of the first 24 h)

**Differential Diagnosis**
Infection of perineum, vagina, cervix
Endometritis
Salpingitis
Peritonitis
Septicemia
Thrombophlebitis
UTI
Mastitis

**F**

**Common Pathogens**
GBS
CT/GC
Mycoplasma hominis
Gardnerella

*Assoc. w/ Increased Risk of Postpartum Infection*
Group A and D streptococci
Enterococcus
E. coli
Klebsiella
Proteus
Staph
Anaerobes
Peptococcus
Peptostreptococcus
Bacteroides fragilis
Clostridium
Fusobacterium
Mobiluncus

**Risk Factors**
C/S
Multifetal gestation
Young maternal age
Nulliparity
Coagulation disorders
Smoking
HPV
Episiotomy/laceration breakdown

**Endometritis**
Polymicrobial infection that travels from the vagina or incision into the uterus
Reduced with hand washing and aseptic technique
Serious infection is more likely in women who sustain a fourth-degree laceration

**SOURCES**
Anderson, D., Novak, P., Keith, J. & Elliott, M. (2007). *Dorland's medical dictionary* (30th ed.). Retrieved April 24, 2008, from http://www.dorlands.com
Cunningham, G., Leveno, K. J., Bloom, S. L., Hauth, J. C., Gilstrap, L. C., & Wenstrom, K. D. (2005). *Williams obstetrics* (22nd ed.). New York: McGraw-Hill Professional.
Tharpe, N. (2008). Postpregnancy genital tract and wound infections. *Journal of Midwifery & Women's Health, 53*(3), 236–246.
Varney, H., Kriebs, J. M., & Gegor, C. L. (2004). *Varney's midwifery* (4th ed.). Sudbury, MA: Jones and Bartlett.

## FIBROIDS: LEIOMYOMATAS

### Definition
Benign tumors associated with the smooth muscle of the uterus

### Statistics
25–50% of women
Incidence increases with age

### Signs and Symptoms
| | |
|---|---|
| Increased uterine bleeding with menses | Increased abdominal girth |
| Pelvic pressure or pain | Urinary difficulties |
| Infertility | Rectal pain or pressure |
| Pregnancy complications | |

### Diagnosis
History of change in menstrual cycle characteristics
Abdominal/bimanual exam irregularities
U/S

### Types
Subserous—pedunculated fibroid that grows outside the uterus, under the uterine
    serosa, easily palpated on abdominal exam
Intramural—located in the uterine myometrium; on exam uterus feels misshapen
Submucosal—pedunculated fibroid that grows from the endometrium and extends
    into the uterine cavity; on exam the uterus feels enlarged

### Differential Diagnosis
| | |
|---|---|
| Endometrial cancer | UTI |
| Endometriosis | Ovarian mass |
| Adenomyosis | Ascites |
| Constipation | Abdominal or pelvic masses |
| IBS | |

### Treatment

*Asymptomatic:* No tx

*Symptomatic*
GnRH agonists (Lupron, Synarel, Zoladex) reduce size by 35–60% in 3 mo
Mirena IUD
COC
NSAIDs
Surgery
Uterine artery embolization

### Pregnancy Complications
| | |
|---|---|
| S > D | Placental abruption |
| Spontaneous abortion | Malpresentation |
| Preterm labor | Arrest of labor |
| Fetal growth restriction | Retained placenta |

**Postpartum Complications:** Fibroids degenerate quickly so there is often pain and
bleeding

**Postmenopause:** HRT can cause fibroids to regrow

#### SOURCES
NorthPoint Domain. (2008). *UFEinfo*. Retrieved January 2, 2008, from http://www.ufeinfo.com
Schuiling, K. D., & Likis, F. E. (2006). *Women's gynecologic health.* Sudbury, MA: Jones and Bartlett.

# GENETICS: PRENATAL TESTING OPTIONS

### Understand Prenatal Screening Tests and Results
Pts need to be counseled in the difference between a test used for screening and one used for diagnosis. Multiple marker screening (Quad screen) is a prenatal test that assesses the *risk* of having an affected fetus. These tests do not diagnosis a woman as carrying an affected fetus. Further testing must be done to determine if the results of the screen are a true positive.

### Benefits and Risks of Prenatal Testing
Information used to determine whether or not to continue the pregnancy
Results affect the management of the pregnancy
Plan for possible complications w/ the birth process
Plan for problems that may occur in the newborn infant
Find conditions that may affect future pregnancies
Increase anxiety associated w/ pregnancy regardless of outcome

### Understand the Patient's Perspective
Anchoring—Everyone has preconceived notions of their own "risk," and that will affect how they interpret their "true" risk
Framing—The delivery of information can change the interpretation (e.g., % who die, % affected, and % who survive can all be evaluated differently by the pt)
Representativeness—Context in which someone makes a judgment about an outcome affects how the risk is perceived: Do they have a family member w/ the disease? Do they only know the disease from media coverage?
Availability—The more familiar a pt is w/ the disease outcome, the more likely they are to perceive their risk as higher

### Effective Use of Risk Information in Counseling
Assess baseline level of literacy and numeracy
Inquire about knowledge of the testing process and its outcomes
Identify preconceptions about personal risk of outcomes in question
Discuss personal experience or familiarity w/ conditions or tests in question
Present numeric risk information
Use rates to describe risk
Frame risk both in terms of the chance of an undesired outcome *and* the chance of an unaffected infant or "successful" outcome
Assess application of risk information provided to the decision at hand
Incorporate personal values
Participate w/ partner or family in decision making

### When to Refer for Counseling
Possible carrier status for a genetic disease
Positive prenatal screen
Mental retardation or developmental delay
Known chromosomal abnormality (fragile X, trisomies, inversions/translocations)
Family history of cleft lip/palate, congenital heart disease, NTDs, mental retardation, hemophilia A or B, Duchenne/Becker MD, fragile X
Stature significantly different from parents or ethnic group
Exposure to teratogens (alcohol, radiation, occupational chemical exposures, toxoplasmosis, rubella, CMV, syphilis, IDDM, epileptic drugs)
Consanguinity
Recurrent SAB
Age 35 yr or older
Hx of previous infant affected by a genetic disorder
Hx of unexplained IUFD or neonatal death
Also consider referral if FOB has a family hx of genetic disease, or offspring w/ a birth defect

### Follow-up for Positive Prenatal Screen
Ensure that EDD is accurate
Level II U/S (standard of care for all positive screens)
Amniocentesis
Genetic counseling

TABLE G-1  Overview of Genetic Testing During Pregnancy

| Test | Procedure | Screen | Counseling | Other |
|---|---|---|---|---|
| Chorionic villus sampling (CVS) (10–12 wk) | Removal of sample of chorion from the developing placenta, transcervically w/ U/S guidance; Rhogam for Rh-neg women | All genetic diseases | Earliest available testing; allows for early termination; may facilitate bonding if genetic anomaly is real concern; postprocedural spotting is common | Risk of Ab 0.6–0.8%; mosaicism requiring F/U amniocentesis |
| First trimester screen (10–14 wk) | Blood sample: βhCG PAPP-A U/S: nuchal fold thickness | Trisomy 21 | If positive, then offer CVS or amnio to confirm diagnosis; test integrated w/ Quad screen in 2nd tri; offer 2nd tri screening to assess NTD risk even if woman desires only 1st tri aneuploidy screening | Noninvasive procedure; integrated 1st/2nd tri screening is more sensitive than 1st tri screen alone |
| Amniocentesis (15–20 wk) | Removal of amniotic fluid (20–30 ml) by needle aspiration transabdominally; Rhogam for Rh-neg women | All genetic diseases; fetal lung maturity (late 2nd–3rd tri) | Reliable test, preliminary results available in 48 h, full results in 1 wk; pts often report cramping for 1–2 h after procedure | Risk of Ab 0.5–1.0% |
| Quad screen (15–20 wk) Optimum = 16 wk | Blood sample: MSAFP βhCG Estriol Inhibin A | NTDs Trisomy 21 Trisomy 18 | High false-positive rate; generally only 5% of positive results are true-positive; if result is positive then level II U/S and/or amnio offered | Screen is noninvasive, but if positive pt may opt for amnio; level II U/S standard of care for positive screens; elevated or decreased MSAFP requires further monitoring |
| Thalassemia (α or β) | Blood electrophoresis | Hemoglobinopathies | Consider if pt exhibits anemia and is nonresponsive to iron therapy and/or is of Asian, African, Mediterranean, Middle Eastern descent | If pt is a carrier, then FOB needs to be screened to assess risk to fetus |
| Cystic fibrosis | Blood sample, genetic testing | CTFR gene mutation | Routinely offered to all patients | If positive, then FOB needs screening |

Sources: Adapted from American College of Obstetricians and Gynecologists. (2001). Prenatal diagnosis of fetal chromosomal abnormalities. 2006 compendium of selected publications (p. 867). Washington, DC: Author. American College of Obstetricians and Gynecologists. (2007). Screening for fetal chromosomal abnormalities (ACOG Practice Bulletin No. 77). Obstetrics and Gynecology, 109(1), 217–228. American College of Obstetricians and Gynecologists. (2005). Update on carrier screening for cystic fibrosis (ACOG Committee Opinion No. 325). In ACOG 2008 compendium of selected publications: Vol. 1. Committee opinions and policy statements (pp. 325, 329). Washington, DC: Author.

| Disease | Screening Test | Carrier Frequency |
|---|---|---|
| **Autosomal Recessive** | | |
| α-Thalassemia | α-Hb gene mutation; screen if Southeast Asian or Chinese descent | 1:25 |
| β-Thalassemia | β-Hb gene mutation; screen if Mediterranean, Asian Indian, Bangladeshi, Pakistani, Middle Eastern descent | 1:30 |
| Cystic fibrosis | CFTR gene mutation; most common in European ancestry, ACOG recommends testing for everyone | 1:29 European ancestry |
| | | 1:29 Ashkenazi Jewish |
| | | 1:48 Hispanics |
| | | 1:65 African ancestry |
| | | 1:150 Asian ancestry |
| Sickle cell trait | β-chain gene mutation; screen if African ancestry | 1:12 |
| Tay-Sachs disease | Hexosaminidase A deficiency; test all patients with Ashkenazi Jewish ancestry | 1:30 |
| Canavan | Aspartoacylase (ASPA) deficiency; test all patients with Ashkenazi Jewish ancestry | 1:40 |
| Nieman/Pick | Acid sphingomyelinase deficiency; test if Ashkenazi Jewish ancestry and family history of disease | 1:90 |
| Gaucher disease type I | Glucocerebrosidase deficiency; test if Ashkenazi Jewish ancestry and family history of disease; type I is a mild disease form, often with no disease manifestations | 1:14 |
| Familial dysautonomia | IKBKAP gene mutation; test if Ashkenazi Jewish ancestry and family history of disease | 1:30 |
| **Disease** | **Screening Test** | **Incidence Frequency** |
| **X-linked Recessive** | | |
| Duchene/Becker muscular dystrophy | Dystrophin gene mutation | 1:3000 male births |
| Fragile X syndrome | CGG repeat number on X chromosome | Risk based on number of maternal repeats |
| **Autosomal Dominant** | | |
| Huntington disease | CAG repeat length | 50% |
| Myotonic dystrophy | CTG expansion of repeats in the DMPK gene | 50% |
| Neurofibromatosis type 1 | NF1 gene mutation | 50% |

Sources: Adapted from Creasy, R. K., & Resnik, R. (2004). *Maternal-fetal medicine* (5th ed.). Philadelphia: Saunders. Varney, H., Kriebs, J. M., & Gegor, C. L. (2004). *Varney's midwifery* (4th ed.). Sudbury, MA: Jones and Bartlett.

G

TABLE G-3   Quad Screen Result Interpretations

| Anomaly | MSAFP | βhCG | Estriol | Inhibin A |
|---|---|---|---|---|
| NTDs | Increased | Normal | Normal | Normal |
| Trisomy 21 | Decreased | Increased | Decreased | Increased |
| Trisomy 18 | Decreased | Decreased | Decreased | Normal |

TABLE G-4   Down Syndrome (Trisomy 21) Risk by Maternal Age

| Maternal Age | Risk for Trisomy 21 | False-Positive Rate (Quad Screen) |
|---|---|---|
| 20 | 1/1527 | 2.4% |
| 25 | 1/1352 | 2.9% |
| 30 | 1/895 | 5.0% |
| 35 | 1/356 | 14.0% |
| 40 | 1/97 | 40.0% |
| 45 | 1/23 | > 40.0% |

Source: Adapted from Gabbe, S. G., Niebyl, J. R., & Simpson, J. L. (Eds.). (2002). Obstetrics: Normal and problem pregnancies (4th ed.). New York: Churchill Livingstone.

TABLE G-5   Frequency, Sensitivity, and False-Positive Rates for Trisomy 21, 18, and NTDs

| Anomaly | Frequency | Detection Rate w/Quad Screen (Sensitivity) (%) | False-Positive Rate (FPR) (%) |
|---|---|---|---|
| Trisomy 21 | ~1/700 | All screens: 79.3<br>< age 35: 68.1<br>≥ age 35: 91.4 | All screens: 7.38<br>< age 35: 5.16<br>≥ age 35: 22.43 |
| Trisomy 18 | ~1/5000 | All screens: 77.8<br>< age 35: 69.5<br>≥ age 35: 86.8 | All screens: 7.5<br>< age 35: 5.23<br>≥ age 35: 22.86 |
| Neural tube defects | ~1/2500 | 75 | ~2.0–4.0 |

Sources: Adapted from Benn, P. A., Ying, J., Beazoglou, T., & Egan, J. F. (2001). Estimates for the sensitivity and false-positive rates for second trimester serum screening for down syndrome and trisomy 18 with adjustment for cross-identification and double-positive results. Prenatal Diagnosis, 21(1), 46–51. Creasy, R. K., & Resnik, R. (2004). Maternal-fetal medicine (5th ed.). Philadelphia: Saunders. Varney, H., Kriebs, J. M., & Gegor, C. L. (2004). Varney's midwifery (4th ed.). Sudbury, MA: Jones and Bartlett.

**Web Resources for Clinicians**

www.acmg.net—American College of Medical Genetics: offers resources regarding genetic screening
www.isong.org—International Society of Nurses in Genetics: defines the role of nurses in the genetics field
www.genome.gov—National Genome Research Institute: links to fact sheets for clinicians and patients
www.genereviews.org—NIH sponsored site offering current information regarding genetic research and a directory for testing laboratories
www.ncbi.nlm.nih.gov/sites/entrez?db=omim—Online Mendelian Inheritance in Man (OMIM): covers FAQs regarding inheritance patterns
www.cdc.gov/genomics—ACCE project from the CDC: explanations of the validity of genetic testing, resources for clinicians and patients
www.ghr.nlm.nih.gov—National Library of Medicine genetics compendium: intended for the lay public

**SOURCES**

American College of Obstetricians and Gynecologists. (2001). Prenatal diagnosis of fetal chromosomal abnormalities. 2006 compendium of selected publications (pp. 867). Washington, DC: Author.
American College of Obstetricians and Gynecologists. (2007). Screening for fetal chromosomal abnormalities (ACOG Practice Bulletin No. 77). Obstetrics and Gynecology, 109(1), 217–228.
American College of Obstetricians and Gynecologists. (2005). Update on carrier screening for cystic fibrosis (ACOG Committee Opinion No. 325). In ACOG 2008 compendium of selected publications: Vol. 1. Committee opinions and policy statements (p. 236–239). Washington, DC: Author.
Benn, P. A., Ying, J., Beazoglou, T., & Egan, J. F. (2001). Estimates for the sensitivity and false-positive rates for second trimester serum screening for Down syndrome and trisomy 18 with adjustment for cross-identification and double-positive results. Prenatal Diagnosis, 21(1), 46–51.
Creasy, R. K., & Resnik, R. (2004). Maternal-fetal medicine (5th ed.). Philadelphia: Saunders.
Gates, E. A. (2004). Communicating risk in prenatal genetic testing. Journal of Midwifery & Women's Health, 49(3), 220.
Little, C. M., & Lewis, J. A. (2005). Genetic resources for midwifery practice. Journal of Midwifery & Women's Health, 50(3), 246.
Varney, H., Kriebs, J. M., & Gegor, C. L. (2004). Varney's midwifery (4th ed.). Sudbury, MA: Jones and Bartlett.

# GENITAL WARTS: CONDYLOMA ACUMINATA

## Cause
HPV types 6 and 11 most common
HPV types 16, 18, 31, 33, and 35 also associated

## Signs and Symptoms
Flat papular or pedunculated growths
Found on the vulva, sometimes on cervix, vagina, urethra, anus, mouth, and penis

## Diagnosis
Visual inspection or confirmed by biopsy

## Treatment
20–30% self resolve w/in 3 mo

### Pt Applied
Podofilox (damages growth process of the wart and enhances immune response)
  0.5% solution/gel applied to warts BID × 3 d followed by 4 d of no therapy and
  then rpt if necessary
Imiquimod (Aldera) (enhances immune response) 5% cream QD at HS 3 × per wk
  for 16 wk, wash treated area w/ soap and water 6–10 h after application

### Provider Applied
Bi/trichloroacetic acid 80–90%
  Causes death of wart tissue
  Wart turns white
  Rpt weekly until resolution
  Protect healthy skin surrounding wart w/ barrier (KY jelly or Vaseline)
  If overtreated apply powdered talc, sodium bicarbonate, or liquid soap to remove
  excess
Cryotherapy causes death of wart tissue by thermolysis—Apply once Q 1–2 wk
Podophyllin resin causes wart tissue necrosis 10–25% applied to wart and air dried
  Rpt weekly
  No open lesions during tx
Surgical removal
Intralesional interferons or laser surgery

## Patient Education
Common infection
Sexually transmitted
Difficult to note time of infection due to variable incubation period
Condoms do not offer complete protection
HPV testing not indicated
Reinfection does not increase incidence of outbreaks

## Follow-up
Recurrence in 3 mo common, pt can return for tx

## Pregnant/Newborn
No imiquimod, podophyllin, or podofilox during pregnancy
Occurrence/number often increases due to decreased immune system suppression
C/S indicated if excessive growth would cause increased bleeding due to tissue
  trauma
Respiratory papillomatosis in the newborn possible, though infection transmission
  rate not known

G

### SOURCES
American College of Obstetricians and Gynecologists. (2005). Human papillomavirus (ACOG Practice
  Bulletin No. 61). In ACOG 2008 compendium (pp. 1231–1243). Washington, DC: Author.
Centers for Disease Control and Prevention. (2006). Sexually transmitted diseases treatment
  guidelines. Morbidity and Mortality Weekly Report, 55(RR-11), 62–66.

## GESTATIONAL DIABETES (GDM)

**Risk-Based Protocol**

*High Risk*
- Glucose testing as soon as possible, if neg rpt at 24–28 wk using average risk protocol
- Marked obesity
- Hx of GDM
- Hx of delivery of LGA infant
- Glycosuria
- PCOS
- Strong family Hx of diabetes (1st degree relatives)

*Average Risk*
- Not high or low risk: test at 24–28 wk w/ either
- One step: 100 g GTT
- Two step: GCT followed by GTT if abnormal GCT

*Low Risk*
- Age < 25 yr
- Normal prepregnancy wt
- No known diabetes in 1st-degree relatives
- No hx of abnormal glucose tolerance
- No hx of poor obstetric outcomes

**Diagnosis**
1. Fasting plasma glucose > 126 mg/dl
2. Casual plasma glucose > 200 mg/dl on two separate days
3. GCT—measure plasma or serum glucose 1 h after 50 g oral glucose load
   If glucose level > 140 mg/dl then perform GTT (80% of GDM detected)
   If glucose level >130 mg/dl then perform GTT (90% of GDM detected)
4. Oral glucose tolerance test (GTT)—measure plasma or serum glucose level at fasting, 1, 2, and 3 h after 100 g oral glucose load
   GDM dx if two or more of the values are > cutoff values

**Important Aspects of Testing**
- Testing should be done in the morning
- Overnight fast for 8–14 h
- No smoking before or during the testing
- Liquid drinks must be consumed in 5 min

**Pregnancy/Delivery Risk Factors**

*Maternal*
- HTN
- Preeclampsia

*Delivery*
- Shoulder dystocia
- Primary C/S

*Fetal/Neonatal*
- Macrosomia
- Hyperbilirubinemia
- Neonatal hypoglycemia
- Impaired lung maturity

**Postpartum Management of GDM Patients**
- Monitor blood glucose levels pre- and postprandial for first 24 h
- Most pts will have complete resolution of blood glucose issues immediately after delivery
- Screen all GDM pts at 6–12 wk postpartum for diabetes
- 22% will have elevated blood glucose levels at 6 wk postpartum requiring further management

TABLE G-6    Summary of Cutoff Values for Diagnosis and Screening for Gestational Diabetes

| | 50 g Load | 75 g Load | | 100 g Load | |
| | ADA USPSTF ACOG (mg/dl) | ADA (mg/dl) | WHO (mg/dl) | National Diabetes Group Data (mg/dl) | ADA and ACOG (mg/dl) |
|---|---|---|---|---|---|
| Fasting | | 95 | 126 | 105 | 95 |
| 1 hour | 140 or 130 | 180 | | 190 | 180 |
| 2 hour | | 155 | 200 | 165 | 155 |
| 3 hour | | | | 145 | 140 |

*Sources:* Adapted from American Diabetes Association. (2004). Gestational diabetes mellitus position statement. *Diabetes Care, 27*(Suppl. 1), 88–90. Desai, S. P. (2004). *Clinician's guide to laboratory medicine: A practical approach* (3rd ed.). Hudson, OH: Lexi-Comp. Frye, A. (1997). *Understanding diagnostic tests in the childbearing years* (6th ed.). Portland, OR: Labrys Press. Hollander, M., Paarlberg, M., & Huisjes, A. (2007). Gestational diabetes: A review of the current literature and guidelines. *Obstetrical and Gynecology Survey, 62*(2), 125. Mulholland, C., Njoroge, T., Mersereau, P., & Williams, J. (2007). Comparison of guidelines available in the United States for diagnosis and management of diabetes before, during, and after pregnancy. *Journal of Women's Health, 16*(6), 790.

G

### Alternative Glucose Loads

18 Branch or Brock jelly beans consumed in 2 min
28 No. 110 jelly beans consumed in 2 min
600 calories mixed-nutrient breakfast

### Treatment

Referral to nutritionist, endocrinologist
Comanagement w/ MD
Diet control
Insulin

### SOURCES

American Diabetes Association. (2004). Gestational diabetes mellitus position statement. *Diabetes Care, 27*(Suppl. 1), 88–90.

Desai, S. P. (Ed.). (2004). *Clinician's guide to laboratory medicine: A practical approach* (3rd ed.). Hudson, OH: Lexi-Comp.

Frye, A. (1997). *Understanding diagnostic tests in the childbearing years* (6th ed.). Portland, OR: Labrys Press.

Hollander, M., Paarlberg, M., & Huisjes, A. (2007). Gestational diabetes: A review of the current literature and guidelines. *Obstetrical and Gynecology Survey, 62*(2), 125.

Mulholland, C., Njoroge, T., Mersereau, P., & Williams, J. (2007). Comparison of guidelines available in the United States for diagnosis and management of diabetes before, during, and after pregnancy. *Journal of Women's Health, 16*(6), 790.

## GONORRHEA (GC)

**Cause**

*Neisseria gonorrhoeae* a gram-negative diplococci

**Statistics**

Estimated 700,000 new infections in the United States each year

**Risk Factors**

| | |
|---|---|
| Age < 29 yr old | New/multiple partners |
| Hx of infection | Sex work |
| Other STIs | Drug use |

**Signs and Symptoms**

*Women*

| | |
|---|---|
| Asymptomatic | Increased vaginal discharge |
| Pain/burning w/ urination | Irregular vaginal bleeding |

*Men*

Asymptomatic or burning sensation during urination
White/yellow/green discharge from penis
Painful or swollen testicles

*Men and Women (Anal)*

| | |
|---|---|
| Asymptomatic | Soreness |
| Discharge | Bleeding |
| Itching | Pain w/ bowel movement |

**Transmission**

| | |
|---|---|
| Penis | Anus |
| Vagina | Ejaculation not required for transmission |
| Mouth | Maternal fetal transmission during delivery |

**Sequelae**

| | |
|---|---|
| PID | Infertility |
| Ectopic pregnancy | Epididymitis |

**Diagnosis**

Endocervical, vaginal, urethral, or urine specimen tested by cultures, nucleic acid
hybridization test, or nucleic acid amplification test (NAAT)
Coinfection w/ CT common, tx for both unless CT is ruled out

**Treatment**

Ceftriaxone 125 mg IM once (Preg Cat B)
Cefixime 400 mg PO once (Preg Cat B)
Ciprofloxacin 500 mg PO once (some strains resistant) (Preg Cat C)
Ofloxacin 400 mg PO once (Preg Cat C)
Levofloxacin 250 mg PO once (Preg Cat C)

**Follow-up**

No TOC needed except in pregnancy and areas of the country with resistant strains
TOC 3 wk after tx
Tx partner

**Patient Education**

| | |
|---|---|
| Safe sex | Not cured until 2 wk after tx |
| Risk of CT infection | Reinfection/other STI testing |

**Newborn**

Acute illness manifests 2–5 d after birth: ophthalmic prophylaxis recommended
Tx w/ ceftriaxone 25–50 mg/kg IV or IM single dose, not to exceed 125 mg

**SOURCES**

Centers for Disease Control and Prevention. (2006). Sexually transmitted diseases treatment
guidelines, *2006. Morbidity and Mortality Weekly Report,* 55(RR-11), 42, 49.
Thompson Healthcare Inc. (2007). *MICROMEDEX healthcare series.* Retrieved August 24, 2008, from
http://www.micromedex.com

## GROUP BETA STREPTOCOCCUS (GBS) GUIDELINES

### Etiology

Beta-hemolytic streptococcus found in the GI tract

10–30% of pregnant and nonpregnant women are colonized either vaginally or rectally

Colonization can be transient, persistent, or intermittent

Colonization during pregnancy increases the risk of chorioamnionitis and postpartum endometritis

GBS bacteriuria increases the incidence of PTL and PROM, and should be treated w/ cephalexin (Keflex) 500 mg BID × 10 d

### Screening

Routinely done between 35–37 wk

Vaginal/rectal culture

Test is valid for 5 wk

May need to repeat if postdates

If pt is PCN allergic, add antibiotic sensitivities to the lab order

TABLE G-7    Intrapartum Indications for Prophylaxis for GBS

G

| Indicated | Not Indicated |
|---|---|
| Previous infant with GBS disease | Previous pregnancy with a GBS+ screen (unless current pregnancy also has a + screen) |
| GBS bacteriuria during current pregnancy | Planned C/S delivery performed in the absence of ROM (regardless of GBS status) |
| Positive GBS screen during current pregnancy in the last 5 wk | Negative GBS screen |
| Unknown GBS status and any of the following risk factors:<br>—Delivery at < 37 wk gestation<br>—Amniotic membrane rupture ≥ 18 hrs<br>—IP temp ≥ 100.4°F | |

*Source:* Adapted from American College of Nurse-Midwives. (2003). Early-onset group B strep infection in newborns: Prevention and prophylaxis (ACNM Clinical Bulletin No. 2). *Journal of Midwifery & Women's Health, 48*(5), 375. Schrag, S. D., Gorwitz, R., Fultz-Butts, K., Schuchat, A. (2002). Prevention of perinatal group B streptococcal disease: Revised guidelines from CDC. *Morbidity and Mortality Weekly Report, 51*(RR-11), 1–22.

**Treatment**

TABLE G-8    Treatment for GBS in Labor

| GBS IP Antibiotic Prophylaxis | IV Dose | Pregnancy Category |
|---|---|---|
| Penicillin G | 5 million units, load | B |
|  | 2.5 million units Q 4 h |  |
| Ampicillin | 2 g, load; 1 g Q 4h | B |
| Cefazolin | 2 g, load; 1 g Q 8 h | B |
| Clindamycin | 900 mg Q 8 h | B |
| Erythromycin | 500 mg Q 6 h | B |
| Vancomycin | 1 g Q 12h | C |
| Gentamicin | 1–2.5 mg/kg/dose | D |
|  | Q 8–12 h |  |

Source: Adapted from Schrag, S. D., Gorwitz, R., Fultz-Butts, K., & Schuchat, A. (2002). Prevention of perinatal group B streptococcal disease: Revised guidelines from CDC. *Morbidity and Mortality Weekly Report, 51*(RR-11), 1–22.

*Antibiotic Choice for GBS Intrapartum Prophylaxis*
   1st line: Penicillin G
   2nd line: Cephalosporin
      Use if PCN allergy manifests as a rash
      *Do not* use if PCN allergy involves anaphylaxis
   3rd line: Clindamycin or erythromycin
   4th line: Vancomycin
   Choice of antibiotic for PCN allergic pts will depend on sensitivity results from the
      GBS culture

**Early Onset Neonatal GBS (EONS)**

*Etiology*
   Vertical transmission from mother to baby

*Incidence*
   0.5/1000 live births (w/ current CDC guidelines treatment protocols being observed)

TABLE G-9    Risk Factors for EONS

| Factors That Influence EONS | Incidence per 1000 Live Births |
|---|---|
| ROM > 18 h | 14.0 |
| Intra-amniotic infection | 14.0 |
| Colonization status: |  |
|    Lightly colonized | 4 |
|    Heavily colonized | 50 |
| Gestational age < 28 wk | 27.8 |
| Birth weight: |  |
|    < 1500 g | 5.99 |
|    1500–2400 g | 2.51 |
|    > 2500 g | 0.89 |
| GBS negative, no risk factors | 0.2 |
| GBS negative and risk factors (prolonged ROM, IP fever, gestational age < 37 wk) | 0.9 |
| GBS positive, no risk factors | 5.1 |

Source: Adapted from Jolivet, R. (2002). Early-onset neonatal group B streptococcal infection: 2002 guidelines for prevention (Abstract). *Journal of Midwifery & Women's Health, 47*(6), 435–446.

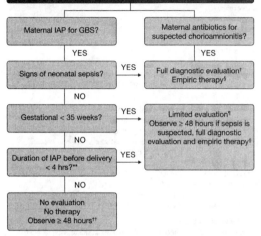

Sample algorithm for management of a newborn whose mother received intrapartum antimicrobial agents for prevention of early-onset group B streptococcal disease* or suspected chorioamnionitis. This algorithm is not an exclusive course of management. Variations that incorporate individual circumstances or institutional preferences may be appropriate.

* If no maternal intrapartum prophylaxis for GBS was administered despite an indication being present, data are insufficient on which to recommend a single management strategy.

† Includes complete blood cell count and differential, blood culture, and chest radiograph if respiratory abnormalities are present. When signs of sepsis are present, a lumbar puncture, if feasible, should be performed.

§ Duration of therapy varies depending on results of blood culture, cerebrospinal fluid findings, if obtained, and the clinical course of the infant. If laboratory results and clinical course do not indicate bacterial infection, duration may be as short as 48 hours.

¶ CBC with differential and blood culture.

** Applies only to penicillin, ampicillin, or cefazolin and assumes recommended dosing regimens (Box 2).

†† A healthy-appearing infant who was ≥ 38 weeks' gestation at delivery and whose mother received ≥ 4 hours of intrapartum prophylaxis before delivery may be discharged home after 24 hours if other discharge criteria have been met and a person able to comply fully with instructions for home observation will be present. If any one of these conditions is not met, the infant should be observed in the hospital for at least 48 hours and until the criteria for discharge are achieved.

FIGURE G-1 Assessment Algorithm for EONS. *Source:* Reprinted from Schrag, S. D., Gorwitz, R., Fultz-Butts, K., Schuchat, A. (2002). Prevention of perinatal group B streptococcal disease: Revised guidelines from CDC. *Morbidity and Mortality Weekly Report, 51*(RR-11), 1–22.

**SOURCES**

American College of Nurse-Midwives. (2003). Early-onset group B strep infection in newborns: Prevention and prophylaxis (ACNM Clinical Bulletin No. 2). *Journal of Midwifery & Women's Health, 48*(5), 375.

Jolivet, R. (2002). Early-onset neonatal group B streptococcal infection: 2002 guidelines for prevention (Abstract). *Journal of Midwifery & Women's Health, 47*(6) 435–446.

Schrag, S., Gorwitz, R., Fultz-Butts, K., & Schuchat, A. (2002). Prevention of perinatal group B streptococcal disease: Revised guidelines from CDC. *Morbidity and Mortality Weekly Report, 51*(RR-11), 1–22.

## GYN EXAM

### Getting to Know the Woman
What would you like to be called?
What brought you in today?
Explain the plan for the visit

### GYN Overview
Date of last menstrual period
Age of menarche
Frequency of menses
Duration of menses
Discomforts of menstruation
Pregnancy history (GTPAL—**G**ravida, **T**erm pregnancies, **P**reterm births 20–37 wk, and > 500 g, **A**bortions prior to 20 wk, **L**iving children)

### Sexuality
"Are you currently involved in a sexual relationship?"
"Do you have sex w/ men, women, or both?"
"What kind of sex to you have: oral, vaginal, anal?"
"Do you have any questions or concerns about your sexual relationship?"
"How many partners have you had in the past year?"
"What do you use for contraception?"
"Are you interested in any other methods?"
"Have you ever had a sexually transmitted disease?"
"How do you protect yourself from sexually transmitted diseases?"
"Do you have any problems or questions related to sex or sexuality?"

### Current Medical Problems
"Do you have any current health concerns you would like to address today?"

### Current Medications, Allergies, Herbal Supplements, and Vitamins
Inquire about any medication allergies, current medication use
Discuss with pt the use of any herbal supplements or vitamins

### Personal Habits
Exercise
Sleep
Nutrition

### Substance Use
Tobacco
Alcohol
Illicit substances

### Healthcare History
Any past medical diagnoses (diabetes, thyroid dysfunction, HTN, heart disease, autoimmune disorders, kidney disease/UTI, hepatitis/liver disease, varicosities/phlebitis, neurologic/epilepsy, psychiatric)
Hx of blood transfusions
Immunization history
Surgeries and hospitalizations

### Family History
Illness in first-degree relatives (parents and siblings)
Congenital malformations

### Social/Occupational
Relationship status
School vs. employed
Moving

### Safety
Abuse
Violence

## Review of Systems

General: fever, wt change, sleep patterns
HEENT/Neck: H/A, visual changes, hearing loss, colds
Cardiovascular: chest pain, palpitations
Respiratory: difficulty breathing, shortness of breath
Gastrointestinal: loss of appetite, N/V, constipation, diarrhea
Genitourinary: dysuria, flank pain, frequency, hematuria, incontinence
GYN/genital: pain, abnormal bleeding, discharge
Endocrine: intolerance to heat or cold
Dermatology: rash, itching
Psychiatric: depression, anxiety, mood disturbances, thoughts of hurting self or others
Musculoskeletal: joint pain, swelling, restriction of motion

## Physical Exam

General: alert, oriented, dressed appropriately, signs of trauma
HEENT: hair, facial structure, eyes, ears, thyroid, lymph nodes
Heart: RRR, murmurs
Chest and lungs: breathing pattern and RR, wheezing, rales, crepitus, stridor
Breasts: symmetry, size, contour, edema, venous pattern, nipples, lesions, discharge, palpation, BSE education
Abdomen: bowel sounds, liver, spleen, kidneys
Skin: texture, color, lesions, hair, nails, tattoos
Neurologic: cranial nerve function, deep tendon reflexes
Musculoskeletal: range of motion, joints, edema

## Pelvic Exam

Explain exactly what you will do and ask permission to do it
Never force someone's legs apart, ask pt to move their knees to a specific place
Offer a mirror
Contracting: "Please let me know if you would like me to change what I am doing to make it more comfortable for you or ask me to stop if you would like me to"
Choose a speculum:
  Pederson (flat, narrow bill)
  Graves (wider, curved bill for looser vaginal walls of multiparous women)
External: genital anatomy, hair pattern, secondary sex characteristics, lacerations, scars, condylomata, lesions, varicosities, inflammation, dermatitis, pigmentation changes, vesicles, ulcers, fistulas, fissures, discharge, prolapse
Vagina: tone, rugae, color, secretions, inflammation, foreign bodies, polyps, bleeding, lesions, cysts
Bimanual:
  Cervix—size, shape, consistency, smoothness, CMT
  Uterus—size, shape, position, mobility, pain
  Ovaries—size, shape, pain
  Rectal (if done)—assess retroverted uterus, endometriosis, thickness of rectovaginal wall, occult blood test

**G**

**SOURCES**

Schuiling, K. D., & Likis, F. E. (2006). *Women's gynecologic health.* Sudbury, MA: Jones and Bartlett.
Seidel, H. M., Ball, J., Dains, J., & Benedict, W. (2006). *Mosby's physical examination handbook* (6th ed.). St. Louis, MO; Mosby.

# HEADACHES

## Migraine
Unilateral
Gradual onset
Crescendo pattern
Pulsating
Moderate to severe pain intensity
Aggravated by routine daily activities
Duration 4–72 h
N/V
Photophobia and/or phonophobia
First onset before age 40 yr
Aura—fully reversible visual, sensory, or dysphasic speech that is followed by a migraine within 60 min, symptoms develop gradually over > 5 min

### Menstrual Migraines
Occur 2 d before and up to 3 d after the onset of menstruation
Occurs at least 2 out of every 3 mo
Use of OCPs may increase or decrease severity
Thought to be associated with estrogen withdrawal

## Tension H/A
Bilateral
Last from 30 min to 7 d
Mild to moderate severity
Pressure or tightness not pulsating pain
Does not disturb daily activities
Not associated with N/V, photophobia, or phonophobia

## Cluster H/A
Always unilateral
Starts at eye or temple
Pain begins quickly reaching crescendo within min
Deep, continuous, excruciating, and explosive severe pain
Does not interfere with daily activity
Duration: 15 min to 3 h

### Accompanied by at Least One Associated S/Sx
Ipsilateral lacrimation
Eye redness
Stuffy nose
Rhinorrhea
Pallor
Sweating
Miosis and/or ptosis
Sensitivity to EtOH
Focal neurologic s/sx rare
Refer to neurology if associated sx present

**H/A Differential Diagnosis**

TABLE H-1   Headache Differential Diagnosis

|         | Location   | Character                   | Duration          | Associated S/Sx                  |
|---------|------------|-----------------------------|-------------------|----------------------------------|
| Migraine | Unilateral | Throbbing moderate to severe | Minutes to days | N/V Photophobia Phonophobia |
| Tension | Bilateral  | Constant mild to moderate   | 4–72 h            | None                             |
| Cluster | Unilateral | Excruciating severe         | < 3 h             | Tearing, sweating, swelling      |

*Source:* Adapted from Loder, E., & Martin, V. (Eds.). (2004). *Headaches.* Philadelphia: American College of Physicians.

**Assessment**
   Have pt keep H/A diary
   www.headaches.org—sample diaries

**Red Flags**
   SNOOP
      **S**ystemic symptoms/risk factors: fever, weight loss, HIV, cancer, HTN, endocrine disorders
      **N**eurologic s/sx: confusion, change in consciousness or personality
      **O**nset: sudden, abrupt, split second
      **O**lder: new onset or progression after age 40–50 yr
      **P**revious H/A hx: change in frequency, severity, clinical features

**H**

**Treatment**
   Doses vary depending on type
   *See* Table H-2.

**Nonpharmacologic Treatments**
   Exercise
   Biofeedback
   Massage
   Nicotine and caffeine cessation
   Hydration
   Stress and trigger reduction

**Natural Treatments**
   Feverfew 0.2% for migraines
   Butterbur 50 mg BID for migraines
   Magnesium and vitamin B supplementation for migraines

**SOURCES**

Arcangelo, V. P., & Peterson, A. M. (Eds.). (2006). *Pharmacotherapeutics for advanced practice: A practical approach* (2nd ed.). Philadelphia: Lippincott Williams and Wilkins.
Epocrates, I. (2008). Epocrates online. Retrieved May 27, 2008, from http://www.epocrates.com
Graves, B. (2006). Management of migraine headaches. *Journal of Midwifery & Women's Health, 51*(3), 174–184.
Hale, T. W. (2008). *Medications and mothers' milk* (13th ed.). Amarillo, TX: Hale Publishing.
Loder, E., & Martin, V. (Eds.). (2004). *Headaches.* Philadelphia: American College of Physicians.
Schuiling, K. D., & Likis, F. E. (2006). *Women's gynecologic health.* Sudbury, MA: Jones and Bartlett.
Von Wald, T., & Walling, A. (2002). Headaches during pregnancy. *Obstetrics and Gynecology Survey, 57*(3), 179–185.

TABLE H-2  Headache Treatments

| Medication Information | Primarily Treats* | Dose | Pharmacology |
|---|---|---|---|
| Aspirin<br>Preg Cat C during 1st and 2nd trimester; Preg Cat D during 3rd trimester<br>Lact Cat L3 | MI, C, T | 325–650 mg PO Q 4 h PRN (Max 4 g/24 h PO) | Salicylate analgesic |
| Acetaminophen (Tylenol)<br>Preg Cat B<br>Lact Cat L1 | MI, C, T | 325–1000 mg PO/PR Q 4–6 h (max 4 g/24 h) | Analgesic |
| Ibuprofen (Motrin, Advil)<br>Preg B in 1st and 2nd trimesters, D in 3rd trimester<br>Lact Cat L1 | MI, C, T | 200–400 mg PO Q 4–6 h (Max 1200 mg/24 h) | Analgesic<br>Antipyretic |
| Caffeine<br>Preg Cat C<br>Lact Cat L2 | MI, T | | CNS stimulant |
| Fiacetaminophen/butalbital/caffeine (Fioricet)<br>Preg Cat D<br>Lact Cat L3 | T | 50–100 mg Q 4 h | Mild analgesic, sedative |
| Codeine<br>Preg Cat C<br>Lact Cat L3 | C, MI | | Analgesic |
| Oxycodone<br>Preg Cat B<br>Lact Cat L3 | C, MI | 5–30 mg PO Q 4 h PRN | Narcotic, analgesic |

| Contraindications/Cautions | Side Effects | |
|---|---|---|
| Hypersensitivity to drug class | Anaphylaxis | Nephrotoxicity |
| GI bleed | Angioedema | Hepatotoxicity |
| G6PD deficiency | Bronchospasm | Salicylism |
| Bleeding problems | Bleeding | Reye's syndrome |
| Anticoagulant use | GI bleed | Dyspepsia |
| | Anemia | N/V |
| | Thrombocytopenia | Abdominal pain |
| | Leukopenia | Rash |
| Hypersensitivity to drug/class | Hepatotoxicity | Neutropenia |
| Chronic alcohol use | Neuropathy | Angioedema |
| Impaired liver function | Anemia | Anaphylaxis |
| G6PD deficiency | Pancytopenia | Nausea |
| | Thrombocytopenia | Rash |
| | Leucopenia | |
| Hypersensitivity to drug/class | GI bleed | Anemia |
| 3rd trimester pregnancy | Thromboembolism | Dyspepsia |
| Cardiac problems | Kidney problems | Nausea |
| Fluid retention | Liver problems | Abdominal pain |
| Anticoagulant use | Stevens-Johnson | Constipation |
| Bleeding/clotting problems | syndrome | Headache |
| Impaired renal/liver function | | |
| Hypersensitivity to drug/class | Insomnia | GI problems |
| Heart disease | Heart problems | Increased intraocular |
| GI disease | CNS problems | pressure |
| Impaired liver/renal function | Urticaria | Diuresis |
| Seizure disorder | | |
| Hypersensitivity to drug/class | Agranulocytosis | Lightheadedness |
| Porphyria | Thrombocytopenia | Dizziness |
| Impaired liver/renal function | Respiratory depression | Sedation |
| Drug abuse | Stevens-Johnson | Dyspnea |
| Pregnancy | syndrome | Nausea |
| | Erythema multiforme | Vomiting |
| | Drowsiness | Abdominal pain |
| Hypersensitivity to drug/class | Increased LFTs | Dyspnea |
| CNS depression | Drowsiness | Histamine release |
| Hypotension | Constipation | Convulsions |
| Abdominal conditions | Hypotension | Depression |
| Impaired liver/renal function | CNS symptoms | Nightmares |
| Morbid obesity | Rash | Paralytic ileus |
| Respiratory compromise | N/V | Biliary spasm |
| | Decreased urination | Muscle rigidity |
| | Weakness | Trembling |
| | Blurred vision | |
| Hypersensitivity to drug/class | Respiratory depression | Paralytic ileus |
| Respiratory depression | Cardiac arrest | Constipation |
| Asthma | Apnea | N/V |
| Hypercarbia | Hypotension | H/A |
| Paralytic ileus | Dependency/abuse | Itching |
| Increased intracranial pressure | Seizure | Insomnia |
| Alcohol abuse | Biliary spasm | |
| Seizures | | |
| Impaired liver/renal function | | |
| Drug abuse | | |

**H**

/ continues

TABLE H-2 Headache Treatments (continued)

| Medication Information | Primarily Treats* | Dose | Pharmacology |
|---|---|---|---|
| Sumatriptans<br>Preg Cat C<br>Lact Cat L3 | MI | 25–100 mg<br>PO x 1<br>(max 200<br>mg/24 h) | |
| Ergotamine<br>Preg Cat X<br>Lact Cat L4 | MI | One tablet<br>sublingual<br>then 1 tab<br>Q 30 min<br>PRN (max 3<br>tab/24 h or<br>5 tab/wk) | |

| Contraindications/Cautions | Side Effects | |
|---|---|---|
| Hypersensitivity to drug/class | Heart problems | Blindness |
| HTN | Stroke | Seizures |
| Heart disease | Ischemia | Fatigue |
| Cerebrovascular disease | | |
| Migraine basilar/hemiplegic | | |
| PVD | | |
| Avoid breastfeeding x 12 h after dose | | |
| Impaired liver/renal function | | |
| Hypersensitivity to drug class | Cardiovascular problems | Numbness |
| Cardiac problems | Vertigo | Paresthesia |
| Not to be used for headaches in pregnancy | Itching | Weakness |
| | N/V | Pleuropulmonary fibrosis |
| | Retroperitoneal fibrosis | Cold extremities |
| | Muscle pain | |

*MI = migraines; C = cluster; T = tension.

*Sources:* Adapted from Epocrates, I. (2008). Epocrates online. Retrieved May 27, 2008, from http://www.epocrates.com. Hale, T. W. (2008). *Medications and mothers' milk* (13th ed.). Amarillo, TX: Hale Publishing.

H

## HEARTBURN (INDIGESTION)

### Prevention
Eat small frequent meals
Limit fluid intake with meals
Avoid spicy, fatty foods, coffee, and alcohol
Drink 8 oz of milk 30–45 min after meal to neutralize acids
Take antacids after meals
Do not lie down for 2 h after meals

TABLE H-3  Heartburn Treatments

| Class | Medication Information | Dose | Pharmacology |
|---|---|---|---|
| Antacids | Sodium bicarbonate | 325–1300 mg PO Q 4 h PRN (max 15.6 g/24 h) | |
| | Calcium carbonate (Tums) | 1–2 tab PO QID | |
| | Aluminum hydroxide/ Magnesium hydroxide/ simethicone (Maalox/ Mylanta) | 10–50 ml PO QID (max 500 mg/24 h) take 1–3 h after meals, before bedtime | |
| Histamine-2 blockers | Cimetidine (Tagamet) Preg Cat B Lact Cat L2 | 300 mg PO QID or 400 mg PO BID (Max 2400 mg/24 h) | Reduces gastric acid secretion |
| | Famotidine (Pepcid) Preg Cat B Lact Cat L1 | 20 mg BID or 40 mg QHS | Reduces gastric acid secretion |
| | Ranitidine (Zantac) Preg Cat B Lact Cat L2 | 75 mg PO QD | |

Elevate head at least 6 inches when lying down
Quit smoking
Lose weight (if indicated)
See Table H-3.

**SOURCES**
Epocrates, I. (2008). *Epocrates online*. Retrieved May 27, 2008, from http://www.epocrates.com
Hale, T. W. (2008). *Medications and mothers' milk* (13th ed.). Amarillo, TX: Hale Publishing.
Varney, H., Kriebs, J. M., & Gegor, C. L. (2004). *Varney's midwifery* (4th ed.). Sudbury, MA: Jones and Bartlett.

| Contraindication | Side Effects | |
|---|---|---|
| Hypersensitivity to drug/class | Metabolic alkalosis | Hypernatremia |
| Alkalosis | Cardiac problems | Constipation |
| Electrolyte abnormailities | Flatulence | Diarrhea |
| CHF | Edema | Rebound acidity |
| Hypovolemia | | |
| Renal dysfunction | | |
| Hypersensitivity to drug/class | Milk-alkli syndrome | N/V |
| Hypercalciuria | Hypercalcemia | Abdominal pain |
| Renal calculi | Constipation | H/A |
| Hypophosphatemia | Anorexia | Confusion |
| Impaired renal function | | |
| Hypersensitivity to drug/class | Seizures | Aluminum toxicity |
| Impaired renal function | Diarrhea | Magnesium toxicity |
| Impaired bowel motility | Constipation | Hypophosphatemia |
| Volume depletion | | |
| Hypersensitivity to drug/class | CNS side effects | Hallucinations |
| Impaired renal/liver function | Blood problems | Diarrhea |
| Pulmonary disease | Pneumonia | Gynecomastia |
| Diabetes | Depression | N/V |
| Immunocompromised | Psychosis | |
| Hypersensitivity to drug/class | Anaphylaxis | HA |
| Impaired renal function | Angioedema | Dizziness |
| | Blood problems | Constipation |
| | Heart problems | Diarrhea |
| | CNS toxicity | Taste changes |
| Hypersensitivity to drug/class | Hepatotoxicity | H/A |
| Porphyria | Pneumonia | Diarrhea |
| Impaired liver/renal function | Interstitial nephritis | Constipation |
| Pulmonary disease | Thrombocytopenia | Muscle aches |
| Diabetes | Granulocytopenia | Vertigo |
| Immunocompromised | Leucopenia | Malaise |
| | Agrnaulocytosis | Dizziness |
| | Pancytopenia | Dry mouth |
| | Mental confusion | Dry skin |
| | Hallucinations | N/V |
| | Pancreatitis | Rash |
| | Hypersensitivity | Confusion |
| | Erythema multiforme | Fatigue |
| | Arrhythmias | |

/ continues

TABLE H-3    Heartburn Treatments (continued)

| Class | Medication Information | Dose | Pharmacology |
|---|---|---|---|
| Proton pump inhibitors | Omeprazole (Prilosec)<br>Preg Cat C<br>Lact Cat L2 | 20 mg PO QD | Reduces gastric acid secretion |
| | Lansoprazole (Prevacid)<br>Preg Cat B<br>Lact Cat L3 | 15–30 mg PO QD-BID | Reduces stomach acid secretion |
| | Esomeprazole (Nexium)<br>Preg Cat C<br>Lact Cat L2 | 20–40 mg PO QD | Reduces gastric acid secretion |
| Other | Sucralfate (Carafate)<br>Preg Cat B<br>Lact Cat L2 | 1g PO QD | |

| Contraindication | Side Effects | |
|---|---|---|
| Hypersensitivity to drug/class<br>Impaired liver function | Blood dyscrasias<br>Hepatic dysfunction<br>Stevens-Johnson<br>  syndrome<br>Toxic epidermal<br>  necrosis<br>Erythema multiforme | Pancreatitis<br>Interstitial nephritis<br>H/A<br>Diarrhea<br>Abdominal pain |
| Hypersensitivity to drug/class<br>Impaired liver function | Blood dyscrasias<br>Hepatic dysfunction<br>Stevens-Johnson<br>  syndrome<br>Toxic epidermal<br>  necrosis<br>Erythema multiforme<br>Pancreatitis | Anaphylactoid reaction<br>Interstitial nephritisa<br>H/A<br>Diarrhea<br>Constipation |
| Hypersensitivity to drug/class<br>Impaired liver function | Blood dyscrasias<br>Hepatic dysfunction<br>Stevens-Johnson<br>  syndrome<br>Toxic epidermal<br>  necrosis<br>Erythema multiforme<br>Pancreatitis<br>Interstitial nephritis<br>Esophageal stricture<br>Esophageal laceration | Esophageal varices<br>Barrett's esophagus<br>Gastric ulcer<br>Hernia<br>H/A<br>Diarrhea<br>Abdominal pain<br>Nausea |
| Hypersensitivity to drug/class<br>Dysphagia<br>GI obstruction<br>Chronic renal failure | Constipation | Bezoar formation |

Sources: Adapted from Epocrates, I. (2008). Epocrates online. Retrieved May 27, 2008, from http://www.epocrates.com. Hale, T. W. (2008). Medications and mothers' milk (13th ed.). Amarillo, TX: Hale Publishing.

**H**

## HELLP

### Definition
**H**emolysis—RBC destruction
**E**levated **l**iver enzymes—secondary to liver damage
**L**ow **p**latelets—due to increased platelet aggregation and destruction

### Statistics
0.2–0.6% of all pregnancies
Occurs in 10–20% w/ preeclampsia

### Risk Factors
Multiparous
Maternal age > 25 yr
White race
Hx of preeclampsia
PIH

### Signs and Symptoms
RUQ pain (right chest or midepigastric pain)
PIH
Proteinuria
N/V
H/A
Visual changes
Jaundice
Malaise

### Diagnosis
Based on lab results (CBC & LFTs)
Any patient in the 3rd trimester c/o RUQ pain should be evaluated immediately
   regardless of BP or proteinuria

### Labs

TABLE H-4   HELLP Lab Findings

| | |
|---|---|
| Hb/HCT | Decreased |
| Bilirubin | Elevated (> 1.2 mg/dL) |
| AST (SGOT) | Elevated (> 70 IU/L) |
| ALT (SGPT) | Elevated (> 70 IU/L) |
| Uric Acid | Elevated (above 6.0 mg/dL of concern in pregnancy) |
| Creatinine | Elevated |
| LDH | Elevated (> 600 IU/L) |
| PT/PTT | Normal |
| Fibrinogen | Normal |
| PLT | < 100,000/ml |

*Sources:* Adapted from Burrow, G., Duffy, T., & Copel, J. (2004). *Medical complications during pregnancy* (6th ed.). Philadelphia, PA: Elsevier Saunders. Desai, S. P. (2004). *Clinician's guide to laboratory medicine: A practical approach* (3rd ed.). Hudson, OH: Lexi-Comp.

### Differential Diagnosis

*Based on Symptoms*
Pyelonephritis
Kidney stones
Gall bladder disease
Gastroenteritis
Appendicitis
Peptic ulcer

*Based on Lab Values*

Decreasing plt count in 3rd trimester is key to differentiating HELLP from other pathologies

Viral hepatitis

Acute fatty liver of pregnancy (AFLP)

Cholestasis of pregnancy

Thrombotic thrombocytopenia purpura (TTP)

Hemolytic-uremic syndrome (HUS)

Sepsis

DIC

Connective tissue disease

Antiphospholipid syndrome (APS)

*See* Table H-5.

## Treatment

Control HTN (Apresoline/Aldomet)

Control bleeding (albumin, volume expanders)

Expedite delivery

$MgSO_4$ seizure precaution

High-dose steroid Tx (unknown mechanism, may reduce endothelial destruction in liver)

Blood transfusion

Plasma exchange postpartum

LDH and plts best indicators of worsening condition during intrapartum and postpartum

## Outcomes

Most patients stabilize within 24–48 h of delivery

3–5% mortality rate d/t cerebral hemorrhage, cardiopulmonary arrest, DIC, ARDS, hypoxic ischemic encephalopathy, intra-abdominal bleeding, subcapsular liver hematomas/liver rupture

Renal impairment—transient elevation of serum creatinine, acute renal failure, hyponatremia, and nephrogenic diabetes insipidus

Pulmonary impairment—pleural effusions, pulmonary edema, and ARDS

Retinal detachment

Postictal cortical blindness

Hypoglycemic coma

## Counseling for Future Pregnancies

20% risk of preeclampsia in subsequent pregnancies

< 5% risk of HELLP in subsequent pregnancies

Overall increase risk for poor pregnancy outcome

## SOURCES

Barton, J., & Sibai, B. (2004). Diagnosis and management of hemolysis, elevated liver enzymes, and low platelets syndrome. *Clinics of Perinatalogy, 31*(4), 807–833.

Baxter, J., & Weinstein, L. (2004). HELLP syndrome: The state of the art. *Obstetrics and Gynecology Survey, 59*(12), 838–845.

Burrow, G., Duffy, T., & Copel, J. (2004). *Medical complications during pregnancy* (6th ed.). Philadelphia: Elsevier Saunders.

Cunningham, G., Leveno, K. J., Bloom, S. L., Hauth, J. C., Gilstrap, L. C., & Wenstrom, K. D. (2005). *Williams obstetrics* (22nd ed.). New York: McGraw-Hill Professional.

Desai, S. P. (Ed.). (2004). *Clinician's guide to laboratory medicine: A practical approach* (3rd ed.). Hudson, OH: Lexi-Comp.

Norwitz, E., & Schorge, J. (2001). *Obstetrics and gynecology at a glance.* Oxford, UK: Blackwell Science.

O'Brien, J., & Barton, J. (2005). Controversies with the diagnosis and management of HELLP syndrome. *Clinical Obstetrics and Gynecology, 48*(2), 460–477.

Padden, M. (1999). HELLP syndrome: Recognition and perinatal management. *American Family Physician, 60*(3). 829–839.

Varney, H., Kriebs, J. M., & Gegor, C. L. (2004). *Varney's midwifery* (4th ed.). Sudbury, MA: Jones and Bartlett.

H

**TABLE H-5** HELLP Differential Diagnosis

| Condition | ↓ PLT Count | Coagulopathy | HTN | Renal Disease | CNS Disease | Hemolytic Anemia | Peak Time of Onset |
|---|---|---|---|---|---|---|---|
| Preeclampsia | Mild | Variable | Severe | Mild | Mild | Mild | 3rd trimester |
| HELLP | Severe | Mild | Variable | Mild | Variable | Moderate | 3rd trimester |
| HUS | Moderate | Variable | Variable | Severe | Variable | Moderate | Postpartum |
| TTP | Severe | Variable | Variable | Mild/Variable | Severe | Severe | 2nd trimester to term |
| SLE | Mild | Variable | Variable | Mild/Moderate | Mild | Mild | Anytime |
| APS | Mild | Variable | Variable | Variable | Mild | Variable | Anytime |
| AFLP | Variable | Severe | Variable | Variable | Mild | Mild | 3rd trimester |

Sources: Adapted from Desai, S. P. (Ed.). (2004). *Clinician's guide to laboratory medicine: A practical approach* (3rd ed.). Hudson, OH: Lexi-Comp. Varney, H., Kriebs, J. M., & Gegor, C. L. (2004). *Varney's midwifery* (4th ed.). Sudbury, MA: Jones and Bartlett.

# HEMORRHAGE: POSTPARTUM

## Definition
Older definition: > 500 cc blood loss within first 24 h
Newer definition: > 1000 ml of blood lost within the first 24 h or hemodynamically
   unstable

## Cause

*Atony*
   Grand multiparity
   Uterine overdistension
   Prolonged labor with pitocin
   Chorioamnionitis
   General anesthesia
   $MgSO_4$
   Rapid labor
   Uterine myomas
   Full bladder

*Retained Placental Tissue or Clots*
   Placenta accrete
   Succenturiate lobe
   Cord avulsion

## Genital Tract Laceration
   Precipitous delivery
   Episiotomy
   Operative vaginal delivery
   Uterine Inversion

## Management
   Call for MD backup
   Deliver placenta ASAP (consider maternal pain relief if manual extraction)
   Check for retained products of conception and/or clots in the lower uterine
      segment or cervical os
   IV placement/check for patency if in place
   Pitocin 10 units IM immediately or 20 units IV after placenta is delivered
   Assess uterine atony
   Check for full bladder
   Bimanual compression
   Uterotonics as necessary
   Assess for lacerations and start repair
   Clamp bleeding vessels quickly
   Verify type and screen
   Monitor VS for s/sx of shock

## Medications

*Pitocin (Oxytocin, Syntocinon, Pit)*
   IM: 10 IU/ml
   IV: 10–40 units/1000 ml
   Never IV push
   Effective 2–3 min after injection
   Contraindicated: uterine hyperstimulation

*Methergine (Ergonovine/Methylergonovine, Ergotrate, Ergometrine Methylergometrine,
Methylergonovine Maleate)*
   IM: 0.2 mg
   Never give IV
   Oral: 0.2 to 0.4 mg Q 6–12 h for max of 48 h
   Do not administer prior to birth of baby
   Contraindicated: HTN, preeclampsia, eclampsia
   *See also* Methergine

H

*Misoprostol (Cytotec, Miso)*
   PR/PV/PO: 600 to 1000 mcg

*Hemabate (Carboprost, Carboprost Tromethamine, Prostin/15M in Canada)*
   IM: 250 mcg Q 15–90 min PRN for max of 2 mg
   May work when other oxytocolytics are not controlling uterine bleeding
   Contraindicated: asthma

*Prostin (Dinoprostone, Prostaglandin E2, Cervidil, Prepidil)*
   Vaginal suppository 20 mg

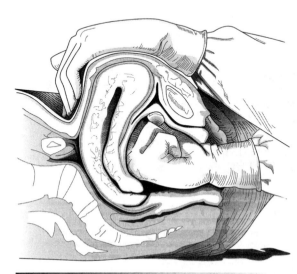

FIGURE H-1   Image of Bimanual Compression. *Source:* Reprinted from
Cunningham, G., Leveno, K. J., Bloom, S. L., Hauth, J. C., Gilstrap, L. C., &
Wenstrom, K. D. (2005). *William's obstetrics (22nd ed.).* New York: McGraw-Hill
Professional.

**SOURCES**

Alfirevic, Z., & Mousa, H. (2007). Treatment for primary postpartum haemorrhage. *Cochrane Database
   of Systemic Review,* (3), CD003249.
Thompson Healthcare Inc. (2007). *MICROMEDEX: Healthcare series.* Retrieved August 24, 2008, from
   http://www.micromedex.com

# HEMORRHOIDS

## Definition

Varicosities of the veins around the anus or lower rectum

Form as a result of straining to defecate or pushing intrapartum

## Risk Factors

Aging

Chronic constipation or diarrhea

Anal intercourse

Erect posture

Lack of venous valves

Pregnancy d/t pressure on the lower GI tract vessels preventing adequate blood return

Defects in drainage due to overly tense anal sphincter muscles

| Signs and Symptoms | Diagnosis | Differential Diagnosis |
|---|---|---|
| Rectal Bleeding | Visual inspection | Colorectal cancer |
| Pain | Digital rectal exam | IBS |
| Irritation | Possible anoscopic or | Crohn's disease |
| Itching | proctoscopic exam | |
| Swelling | Sigmoid or colonoscopy | |
| Hard round lump near anal opening | | |

H

### HEMORRHOID TREATMENT

Witch hazel or white oak bark infused cloths

    Pour 1 pint boiling water over 1 oz of herbs and steep for 10 hours

    Refrigerate the infusion for preservation

    Apply several times per day either hot or cold

Tub baths several times/d in plain warm water for approx 10 min

Application of hemorrhoid cream or suppositories

Elevation of the feet on a stool while sitting on the toilet

Lubrication with olive oil or water-based lubrication

Replacement back inside the rectum

Vitamin E capsules 400 IU placed inside the anus at night

Yellow dock root tincture (1/2 drop PO TID)

Nettle infusion or freeze-dried nettles

Collinsonia root tincture or tablets

Vitamin C 500 mg doses with up to 3 g QD (divided doses)

## Surgical Removal

Rubber band ligation—removal of circulation to internal hemorrhoid such that it resolves in a few days

Sclerotherapy—injection of chemicals into blood vessels surrounding hemorrhoid to cause shrinking

Infrared coagulation—burning hemorrhoidal tissue

Hemorrhoidectomy—excision of internal or external hemorrhoids

## Prevention

Relief of diarrhea or constipation

Drinking 6–8 glasses of water QD

Increase fiber in diet (fruits, vegetables, whole grains, or supplements)

Stool softeners to eliminate straining

Exercise

Avoid heaving lifting and prolonged periods of standing

Elevate legs and bottom when resting

Avoid restrictive pants or stockings

**SOURCES**

Frye, A. (2004). Holistic midwifery: A comprehensive textbook for midwives in homebirth practice. Portland, Oregon: Labrys Press.

National Institute of Diabetes and Digestive and Kidney Diseases. (2004). Hemorrhoids (Patient Information No. 07-3021). Bethesda, MD: NIH.

## HERBS

### Statistics
38.2 million adults use some type
Women more than men
Increased education increases frequency of use

### Overview
They do have side effects
They are medications
They come in different forms

### Resources
www.naturalstandard.com
nccam.nih.gov

### Disease-Specific Treatment

*Dysmenorrhea*
Indicated for pain relief
Vitamin $B_1$ 100 mg QD (better alone than $B_6$ or magnesium)
Magnesium QD (better alone than in combination)
Vitamin $B_6$ QD (better alone than magnesium or the combination)
TSS (Japanese herbal supplement) daily
Contraindicated
Fish oil—side effects outweighed benefits
Vitamin E—no pain relief compared to placebo

*Decrease Inflammation*
Black cohosh
Chaste tree
Dong quai
Black haw
Omega-3 fatty acids
Vitamin E
Thiamine ($B_1$)
Niacin ($B_3$)
Magnesium

*Menopause*
Black cohosh
Phytoestrogens
Kava kava
St.-John's-wort
*Also see* Menopause

*PMS/Mastalgia*
$B_6$
Chaste tree berry
Calcium
Evening primrose oil

### Commonly Used Herbs

*Ginkgo biloba*
120–240 mg QD divided into 2–3 doses/d—flavinoid
Act as an antioxidant to reduce capillary fragility, induce platelet aggregation,
degranulation of neutrophils, and production of oxygen radicals
Used for decrease in cerebral function (concentration, fatigue, anxiety, dizziness,
H/A, memory), and altitude sickness

*St.-John's-Wort*
Acts as an atypical antidepressant (similar to a weak monoamine oxidase inhibitor)

*Ginseng*
  1–2 g crude herb daily
  100–300 mg extract TID
  Includes 18 ginsenosides or steroidal saponins
  Increases the body's defense against stress
  Tx anxiety, weakness, dyspnea, forgetfulness, fatigue, decreased libido, and
    nausea
  Improves vitality, immune function, fertility, sexual function, and performance
  Contraindications: pregnancy, HTN, emotional imbalance, H/A, heart palpitations,
    insomnia, asthma, high fever

*Garlic*
  2–4 g fresh QD (approx 1 clove)
  Decreases lipid levels and prevent atherosclerosis
  Raw garlic contains allicin, which inhibits MHG Co A reductace, activates
    fibrinolysis, and inhibits platelets
  Side effects: GI discomfort, bloating, H/A, sweating, lightheadedness,
    menorrhagia, odor
  Caution when taken with any other antiplatelet medication/supplement

*Echinacea*
  Start at first onset of symptoms and continue for 10–14 days
  Nonspecific immunostimulant
  Treats URIs, UTIs, and superficial wounds/ulcers
  Contraindicated for people with ragweed or yarrow allergies, and individuals taking
    hepatotoxic drugs
  Side effects: GI upset, diarrhea, constipation, skin rash

*Valerian*
  450 mg Qhs
  Treats sleep disturbances of all types without morning drowsiness
  Contraindicated in pregnancy and individuals using barbiturates, benzodiazepines,
    opiates, and alcohol
  Side effects: H/A, hangover, paradoxical stimulation, restlessness, cardiac
    disturbances

*Chaste Tree Berry (Vitrex)*
  Iridoid glycosides—agnuside and aucubin, flavonoids, essential oils
  Binds to dopamine receptors in pituitary
  Decreases prolactin level, which decreases the LH surge allowing the luteal phase
    to occur more quickly resulting in increased progesterone and decreasing PMS
  Side effects: GI distress, skin rash, increased acne, H/A, increased menstrual
    volume
  Contraindicated in pregnancy and lactation as well as in individuals taking dopamine
    agonists or antagonists
  May decrease contraception effectiveness

## Pregnancy

*General Daily Maintenance*
  Red raspberry leaf
  Nettles infusion 1 cup QD
  Rescue remedy PRN

*Morning Sickness*
  Red raspberry leaf and mint combo infusion before rising
  Fennel or anise seed—tea before rising

*Heartburn*
  Dandelion 10 drops tincture
  Slippery elm tea PRN

H

*Constipation*
Slippery elm tea PRN
Amaranth eaten steamed or in an infusion
Increased green leafy vegetable intake

*Fatigue/Mood Swings*
Red raspberry leaf infusion BID–TID PRN
Skullcap 30 drops tincture or 2 cup infusion QD

*Insomnia*
Skullcap 30 drops tincture or 2 cup infusion QD

*Bleeding Gums*
Myrrh gum, toothpaste, dip floss in myrrh tincture

*Ptyalism*
Cinnamon: chew naturally flavored gum

*Leg Cramps*
Nettles: 1 cup infusion QD or eat steamed greens

*Varicosities*
Nettles
Oat straw: 1 cup infusion QD
Comfrey: poultice applied to area PRN

*Hemorrhoids*
Yellow dock ointment applied PRN
Yarrow and plantain combo ointment QD, BID, or PRN
Witch hazel bark sitz bath made from infusion

## Fertility and Regulating Menses

*Red Clover (Trifolium pratense)*
Exceedingly high in calcium and magnesium, which promotes nervous system
relaxation and therefore increases fertility
Considered the best fertility promoter
Infuse 1 oz dried flowers with 1 tsp dried mint leaves (any kind) in a quart of boiled
water for 4 h
Drink freely throughout the day, for several months continuously
Alfalfa is a substitute for red clover but it is not as effective

*Nettles (Urtica dioica)*
Nourishes and tones uterus, balances hormones through strengthening the kidneys
and adrenal glands
Drink 1+ cups infusion (made from dried leaves) QD for several months

*Red Raspberry Leaf (Rubus)*
High in calcium and therefore a uterine tonic
One or more cups of infusion QD for months
Infuse 0.5 oz red clover and 0.5 oz red raspberry leaf in a quart of water for 4 h
Add 5–15 drops of dong quai root or false unicorn root to tea

*Dong Quai Root*
Tang Kwei Gin—water-based combination extract sold in Chinatown stores
Take on days between ovulation and menstruation

### SOURCES

Dennehy, C. E. (2006). The use of herbs and dietary supplements in gynecology: An evidence based
review. *Journal of Midwifery & Women's Health, 51*(6), 402.
Proctor, M., & Murphy, P. (2001). Herbal and dietary therapies for primary and secondary
dysmenorrhea. *Cochrane Database of Systematic Reviews, CD002124*(2), 1–11.
Tesch, B. J. (2001). Herbs commonly used by women: An evidence-based review. *American Journal of
Obstetrics and Gynecology, 1,* 89–102.
Weed, S. S. (1985). *Wise women herbals for the childbearing year.* Woodstock, NY: Ash Tree.

# HERPES SIMPLEX VIRUS (HSV)

## Statistics
1 in 5 adolescents/adults has genital HSV
1 in 4 women
1 in 8 men

## Signs and Symptoms
Ranges from nothing to obvious "cold sores"
Painful sores that eventually crust over and form a scab while healing
Red patches of skin
Tiny sores that appear like pimples or ingrown hairs
Fissures
Anal irritation similar to hemorrhoids
Vaginal itching/irritation similar to yeast infection
Urethral pain similar to a UTI

*Primary Outbreak*
Often the most severe
Lasts 3–4 wk
Can include flulike symptoms (sore throat, fever, swollen glands, headaches, fatigue)

*Recurrences*
HSV-2 average of 4/yr with more often in the 1st yr after infection
1/3 can pass undetected because there are no s/sx

## Dx
Sex hx: Number of partners, personal protection, STI history
GU hx: infections, discharges, skin changes, irritations, lumps/bumps, sores

*PE*
Women: pelvic exam with detailed internal/external visual inspection and lymph nodes
Men: visual inspection with close attention to skin and urethral discharge and lymph
   nodes

*Labs*
General viral culture
   Swab lesion within 3 d after appearance of lesion, but no more than 7 d,
      refrigerate and transport at 4°C
   Highly specific and widely available
   Virus must be kept alive during transport
   Sensitivity affected by specimen quality/timing
ELVIS (enzyme-linked virus-inducible system) culture
   Swab lesion within 3 d after appearance of lesion, but no more than 7 d,
      refrigerate and transport at 4°C
   Highly specific and rapid (1–2 d)
   Expensive
   Risk of false negatives
Antigen detection
   Swab lesion within 3 d after appearance of lesion, but no more than 7 d,
      refrigerate and transport at 4°C
   Rapid results
   Inexpensive
   Lower sensitivity than culture
Serology
   Requires blood draw (or finger stick for some kits)
   Measures HSV antibodies
   Current lesions not required
   Detects established HSV infection
   Type-specific tests available
   Recent infection may give a false negative due to delay of antibody up-regulation,
      earliest positive result ~12 d postinfection

**H**

FDA-approved glycoprotein G-based type specific tests for HSV antibodies:

HerpesSelect ELISA—96–97% sensitive and 98% specific testing for HSV-2

HerpesSelect immunoblot—more sensitive and specific but more expensive than Elisa

Biokit HSV-2—93% sensitive and 98% specific for HSV-2; done in office by finger stick

Captia EIA—ELISA testing for both HSV-1 and HSV-2

## Treatment

*First Outbreak*

Acyclovir 400 mg PO TID × 7–10 d (Preg Cat B, Lact L2)

Acyclovir 200 mg PO 5 times daily × 7–10 d (Preg Cat B, Lact L2)

Famciclovir 250 mg PO TID × 7–10 d (Preg Cat B, Lact L2)

Valacyclovir 1 g PO BID × 7–10 d (Preg Cat B, Lact L1)

*Episodic*

Acyclovir 400 mg PO TID × 5 d

Acyclovir 800 mg PO BID × 5 d

Acyclovir 800 mg PO TID × 2 d

Famciclovir 125 mg PO BID × 5 d

Famciclovir 1000 mg PO BID × 1 d

Valacyclovir 500 mg PO BID × 3 d

Valacyclovir 1000 mg PO QD × 5 d

## Suppression Treatment Considerations

Outbreaks Q month or > 6/yr

Individuals in a sexual relationship with an uninfected partner

*Treatment (Reevaluate Need Annually)*

Acyclovir 400 mg PO BID

Famiciclovir 250 mg PO BID

Valacyclovir 500 mg PO QD

Valacyclovir 1 g PO QD

## Pregnancy

Transmission rate high if infected during end of pregnancy (30–50%) but low if recurrence occurs (< 1%)

No sex with infected partner during 3rd trimester

No new partners late in pregnancy

No oral sex

S/sx and visual inspection at onset of labor

Suppression therapy not highly studied during pregnancy

Vaginal birth OK without lesions

Always consult most recent tx guidelines

## Patient Education

Hx of disease

Dormancy and recurrence

Asymptomatic shedding

Partner notification

Further STI testing

Coping with infection

Sexual and perinatal transmission

Eat foods high in lysine: yogurt, cheese, fruits, milk, meat, or take a lysine supplement

Avoid arginine-rich foods: chocolate, cola, beer, grain cereals, chicken soup, gelatin, seeds, nuts, lentils/peas

## Follow-up

After tx with 1st outbreak

Episodically for evaluation of tx

During pregnancy

## Resources

www.ashastd.org

www.ihmf.org

### SOURCES

Centers for Disease Control and Prevention. (2006). *Sexually transmitted diseases treatment guidelines, 2006. Morbidity and Mortality Weekly Report, 55*(RR-11), 16–20.

DAC Consultants. (2001). *Herpes diagnosis.* Retrieved May 25, 2008, from http://www.herpesdiagnosis.com

# HOME BIRTH

## Statistics

< 1% of births in the United States occur at home

Many women seek dual care with a midwife with hospital privileges to compliment the care she receives from a home birth midwife in communities where home birth is not fully supported by the medical establishment. This facilitates a seamless transfer of care, if necessary, during any stage of the pregnancy or delivery.

TABLE H-6    Antepartum Assessment Criteria for Birth Site Selection

### General Criteria

- Woman physically and mentally healthy and well-nourished
- Adequate social support before and during birth
- Primary participants mature and able to accept responsibility for self-care
- Commitment to maintaining a positive emotional environment for mother throughout process
- Arrangements made for emergency transport
- Childbirth, home birth, and breastfeeding education secured (books/classes)
- Preparation of persons planning to be present at the birth
- Complete records from previous provider for current and/or past pregnancies
- Pediatric care arranged before 36 weeks of pregnancy
- Obstetric consultant identified by 36 weeks
- Help available in home 24 hours a day for at least 1 week after the birth
- Commitment to birth without pharmacologic analgesia or anesthesia
- Understanding of and agreement to the screening criteria
- Open and clear communication with the midwife

### Recommended Indications for Consultation, Collaboration, and/or Referral of Care

- Anemia refractory to treatment
- Chronic hypertension and/or preeclampsia requiring management with medication
- Current mental illness that the midwife deems would have a harmful effect on the perinatal course
- Thromboembolic disease (event) requiring heparin
- Insulin-dependent diabetes
- Placenta previa at term
- Rh isoimmunization or positive antibody screen during current pregnancy
- Active preterm labor that cannot be stopped
- Evidence of chromioamnionitis
- Multiple gestation diagnosed before labor
- Substance abuse
- Nonreassuring fetal surveillance results

*Source:* Reprinted with permission from Vedam, S., Goff, M., & Nolan-Marnin, V. (2007). Closing the theory-practice gap: Intrapartum midwifery management of planned homebirths [Abstract]. *Journal of Midwifery & Women's Health, 52*(3), 291–300.

**H**

## From the ACNM Home Birth Position Statement

The ACNM has established clear guidelines for home birth and publishes a handbook that addresses selection criteria for home birth clients, mechanisms for medical consultation and transfer, and the establishment of quality management systems. The informed consent process for home birth includes the delineation of potential risks and benefits of each available birth site and provision for transport if conditions require personnel and/or equipment available only in the hospital setting.

The home birth setting provides an unparalleled opportunity to study and learn from normal, undisturbed birth. Medical and midwifery students who understand the characteristics of normality are better equipped to recognize deviations from normal. Insights into effective care in pregnancy and childbirth may be derived from clinical experiences with home birth families or from the study of normal birth at home.

## In Accordance with Evidence-Based and Ethical Practice, the ACNM Does the Following

Supports the right of women who meet selection criteria to choose home birth

Recognizes CNMs and CMs as providers who are qualified to attend planned home births

Encourages the promotion of clinical experiences with home birth in education programs

Encourages third-party payors to reimburse qualified providers for home birth services

Urges professional liability insurance carriers to provide coverage for qualified providers who attend home births

Urges all healthcare providers and institutions to collaborate in the creation of seamless systems of care when transfer is needed from the home to the hospital setting

Recommends that further studies focus on the characteristics and management of normal birth, markers of morbidity as they relate to birth site, and qualitative assessments of client satisfaction

**SOURCES**

American College of Nurse-Midwives. (2005). *Homebirth* (Position Statement). Washington DC: Author. Retrieved August 28, 2008, from http://www.midwife.org

Martin, J. A., Hamilton, B. E., Sutton, P. D., Ventura, S. J., Menacker, F., Kirmeyer, S., et al. (2007). Births: Final data for 2005. *National Vital Statistics Report, 56*(6), 1–124.

Vedam, S., Goff, M., & Nolan-Marnin, V. (2007). Closing the theory-practice gap: Intrapartum midwifery management of planned homebirths (Abstract). *Journal of Midwifery & Women's Health, 52*(3) 291–300.

# HOMEOPATHIC REMEDIES

### Definition

Tx of illness by giving very dilute amounts of a substance that produces similar symptoms

Goal is to rebalance "the vital force" or energy in the body

The more dilute the dose the more potent it is considered to be

It is important to be trained and to take a careful hx for accurate prescribing and tx

Evaluate whole picture and discuss both symptoms and emotions

Evaluate severity to choose potency and frequency

Remedies should not be touched with fingers; place under tongue by shaking pellet from vial

### Commonly Used Treatment

*Accidents and Injuries*

Aconite—shock with fear, any complaint that starts suddenly, especially after a shock, or exposure to the cold or cold wind

Apis—bites or stings with swelling, hives, general inflammations (coughs, colds, flu, fevers, earaches, sore throats, etc.)

Arnica—delayed shock, injury with bruising, head injury, sprains with swelling, jet lag

Calendula—cuts and wounds, bites

Cantharis—burns with or without blisters, cystitis

Hepar sulphuricum—inflamed cuts and wounds, general inflammations

Hypericum—painful injuries to nerves, in areas such as the coccyx, fingers, toes

Ledum—puncture wounds, bites; prevents infection

Rhus tox—sprains and strains, joint pain, and inflammation

Ruta—sprains and strains, eye strain

*Everyday Complaints*

Arsenicum—food poisoning; anxious, restless, thirsty for sips, burning pain, better for heat

Belladonna—complaints start suddenly; delirious, dry heat, great pain

Bryonia—sprains, joint pain; complaints start slowly, worsen with slightest movement

Chamomilla—teething; unbearable pain; very angry

Gelsemium—complaints start slowly; apathetic, thirstless, increase urination

Magnesia phosphorica—homeopathic "aspirin," better for heat and pressure

Mercurius solubilis—sweaty and smelly, an increase of saliva, glands swollen

Nux vomica—food poisoning, gastric disorders (bilious), insomnia; IBS

Pulsatilla—teething, food poisoning; weepy, thirstless, better for fresh air

Sulphur—teething, sunburn, restless, thirsty, worse for heat

*Labor*

Aconite—labor is fast and violent, with great fear/anxiety of death

Arnica—take throughout to prevent bruising, Q 4 h or more frequently if there is relief from pain

Caulophyllum—induction for postdates; take 1 Q 4 h for up to 2 d—if no effect, then baby or mother may not be ready for the birth

Arsenicum—vomiting in labor; with typical anxiety and fussiness

Chamomilla—labor exceedingly painful; backache labor; generally obnoxious, angry, impossible to please, asks for things and then doesn't want them

Coffea—contractions are ineffective or stop and/or are extremely painful; fear alternating with excitement, restless, makes jokes, laughs, is generally talkative and hilarious; sensitive to noise

Gelsemium—backache labor, lethargic, lifeless, dazed, thirstless

Kali carbonicum—back labor; irritable, anxious, bossy

Kali phosphoricum—high potency dose (6x) is best for this remedy; use for simple tiredness in labor with no other symptoms

**H**

Pulsatilla—gives up during labor; weepy, clingy, pathetic, looses courage, thirstless, hot and craves fresh air or is better for it

Sepia—gives up in labor; very exhausted—sags on every level

*Rescue Remedy*

Keep a glass of water with 5 drops of rescue remedy at hand at all times; give at any time if panicky or fearful

*Postnatal Kit for the Mother*

Aconite—shock

Arnica—heal bruised muscles; cramping

Belladonna—engorged breasts; throbbing pains, red streaks, breasts hot

Bellis perennis—bruised soreness not helped by arnica

Bryonia—engorgement, painful stitches

Calendula—speeds the healing of a tear or episiotomy

Castor—sore, cracked nipples

China—exhaustion from breastfeeding, anemia

Hypericum—pain in coccyx after the birth especially after forceps, painful hemorrhoids

Magnesia—phosphorica cramping

Nitric acid—exhaustion; irritable

Phosphoric acid—exhaustion from breastfeeding, apathetic

Phytolacca—cracked nipples, plugged duct, abscess/mastitis

Pulsatilla—cramping, weepy, and pathetic

Secale—if methergine injection administered, take one dose after the birth

Silica—cracked nipples

Staphysagria—cramping, administer if mother expresses "resentment and a feeling of assault"

*Source:* Reproduced with permission from Castro, M. (1992). *Homeopathy for pregnancy, birth, and your baby's first year.* New Yrk: St. Martin's Press.

**SOURCES**

Beal, M. W., Steinberg, S. (2003). Homeopathy and women's health care. *Journal of Obstetric, Gynecologic, and Neonatal Nursing, 32*(3), 207–214.

Castro, M. (1992). *Homeopathy for pregnancy, birth, and your baby's first year.* New York: St. Martin's Press.

# HORMONES: HYPERANDROGENISM

### Definition
Androgen excess in women
Adrenal glands and ovaries both produce androgens

### Pharmacology
Dehydropinadrosterone sulfate (DHES), dehydroepiandrosterone (DHEA), and androstenedione are all precursors to testosterone, which is solely androgenic

Androstenediol has both androgenic and estrogenic activity

Testosterone circulates bound to sex hormone-binding globulin (SHBG) (~80%), bound to albumin (~19%), and free (~1%)

Unbound and albumin-bound testosterone contributes to androgenicity; hence, changing levels of SHBG affects the bioavailability of testosterone

TABLE H-7   Factors Affecting the Circulating Levels of SHBG

| Increased SHBG | Decreased SHBG |
|---|---|
| Estrogens | Androgens |
| Thyroid hormone | Synthetic progestins |
| Pregnancy | Glucocorticoids |
| | Growth hormone |
| | Hyperinsulinemia |
| | Obesity |
| | Hypothyroidism |

Source: Schuiling, K. D., & Likis, F. E. (2006). Women's gynecologic health. Sudbury, MA: Jones and Bartlett.

### Signs and Symptoms
Acne
Hirsutism
Clitoromegaly
Polycystic ovaries
Obesity
Oligomenorrhea/amenorrhea
Infertility

### Labs
FSH
Total and free testosterone
17-hydroxyprogesterone (17-OHP)
DHEAS
SHBG
Prolactin
Fasting glucose and insulin
Samples obtained in morning most accurate

H

TABLE H-8   Differential Diagnoses for Hyperandrogenism

| | |
|---|---|
| PCOS | • Most common cause of hyperandrogenism, accounts for 75–90% of cases<br>• Clinical and/or biochemical evidence of hyperandrogenism<br>• Oligo- and/or anovulation<br>• Polycystic ovaries<br>• Exclusion of other etiologies |
| CAH—late onset/ nonclassic | • Occurs in 1–5% of women with hirsutism<br>• Clinically indistinguishable from PCOS<br>• Elevated 17-OHP above 200 ng/dL |
| HAIR-AN syndrome | • Occurs in 3% of cases<br>• Severe hyperandrogenism, possible virilization<br>• Acanthosis nigricans<br>• Severe hyperinsulinemia/insulin resistance |
| Virilizing tumors (ovarian or adrenal) | • Very rare (occurring in 1/300 to 1/1000 patients with hirsutism)<br>• Acute rapid course of virilizing symptoms<br>• Testosterone usually elevated above 200 ng/dL in premenopausal women, or 100 ng/dL in postmenopausal women<br>• Palpable adnexal mass, or mass on imaging of ovaries and/or adrenal glands |
| Idiopathic hirsutism | • Occurs in 5–15% of cases<br>• Biochemical hyperandrogenism is not present<br>• Normal ovulation by basal body temperature charting or luteal phase progesterone measurements |
| Cushing's syndrome | • Frequent referral diagnosis, one of the least common final diagnoses<br>• Evidence of striae over abdomen, central weight distribution, muscle weakness, altered mood, easy bruisability<br>• Elevated 24-hour urinary cortisol or failure of cortisol suppression after overnight dexamethasone suppression test |
| Thyroid disorders | • Palpable thyroid enlargement or mass<br>• Elevated TSH<br>• Suspect with presence of alopecia |
| Androgenic medication use | • May be systemic or topical<br>• Hirsutism |
| Pregnancy | • Virilization occurs during pregnancy<br>• Possible luteoma or theca-lutein cyst |
| Hyperprolactinemia | • Galactorrhea<br>• Elevated PRL |

*Sources:* Goodarzi & Korenman, 2003; Goodman et al., 2001; The Rotterdam ESHRE/ASRM-Sponsored PCOS Consensus Workshop Group, 2004; Speroff & Fritz, 2005.

**SOURCES**

American College of Nurse-Midwives. (2002). Abnormal and dysfunctional uterine bleeding: Clinical bulletin no. 6. *Journal of Midwifery and Women's Health, 47*(3), 207–213.

Goodarzi, M. O., & Korenman, S. G. (2003). The importance of insulin resistance in polycystic ovary syndrome. *Fertility and Sterility, 80*(2), 255–258.

Goodman, N. F., Bledsoe, M. B., Futterweit, W., Goldzeiher, J. W., Petak, S. M., Smith, K. D., et al. (2001). American Association of Clinical Endocrinologists medical guidelines for clinical practice for the diagnosis and treatment of hyperandrogenic disorders. *Endocrine Practice, 7*(2), 120–134.

The Rotterdam ESHRE/ASRM-Sponsored PCOS Consensus Workshop Group. (2004). Revised 2003 consensus on diagnostic criteria and long term health risks related to polycystic ovary syndrome (PCOS). *Human Reproduction, 19*(1), 41–47.

Schuiling, K. D., & Likis, F. E. (2006). *Women's gynecological health.* Sudbury, MA: Jones and Bartlett.

Speroff, L., & Fritz, M. (2005). *Clinical gynecologic endocrinology and infertility* (7th ed.). Baltimore: Lippincott Williams & Wilkins.

# HORMONES: PROGESTERONE

## Definition

Steroid hormone necessary for regulation of menstruation and sustainability of a pregnancy

Progestin is synthetic progesterone

## Common Uses

Birth control (POCP, DMPA, Implanon, Mirena IUD)

Management of oligomenorrhea

DUB

Menometrorrhagia

Polymenorrhea

Tx for amenorrhea or anovulation

Not as effective as estrogen for stopping acute bleeding

## Provera Challenge for Amenorrhea

Medroxyprogesterone (Provera) 5–10 mg PO QD × 10 d

Withdrawal bleeding should occur in 2–7 d after discontinuing progesterone

Pt should RTC in 2 wk for F/U

If no withdrawal bleed occurs or if irregular bleeding persists, diagnostic reevaluation is necessary, including MD consult

Do not start a Provera challenge if pt believes she might be pregnant, even if pregnancy test is negative

**H**

## Treatment for Chronic Anovulation

*Short Term (Not for Contraception)*

Provera 10 mg PO QD × 7–12 d every mo

Norethindrone acetate (Aygestin) 5 mg PO BID × 10 d every mo

*Micronized progesterone (Prometrium) 200 mg PO QD × 10 d

*Preferred choice if patient is at risk for or desires pregnancy

Withdrawal bleeding should occur in 2–7 d after discontinuing progesterone

Instruct patient to call if no withdrawal bleed occurs or if irregular bleeding persists

Implanon (etonogestrel implant 68 mg)

*Long Term (Contraception)*

Levonorgestrel IUD (Mirena)

Medroxyprogesterone acetate (Depo-Provera) 150 mg IM every 3 mo, or 104 mg SQ every 3 mo

## SOURCES

American College of Nurse-Midwives. (2002). Abnormal and dysfunctional uterine bleeding (Clinical Bulletin No. 6). *Journal of Midwifery & Women's Health, 47*(3), 207–213.

Schuiling, K. D., & Likis, F. E. (2006). *Women's gynecologic health.* Sudbury, MA: Jones and Bartlett.

## HORMONES: VAGINAL HORMONE PRODUCTS

TABLE H-9  Vaginal Hormone Products

| Product | Treatment | Active Ingredient | Dose/Route |
|---|---|---|---|
| Estring | Vulvovaginal atrophy; menopausal | Micronized 17-beta-estradiol | 2 mg; 7.5 mcg/24 h<br>Insert vaginal ring for 90 d; remove and reinsert new ring |
| Femring | Vulvovaginal atrophy; vasomotor sx; menopausal | Estradiol acetate | 50 mcg/d or 100 mcg/d<br>Insert vaginal ring PV Q 3 mo |
| Premarin vaginal | Vulvovaginal atrophy; menopausal | Conjugated equine estrogen | 0.5–2 g PV Q d × 3 wk, then 1 wk off<br>Reevaluate symptoms, tapering may be helpful if discontinuation is desired |
| Estrace | Vulvovaginal atrophy; menopausal | Micronized 17-beta-estradiol | 2–4 g PV Q d × 1–2 wk, then 1 g Q d 1–3 times per wk × 1–3 wk. Maintenance: 1 g 1–3 times per wk (3 wk on, 1 wk off). Taper dose or discontinue @ 3–6 mo intervals |
| Vagifem | Vulvovaginal atrophy; menopausal | Estradiol hemihydrate | 1 tab (25 mcg) PV Q d × 2 wk, then twice per wk |
| Progesterone, vaginal (Crinone, Prochieve) | 1. Secondary amenorrhea<br>2. Ovarian failure<br>3. Progesterone-deficient infertility | Progesterone; available as 4% or 8% | 1. 1 app 4% gel QOD × 6 days; if no response, then increase to 8%<br>2. 1 app PV BID<br>3. 1 app PV Q d × 10–12 wk if positive pregnancy test<br>1 app = 90 mg |
| Mirena IUD | Idiopathic menorrhagia<br>Protection from endometrial hyperplasia during ERT | Levonorgestrel | Intrauterine placement, delivers 20 mcg/24 h |

Sources: Schuiling, K.D., Likis, F. E. (2006). Women's gynecologic health. Sudbury, MA: Jones and Bartlett. Varney, H., Kriebs, J. M., & Gegor, C. L. (2004). Varney's midwifery (4th ed.). Sudbury, MA: Jones and Bartlett.

# HUMAN CHORIONIC GONADOTROPIN (hCG)

An hCG level of less than 5 mIU/ml is considered negative for pregnancy
Anything above 25 mIU/ml is considered positive for pregnancy

## hCG Levels in Weeks from LMP (Gestational Age) *

3 wk LMP: 5–50 mIU/ml
4 wk LMP: 5–426 mIU/ml
5 wk LMP: 18–7340 mIU/ml
6 wk LMP: 1080–56,500 mIU/ml
7–8 wk LMP: 7650–229,000 mIU/ml
9–12 wk LMP: 25,700–288,000 mIU/ml
13–16 wk LMP: 13,300–254,000 mIU/ml
17–24 wk LMP: 4060–165,400 mIU/ml
25–40 wk LMP: 3640–117,000 mIU/ml
Nonpregnant females: < 5.0 mIU/ml
Postmenopausal females: < 9.5 mIU/ml

* These numbers are just a *guideline*—every woman's level of hCG can rise
  differently. It is not necessarily the level that matters but rather the change in
  the level.

Urine at 10 d postconception should be positive with approx 15–25 mIU/ml in
serum

**SOURCE**

American Pregnancy Association. (2007). Human chorionic gonadotropin (hCG): The pregnancy
hormone. Retrieved January 5, 2009, from http://www.americanpregnancy.org/duringpregnancy/
hcglevels.html

**H**

# HUMAN IMMUNODEFICIENCY VIRUS (HIV)

HIV results in a weakened immune system and resulting in the development of
acquired immune deficiency syndrome (AIDS)

HIV affects the CD4 cells of the immune system

## Transmission

Sexual: vaginal or anal sex

Blood: transfusion, needle sharing, or needle stick

Vertical: mother to child during pregnancy, delivery, or breastfeeding

## Opportunistic Infections

Brain: meningitis, toxoplasmosis, lymphoma

Eyes: cytomegalovirus retinitis

Skin: Kaposi's sarcoma

Lungs: *Pneumocystis carinii* pneumonia, tuberculosis

## Treatment

Antiretroviral combination therapies to be monitored by a specialist

## Pregnancy

*Screening*

HIV antibody test

Positive: do a Western blot, which has higher sensitivity and specificity

If no test is done prenatally; do rapid test during intrapartum

*Prevention*

Pregnant women should use condoms to prevent new transmission during
pregnancy

*HIV-positive woman*

Transmission rate to baby is 15–25% without maternal tx

With maternal tx using antiretrovirals and careful obstetric planning for risk
reduction, the rate of transmission is decreased to less than 2%

Outcomes are significantly improved if the viral load is less than 1000 copies/ml

A discussion about method of delivery (vaginal vs. C/S) must be held with the
woman based on her clinical situation

Transmission during breastfeeding is 12–14% if the HIV-infected woman
breastfeeds into the second year of life

Avoid invasive procedures to decrease transmission risk: amniocentesis, CVS,
AROM, FSE, IUPC, episiotomy, tears, and fetal abrasions

Decrease maternal viral load with medication

Avoid breastfeeding if formula and potable water available

### SOURCES

American College of Obstetricians and Gynecologists. (2000). Scheduled cesarean delivery and the
prevention of vertical transmission of HIV infection (ACOG Committee Opinion No. 234). Washington,
DC: Author.

Centers for Disease Control and Prevention. (2006). Sexually transmitted diseases treatment
guidelines. *Morbidity and Mortality Weekly Report, 55*(RR-11), 1–12.

# HUMAN PAPILLOMAVIRUS (HPV)

## Statistics
> 100 different types of HPV
> 40 types are sexually transmitted
40% women 14–19 yr infected
50% women age 20–24 yr infected
70% cervical cancer from types 16 and 18
500,000 CIN 1 lesions diagnosed each yr
500,000 new cases of genital warts, 90% from types 6 and 11
Pap screening reduces rates of cervical cancer by 60–90%
50% of college age women have HPV within 4 yr of first intercourse
1/3 of women > 30 yr clear the infection in 1 year
2/3 of women < 24 yr clear the infection in 1 year

## Risk Factors
Multiple partners (high-risk type)
Young age (high-risk type)
Cervical protection (extended exposure of squamocolumnar junction from
    contraception)

## Transmission
Penile-vaginal
Penile-anal
Digital-anal/vaginal/penile
Genito-oral transmission rare
Condoms do not completely eliminate risk of transmission
Tracing infection difficult because it can be dormant for months to years
New partners = exposure to new strains

H

## Diagnosis
Genital warts—see Condaloma
Cervical cancer—see Pap smear guidelines for when to test in relationship to Pap
    smears
Vulvar, vaginal, anal, penile cancer possible though often asymptomatic until
    advanced disease

## Treatment
Genital warts—see page 151
Cervical cancer—refer to oncologist

## Vaccine—Gardasil
Low risk—types 6, 8
High risk—types 16, 18
FDA approved for ages 9–26 yr
Research not published about effectiveness > 26 yr
Most effective in girls who have not yet been sexually active
Contraindicated in pregnancy
100% effective in preventing disease from 4 specific types of HPV
Immunity continued for at least 5 yr
Not FDA approved for men

### Side Effects
Soreness at injection site
Does not contain mercury or thimerosal
Cost $120 per dose (3 doses required = $360)

### Schedule
Dose 1 any time
Dose 2 two months later
Dose 3 six months after dose 1
Dose interval should not be shortened but if it is given late it is okay, no need to
    restart series
Does not eliminate need for cancer screening

**SOURCES**

American College of Obstetricians and Gynecologists. (2005). Human papillomavirus (ACOG Practice Bulletin No. 61). In *ACOG 2008 compendium* (pp. 1231–1243). Washington, DC: Author.

Centers for Disease Control and Prevention. (2007). *Genital HPV.* Retrieved May 26, 2008, from http://www.cdc.gov/std/hpv/default.htm

Centers for Disease Control and Prevention. (2008). *HPV vaccine information for young women.* Retrieved May 26, 2008, from http://www.cdc.gov/std/Hpv/STDFact-HPV-vaccine.htm#hpvvac1

Dunne, E., Unger, E., Sternberg, M., McGuillan, G., Swan, D., Patel, S., et al. (2007). Prevalence of HPV infection among females in the United States. *Journal of the American Medical Association, 297*(8), 813–819.

Saslow, D., Castle, P., Cox, J., Davey, D., Einstein, M., & Ferris, D. (2007). American Cancer Society guidelines for HPV vaccine use to prevent cervical cancer and its precursors. *CA: A Cancer Journal for Clinicians, 57*(1), 7–28.

# INCONTINENCE

**Management**

*History*
  Onset
  Duration
  Patterns (if not clear, use a voiding diary)
  Identify signs of neurological impairment
  Elicit possible psychological causes
  Factors (e.g., surgical history, bowel patterns, medications, birth Hx)

*Reversible Incontinence*
  Need to identify cause—DIAPPERS:
    Delerium
    Infection
    Atrophic vaginitis
    Pharmaceuticals
    Psychological issues
    Excessive urine production
    Reduced mobility
    Stool impaction

**Diary**
  Incontinency diary is an important tool in choosing a treatment and measuring its effectiveness
  Diary should include time and amount of intake of fluids, urination both planned and accidental, and pelvic floor exercises
  When incontinence is recorded there should be a reporting of whether there was an urge to use the bathroom and what activity was being done at that time

**IJ**

**Treatment**
Behavioral methods
Anticholinergics
  Oxybutynin (Ditropan)
    Immediate release—2.5 mg BID or TID titrate up every other wk to max of 5 mg QID
    Extended release—5 mg daily, titrate up every other wk to max dose of 30 mg QD
    Transdermal—1 patch 2×/week, apply to hip/abdomen/buttocks, rotate sites
Tolterodine (Detrol)
  Immediate release—1 mg BID, titrate to max 4 mg/d
  Sustained release—2 mg daily, titrate up to max of 4 mg QD
Pro-Banthine
Bentyl
TCAs
Estrogens
Hycosamine
NSAIDs
Calcium channel blockers
Mipramine
Duloxetin
Pessaries, vaginal weights, Kegels
Surgery

**TABLE I-1**  Classification of Incontinence

| Type of Incontinence | Definition | Description | Associated Conditions of Findings |
|---|---|---|---|
| Stress urinary incontinence | Involuntary leakage with effort or exertion, sneezing, or coughing | Involuntary leakage with effort or exertion, sneezing, or coughing | Hypermobility of bladder neck or insufficient urethral closure pressure |
| Urge urinary incontinence | A strong desire to urinate that is difficult to postpone | Involuntary leakage accompanied by or immediately preceded by urgency | Uninhibited contractions of the detrusor muscle, frequency |
| Mixed urinary incontinence | Involuntary urine leakage associated with symptoms of both stress and urge urinary incontinence | Involuntary leakage with symptoms of both stress and urge incontinence | |
| Continuous urinary incontinence | Continuous urine leakage | Continuous urine leakage | Extremely low urethral closure pressure |
| Extra-urethral urinary incontinence | Leakage of urine from areas other than the urethral meatus | Leakage of urine from areas other than the urethral meatus | Fistula |
| Functional urinary incontinence | Urine loss related to physical conditions outside the urinary tract or cognitive impairment | Involuntary urine leakage related to physical conditions outside the urinary tract or by cognitive impairment | Immobility, often diagnosis of exclusion |
| Uncategorized urinary incontinence | Involuntary urine leakage that cannot be classified by signs and symptoms | Involuntary urine leakage that cannot be classified by signs and symptoms | |

*Sources:* Abrams et al., 2002; Fantl et al., 1996.

**SOURCES**

Abrams, P., Cardozo, L., Fall, M., Griffiths, D., Rosier, P., Ulf, U., et al. (2002). The standardization of terminology of lower urinary tract function: Report from the standardization sub-committee of the International Continence Society. *Neurourology and Urodynamics, 21*, 167–178.

Fantl, J. A., Newman, D. K., Colling, J., et al. (1996). *Urinary incontinence in adults: Acute and chronic management* (AHCPR Publication No. 96-0682). Rockville, MD: U.S. Department of Health and Human Services, Public Health Service, Agency for Health Care Policy and Research.

Schuiling, K. D., & Likis, F. E. (2006). *Women's gynecological health.* Sudbury, MA: Jones and Bartlett.

# INDUCTION OF LABOR

## Indications
Chorioamnionitis
Fetal demise
PIH
PROM
Postdates pregnancy
Pulmonary disease
Chronic HTN
Fetal compromise
Preeclampsia
Eclampsia
HEELP

## Contraindications
Vasa previa/complete placenta previa
Transverse fetal lie
Umbilical cord prolapse
Previous transfundal uterine surgery
Breech presentation

## Special Circumstances
Low transverse C/S
Maternal heart disease
Multiple gestation
Polyhydramnios
Presenting part above pelvic inlet
HTN
Abnormal FHR not requiring C/S
Bishop's score ≤ 5

**I J**

### NATURAL METHODS FOR INDUCTION OF LABOR
Sexual intercourse—encourages cervical ripening d/t prostaglandins present
in semen; female orgasm may up-regulate uterine contractions
Membrane stripping (sweeping)—stimulates prostaglandin release; place
fingers in the os and sweep fingers around, separating the membranes from
the cervix and lower uterine segment (complete 3 full sweeps per exam);
warn pt about cramping/bloody show; very effective w/ Bishop's score ≥ 6;
evidence suggests shorter time to onset of labor at term
Nipple stimulation—massage nipple w/ oiled fingers until ctx is achieved, stop,
wait 5 min and rpt until pattern is established; alternatively breast pump may
be used, 15 min pumping, then 15 min resting

*Herbal Treatments*
Evening primrose oil: 1 capsule PO daily—TID, then 1 capsule (pricked to
release oil) PV QHS
Castor oil: 2–4 T (30–60 ml) diluted in juice, rpt daily × 2 d
Red raspberry leaf: 2–4 oz of infusion (tea) TID
Black cohosh tincture: 10–25 drops TID
Blue cohosh tincture: 5 drops Q 4 h for induction; 10 drops Q 2 h in hot water
for augmentation

## Cervical Ripening

*Prepidil (Dinoprostone Gel)*
0.5 mg PV endocervical Q 6 h
Max 3 doses in 24 h
Remain supine × 15–30 min

*Cervidil (Dinoprostone Vaginal Insert)*
  10 mg insert (0.3 mg/h) PV in posterior fornix
  Remain supine × 30 min
  Remove after 12 h or onset of active labor
  Requires continuous monitoring while in place

*Misoprostol (Cytotec)*
  25 mcg PV in posterior fornix Q 3–6 h
  If no response after 2 doses, then increase to 50 mcg
  Do not exceed 50 mcg per dose, max 200 mcg total
  Not FDA approved for cervical ripening (PGE1 analogue used to treat gastric
    ulcers)
  Contraindicated for VBAC and grand multiparity

*Foley Catheter*
  Insert sterile speculum to visualize os
  Gently introduce Foley catheter bulb through cervix (common use is No. 16 Foley
    catheter w/ 30 ml balloon)
  Ensure that bulb is beyond internal os
  Inflate bulb w/ 10–30 ml of water, depending on catheter
  Remove speculum
  Leave catheter in place for 12 h or start of labor
  Catheter often falls out of cervix at approximately 3–4 cm dilation

## Use of Synthetic Oxytocin
  Pitocin
  10 U per 1000 ml of isotonic IV fluid (10 mU/ml)
  Requires constant monitoring of FHR and uterine contractions
  Half-life is approx 3 min

TABLE 1-2   Low-Dose vs. High-Dose Pitocin Protocol

| Regimen | Starting Dose (mU/min) | Incremental Increase (mU/min) | Dose Interval (min) |
|---|---|---|---|
| Low dose | 0.5–1 | 1 | 30–40 |
|  | 1–2 | 2 | 15 |
| High dose | ~6 | ~6 | 15 |
|  | 6 | 6*, 3, 1 | 20–40 |

*Incremental increase is reduced to 3 mU/min in presence of hyperstimulation and reduced to 1 mU/min with recurrent hyperstimulation

*Source:* Reprinted with permission from American College of Obstetricians and Gynecologists. (1999). Induction of labor (Clinical Management Guidelines No. 10). *2006 compendium of selected publications* (p. 562). Washington, DC: Author.

## Managing Complications
  If nonreassuring FHR → decrease or d/c oxytocin
  Turn woman on side and administer $O_2$
  If hyperstimulation persists → use terbutaline/other tocolytics

### SOURCES
American College of Obstetricians and Gynecologists. (1999). Induction of labor (Clinical Management Guidelines No. 10). *2006 compendium of selected publications* (p. 562). Washington, DC: Author.

Department of Reproductive Health and Research, World Health Organization. (2003). *Managing complications in pregnancy and childbirth: A guide for midwives and doctors.* Geneva: World Health Organization.

Knoche, A., Selzer, C., & Smolley, K. (2008). Methods of stimulating the onset of labor: An exploration of maternal satisfaction (Abstract). *Journal of Midwifery & Women's Health, 53*(4) 381–387.

# INFERTILITY

### Definition

No conception after 12 mo (< age 34 yr) or 6 mo (≥ age 35 yr) of contraceptive-free intercourse

### Statistics

Affects 10–15% of reproductive age couples
40% male
40% female
10–20% unexplained

### Etiology

*Female*

Ovulatory disorders (40%)
Tubal factors (30–50%)
Cervical/uterine factor (10%)
General hormonal imbalance (thyroid disease, hyperprolactinemia, hypogonadotropism, PCOS, hypothalamic disorders)

*Male*

Surgical history
Testicular trauma
Medications
Hx of STIs
Coital frequency and technique
Hx of sexual dysfunction
Number of children fathered

### Semen Analysis

TABLE I-3   Semen Analysis

| Volume | 2–5 ml |
|---|---|
| Motility | > 50% |
| Normal morphology | > 50% |
| Count/ml | 20 million |
| Total count | 40 million |

*Source:* Adapted from Speroff, L., & Fritz, M. A. (2005). *Clinical gynecology, endocrinology, infertility* (7th ed.). Philadelphia: Lippincott Williams & Wilkins.

### Ovulation Abnormalities

Regular menses = regular ovulation
Basal body temperature charting
Documentation of LH surge
U/S visualization of mature follicles
Labs: TSH, prolactin, serum androgens, FSH/LH/Estradiol (d 2, 3, or 4 of cycle)

*Clomid (Clomiphene Citrate) Challenge Test (CCCT)*

Day 5–9—100 mg Clomid PO
Day 10—Measure FSH level
Clomid is a weak synthetic estrogen that binds to estrogen receptors blocking them from binding to endogenous estrogen
This antagonistic function results in increased GnRH pulse amplitude, facilitating ovulation

### Interpreting Results

Day 3 FSH > 9 or FSH/LH ratio > 2.5 = poor ovarian reserve
Day 3 Estradiol > 80 pg/ml (normal 25–75 pg/ml) = low FSH levels
Day 10 FSH >10 = poor prognosis for unassisted pregnancy
If ovulating, consider postcoital testing

I J

### Tubal Abnormalities
Hysterosalpingogram
Sonohysterosalpingogram
Laproscopy

### Cervical/Uterine Abnormalities

*Structural*
Fibroids
Polyps
Congenital anomalies
Scar tissue

*Cervical*
Cervical procedures
Hx of LEEP
Cone biopsy
Cryotherapy
In utero DES exposure

### Treatment
Intrauterine insemination (IUI)
In vitro fertilization (IVF)
Gamete intrafallopian tubal transfer (GIFT)

### Intrauterine Insemination (IUI)

*Uses*
Low sperm count
Decreased sperm motility
Donor sperm
Hostile cervical conditions
Sexual dysfunction
Success rate: 10–20% in one cycle

*Notes*
Providers can only perform this w/ washed sperm
Do during ovulation
Pt should maintain a horizontal position w/ hips slightly elevated for 30 min after
    insemination has occurred
Pt can have a partner do this at home
Fresh semen has a higher rate of success than frozen samples

### In Vitro Fertilization (IVF)
Monitor and stimulate the development of healthy eggs from the ovaries
Collect eggs
Secure sperm
Combine egg and sperm in the laboratory and provide incubation time
Transfer embryo into the uterus

*Success Rates*
35% for women under age 35 yr
25% for women ages 35–37 yr
15–20% for women ages 38–40 yr
6–10% for women over 40 yr

### Web Resources for Infertility
www.womenshealth.gov/faq/infertility.htm
www.americanpregancy.org
www.mayoclinic.com/health/infertility/DS00310
www.asrm.org/Patients/faqs.html

### SOURCE
Speroff, L., & Fritz, M. A. (2005). *Clinical gynecology, endocrinology, infertility* (7th ed.). Philadelphia: Lippincott Williams & Wilkins.
Steele, L. S., & Stratmann, H. (2006). Counseling lesbian patients about getting pregnant. *Canadian Family Physician, 52,* 605–611.

# INTERMITTENT AUSCULTATION (IA)

## Definition

Listening and counting fetal heart sounds heard through the maternal abdomen in a specific pattern

## Auscultation

Fetoscope—combination of a stethoscope and Pinnard horn that allows for the assessment of fetal heart tones, most easily used after 20 wk

Handheld doppler—ultrasound waves detect fetal heart movement assessing rate, rhythm, and changes

External EFM transducer—intermittent sampling of fetal heart movement; data is traced on paper creating a digital reading of the FHR (this not a substitute for audible counting of heart rate for IA)

Fetal heart sounds can be differentiated from the maternal heart rate by comparing the maternal pulse to the FHR

TABLE I-4   Techniques for Performing Intermittent Auscultation

1. After performing Leopold's maneuvers to identify the fetal presentation and position, assist the laboring woman into a position that maximizes audibility and preserves comfort.
2. Assess the uterine contractions by palpation.
3. Determine the maternal pulse rate.
4. Place the fetoscope or Doppler over the fetal thorax or back.
5. Determine the baseline fetal heart rate by listening between contractions and when the fetus is not moving. Verify maternal pulse rate if necessary.
6. Subsequently count the fetal heart rate after a uterine contraction for 30–60 seconds every 15 to 30 minutes in active labor and every 5 minutes in the second stage.
7. Note accelerations or decelerations from the baseline rate by counting and recording the fetal heart rate using a multiple-count strategy agreed upon by practice protocol.

*Source:* Reprinted with permission from American College of Nurse-Midwives. (2007). Intermittent ascultation for intrapartum fetal heart rate surveillance (Clinical Bulletin No. 9). *Journal of Midwifery and Women's Health, 52*(3), 314.

**IJ**

TABLE I-5   Frequency of Auscultation for Women Who Are Low-Risk* During Labor

| Organization | Latent Phase | Active Phase | Second Stage |
|---|---|---|---|
| AWHONN | | 15 min | 5 min |
| ACOG | | 15 min | 5 min |
| SOGC | 30 min | 15–30 min | 5 min |
| RCOG | | 15 min† | 5 min§ |

AWHONN = Association of Women's Health, Obstetric, and Neonatal Nurses, ACOG = American College of Obstetricians and Gynecologists, SOGC = The Society of Obstetricians and Gynaecologists of Canada, RCOG = Royal College of Obstetricians and Gynaecologists.

* None of the professional organization guidelines specifically define "low risk." For the purposes of this bulletin, "low-risk" refers to women who have no medical or obstetric conditions that are associated with utero-placental insufficiency, and/or conditions that are associated with an increased incidence of UA pH of < 7.1 at birth.

† Intermittent auscultation should only be used by experienced practitioners with experience in the technique of auscultation, palpation of contractions, and auditory recognition of pertinent fetal heart rate changes.

§ For a minimum of 60 seconds.

*Source:* Reprinted with permission from American College of Nurse-Midwives. (2007). Intermittent ascultation for intrapartum fetal heart rate surveillance (Clinical Bulletin No. 9). *Journal of Midwifery and Women's Health, 52*(3), 314.

## Documentation
Counted rate (exact number)
Rhythm (terms consistent w/ National Institute of Child Health and Human
    Development Research Planning Group)
Presence/absence of acceleration or deceleration

*If Deceleration Present Document*
Nadir rate
Recurrent or nonrecurrent
Interventions instituted
Labor status
Maternal status

## EFM Compared to IA
EFM has increased risk of incidence of cesarean and operative delivery
IA has no protective effect against cerebral palsy
IA has no difference in perinatal mortality
IA has no difference rate of Apgar < 7 at 5 min
EFM had 50% less neonatal seizures though there were equal rates of cerebral
    palsy at age 4 yr

**SOURCES**

American College of Nurse-Midwives. (2007). Intermittent ascultation for intrapartum fetal heart rate
    surveillance (Clinical Bulletin No. 9). *Journal of Midwifery & Women's Health, 52*(3), 314.
Devane, D., Lalor, J., Daly, S., & McGuire, W. (2005). Cardiotocography versus intermittent
    auscultation of fetal heart on admission to labour ward for assessment of fetal wellbeing (protocol).
    *Cochrane Database of Systematic Reviews*, (1), CD005122.
Feinstein, N. (2000). Fetal heart rate auscultation: Current and future practices. *Journal of Obstetric,
    Gynecologic, & Neonatal Nursing, 29*(3), 306–315.
Goodwin, L. (2000). Intermittent auscultation of the fetal heart rate: A review of general principles.
    *Journal of Perinatal and Neonatal Nursing, 14*(3), 53–61.

# IV FLUIDS

TABLE 1-6  IV Fluid Composition

|  | 0.9% NaCl | Lactated Ringer's | D₅W |
|---|---|---|---|
| Tonicity | Hypertonic | Isotonic | Hypotonic |
| Osmolarity mOsm/l | 304 | 280 | 0 |
| Na+ | 154 mEq/l | 130 mEq/l | 0 |
| Cl- | 154 mEq/l | 109 mEq/l | 0 |
| K+ | 0 | 4 mEq/l | 0 |
| Ca++ | 0 | 3 mEq/l | 0 |
| Lactate | 0 | 28 mEq/l | 0 |
| Dextrose | 0 | 0 | 50 g |

Sources: Adapted from Smeltzer, S., & Bare, B. (2004). In McDonald, Q., & McMahon, D. (Eds.), Textbook of medical surgical nursing (10th ed.). Philadelphia: Lippincott Williams and Wilkins. Corbett, E. C. (2007). Intravenous fluids: It's more than just "fill'er up!" Practical Gastroenterology, Series 52(July), 44–60.

I J

# K

## KICK COUNTS

### Theory
Simple, easy, and universal method of monitoring fetal well-being
No special equipment needed, every woman can do it
Lack of movement or a marked decrease in fetal movement needs further
investigation

### Indication
Maternal reassurance
Maternal-fetal bonding
Gestational age > 28 wks
Maternal report of decreased fetal movement
After trauma (fall, car accident, violence)

### Preparation
Use bathroom
Drink water or juice
Avoid smoking for 2 h before doing kick counts

### Daily Kick Count Methods

*10 by 10*
10 movements in 10 h

*10 by 1*
10 movements in 1 h after you go to the bathroom, drink a glass of water or juice,
and lay down

*Simple Questioning*
"Is your baby moving?"

*ALARMS*
Less than 3 movements in 1 h
No movement for 12 h

### Follow-Up
Pt report of decreased fetal movement with a kick counting session warrants an
immediate NST

#### SOURCES
Christensen, F. C., & Rayburn, W. F. (1999). Fetal movement counts. *Obstetrics & Gynecology Clinics of North America, 26*(4), 607–621.
Varney, H., Kriebs, J. M., & Gegor, C. L. (2004). *Varney's midwifery* (4th ed.). Sudbury, MA: Jones and Bartlett.

# KEGEL

### Definition

Exercises to strengthen the pelvic floor through the contraction and release of the ischiocavernous, transverse perineal, levator ani, pelvic diaphragm, and pubococcygeal muscles.

### Indications

Incontinence
Postpartum
Cystocele
Rectocele
Uterine prolapse
Lax vaginal tone

### Assessment

Encourage woman to tighten her vaginal muscles during an internal exam
May be helpful to observe the introitus while a woman performs a Kegel contraction to ensure that she is tightening those muscles and not inadvertently performing a Valsalva maneuver.

### Patient Education

1. Empty bladder
2. Tighten pelvic floor muscles and hold for 10 sec
3. Relax pelvic floor muscles for 10 sec
4. Repeat exercise 10 times TID

Encourage patient to involve partner or use her own fingers inserted in the vagina to assess her vaginal tone and strength of Kegel contractions
Do kegels while you wait at a stoplight
Do kegels after each trip to the bathroom
Do kegels right after changing your baby's diaper or during each feeding

**K**

### Physical Therapy

Some physical therapists specialize in female pelvic floor dysfunction. Many women benefit from guided biofeedback to properly contract their pelvic floor, thus improving tone and rectifying problems with stool and urine incontinence.

**SOURCES**
Varney, H., Kriebs, J. M., & Gegor, C. L. (2004). *Varney's midwifery* (4th ed.). Sudbury, MA: Jones and Bartlett.

## LABOR: ACTIVE MANAGEMENT OF THE 1ST STAGE

### Statistics

Does not decrease risk of C/S

Does shorten first stage of labor; 2nd and 3rd stages remain unchanged

Results unchanged with epidural use

### Definition (Dublin Protocol)

Labor = painful ctx + complete effacement or bloody "show" or SROM

Must deliver within 12 h after labor dx

Pelvic exams Q 1 hour for first 3 h

If no change in dilation after 1 h then AROM

Pelvic exams Q 2 h rest of labor

Minimum dilation 1 cm/h

If inadequate progress after AROM + 2 h then add pitocin per high-dose protocol

If SROM occurred prior to admission and no progress is observed by 1 h after admission then add pitocin

Midwives manage labor with physician consults when warranted

Midwives offer continuous labor support

Pain medications available, but discouraged

### SOURCES

Cunningham, G., Leveno, K. J., Bloom, S. L., Hauth, J. C., Gilstrap, L. C., & Wenstrom, K. D. (2005). *Williams obstetrics* (22nd ed.). New York: McGraw-Hill.

Rogers, R., Gilson, G. J., Miller, A. C., Izquierdo, L. E., Curet, L. B., & Quails, C. R. (1997). Active management of labor: Does it make a difference? *American Journal of Obstetrics and Gynecology, 177*(3), 599–605.

# LABOR: ACTIVE MANAGEMENT VS. EXPECTANT MANAGEMENT OF THE 3RD STAGE

Risk for PPH increases when placenta is retained for more than 30 min after delivery

## Active Management
Early cord clamping
Gentle cord traction
Administration of exogenous oxytocin
Modified Brandt-Andrews maneuver to check for separation

## Advantages
Maternal blood loss reduced by 79.33 ml
Length of 3rd stage decreased by 9.8 min
Decreased risk of PPH, anemia, and therapeutic oxytocics
Reports of increased maternal pain over expectant management
Overall there was no change in need for manual extraction or secondary PPH
Cord drainage in conjunction with active management decreases overall amount of blood loss, and length of 3rd stage

## Expectant Management
1. Watching for signs of placental separation, and allow for spontaneous expulsion
2. If there is excessive bleeding, interventions such as position change to facilitate expulsion (squatting) or nipple stimulation or breastfeeding to promote endogenous oxytocin production can facilitate faster expulsion

### SOURCES
Brucker, M. (2001). Management of the third stage of labor: An evidence based approach. *Journal of Midwifery & Women's Health, 46*(6), 381.

Cunningham, G., Leveno, K. J., Bloom, S. L., Hauth, J. C., Gilstrap, L. C., & Wenstrom, K. D. (2005). *Williams obstetrics* (22nd ed.). New York: McGraw-Hill.

Giacalone, P. L., Vignal, J., Daures, J. P., Boulot, P., Hedon, B., & Laffargue, F. (2000). A randomised evaluation of two techniques of management of the third stage of labour in women at low risk of postpartum hemorrhage. *British Journal of Obstetrics Gynaecology, 107,* 396–400.

Prendiville, W. J., Elbourne, D., & McDonald, S. (2000). Active versus expectant management in the third stage of labour. *Cochrane Database of Systematic Reviews,* (3), 000007. PMID: 10796082.

L

## LABOR: ARREST DISORDERS

**Prolonged Deceleration Phase**
   3 h primiparous
   1 h multiparous

*Etiology*
   CPD
   Malpresentation
   Excess sedation
   Anesthesia
   Response to pitocin determines outcome
   50% will deliver if no tx

**Secondary Arrest of Dilation**
   Cessation of active phase dilation of > 2 h (per same examiner)

*Etiology*
   Conduction anesthesia
   Excess sedation
   50% CPD will arrest in early active phase
   Consider malposition as reason for arrest after 6 cm dilitation

*Treatment*
   Clinical pelvimetry
   Avoid epidural
   Pitocin augmentation
   Position changes
   Assess contractions with IUPC

**Arrest of Descent**
   No descent ≥ 1 h (per same examiner)
   Do not be fooled by caput and molding

*Etiology*
   CPD
   Malposition

*Treatment*
   Pitocin augmentation
   C/S

**Failure of Descent**
   No descent in deceleration phase of second stage

*Treatment*
   C/S

**Montevideo Units (MVU)**
   Requires IUPC placement
   Measures strength of contractions per mmHg x 10 mm by IUPC over a 10 min
      period
   > 200 MVU/10 min defined as adequate
   Must be > 200 MVU for 2 h without cervical change to be considered arrest
      disorder

**SOURCES**

Cunningham, G., Leveno, K. J., Bloom, S. L., Hauth, J. C., Gilstrap, L. C., & Wenstrom, K. D. (2005). *Williams obstetrics* (22nd ed.). New York: McGraw-Hill.

Varney, H., Kriebs, J. M., & Gegor, C. L. (2004). *Varney's midwifery* (4th ed.). Sudbury, MA: Jones and Bartlett.

# LABOR: FIRST STAGE DYSTOCIA

## Alternative Diagnosis

Asynclitism
Malpresentation
Pelvic type incompatible
Bandel's ring
Oblique lie
Inefficient ctx
OP presentation
Full bladder
Uterine anomalies

## Definitions

Prolonged latent phase dilation, < 0.5 cm/h (> 20 h primip, > 14 h multip)
Protracted active phase (< 1.2 cm/h primip, < 1.5 cm/h multip)
Protracted descent (< 1 cm/h primip, < 2 cm/h multip) descent arrests after it started
Prolonged deceleration phase (> 3 h primip, > 1 h multip) arrest of dilation around 8 cm
Secondary arrest of dilation, no change in dilation > 2 h with same examiner
Arrest of descent—no descent for 1 h with same examiner
Failure of descent—no descent ever

## Where Is the Problem?

*Passenger*
Weight
Position
Attitude (head to shoulder ratio, e.g., baby of diabetic mother, presentation, nuchal cord)

*Passage*
Pelvic type
Hx of pelvic injury or surgery
Full bladder
Prolapsed bladder
Rectocele

*Powers*
Inadequate contractions
Infection
Overdistension

*Psyche*
Primip
Teen
Hx of abuse
Pain
Anxiety
Hx of traumatic birth
PTSD

**L**

## SOURCE

Frye, A. (2004). *Holistic midwifery: A comprehensive textbook for midwives in homebirth practice.* Portland, OR: Labrys Press.

## LABOR: LENGTH

### Latent Phase
Onset of regular contractions up to 3–5 cm
Little descent of presenting part occurs during this phase
*See* Table L-1.

### Second Stage
Friedman: 2.9 h (nullip), 50 min (multip)
Zhang et al. (2002): 2nd stage: 95th percentile—3 h (nullip)
Janni et al. (2002): 2 h in 20.1%
O'Connell et al. (2003): 2nd stage > 2 h in 48% (nullip)

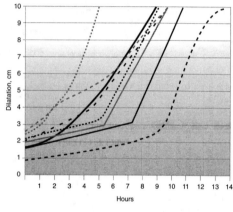

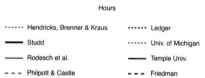

*When the starting point on the abscissa begins with admission to the hospital, a latent phase is not observed.

FIGURE L-1    Progress of Labor in Primigravid Women from the Time of Admission. *Source:* Reprinted with permission from Cunningham, G., Leveno, K. J., Bloom, S. L., Hauth, J. C., Gilstrap, L. C., & Wenstrom, K. D. (2005). *Williams obstetrics* (22nd ed.). New York: McGraw-Hill Professional.

### SOURCES
Cunningham, G., Leveno, K. J., Bloom, S. L., Hauth, J. C., Gilstrap, L. C., & Wenstrom, K. D. (2005). *Williams obstetrics* (22nd ed.). New York: McGraw-Hill.
Greulich, B., & Tarrant, B. (2007). The latent phase of labor: Diagnosis and management. *Journal of Midwifery & Women's Health, 52,* 190–198.
Janni, W., Schielle, B., Peschers, U., Huber, S., Strobi, B., et al. (2002). The protagonistic impact of a prolonged second stage of labor on maternal and fetal outcome. *Acta Obstretica et Gynecologica Scandinavica, 81,* 214–221.
O'Connell, M. P., Hussian, J., Maclennan, F. A., & Lindow, S. W. (2003). Factors associated with a prolonged second state of labor—a case controlled study of 364 nulliparous labours. *Journal of Obstretics and Gynecology, 23,* 255–257.
Varney, H., Kriebs, J. M., & Gegor, C. L. (2004). *Varney's midwifery* (4th ed.). Sudbury, MA: Jones and Bartlett.
Zhang, J., Troendle, J. F., & Yancey, M. K. (2002). Reassessing the labor curve in nulliparous women. *American Journal of Obstetrics and Gynecology, 187,* 824–828.

**TABLE L-1** Summary of Projected Lengths of Active Phase of First Stage of Labor

| Author | Primiparas Mean (h) | Primiparas *Upper Limit (h) | Multiparas Mean (h) | Multiparas *Upper Limit (h) | Notes |
|---|---|---|---|---|---|
| Friedman (1956, 1967) | 4.9 | 11.7 | 2.2 | 5.2 | Measured from 3–4 cm to 10 cm |
| Kilpatrick & Laros (1989) | 8.1, no epidural / 10.2, epidural | 16.6, no epidural / 19.0, epidural | 5.7, no epidural / 7.4, epidural | 12.5, no epidural / 14.9, epidural | Measured from regular, painful ctx Q 3–5 min by history to 10 cm |
| Albers et al. (1996) | 7.7 | 19.4 | 5.7 | 13.7 | Measured from 4 cm to 10 cm |
| Albers (1999) | 7.7 | 17.5 | 5.6 | 13.8 | Measured from 4 cm to 10 cm |
| Zhang et al. (2002) | 5.5 | - | - | - | Measured from 4 cm to 10 cm |

*Upper Limit = 2 SD above the mean (95th percentile)

*Sources:* Adapted from Cunningham, G., Leveno, K. J., Bloom, S. L., Hauth, J. C., Gilstrap, L. C., & Wenstrom, K. D. (2005). *Williams obstetrics* (22nd ed.). New York: McGraw-Hill Professional. Greulich, B., & Tarrant, B. (2007). The latent phase of labor: Diagnosis and management. *Journal of Midwifery & Women's Health, 52,* 190–198. Varney, H., Kriebs, J. M., & Gegor, C. L. (2004). *Varney's midwifery* (4th ed.). Sudbury, MA: Jones and Bartlett.

## LABOR: PAIN MANAGEMENT

**TABLE L–2**  Medication for Labor Pain Management

| Name | Class | Usual Dose | Pharmacokinetics | Comments |
|------|-------|-----------|------------------|----------|
| Nubain (Nalbuphine HCL) | Opioid agonist-antagonist analgesic | 10–20 mg IM 5–10 mg IV | Onset: IM 45 min/IV 2–3 min Peak: IM 30–60/IV 15–20 min Dur: 3–6 h | Contraindicated in women who are narcotic tolerant ↓ FHR variability |
| Stadol (Butorphanol tartrate) | Opioid agonist-antagonist analgesic | 1–2 mg IM or IV | Onset: IM 10–15 min IM/IV rapid Peak: 30–60 min Dur: 3–4 h | Contraindicated in women who are narcotic tolerant ↓ FHR variability |
| Morphine | Opioid agonist analgesic | 2–5 mg IV 10–15 mg IM | Onset: IV rapid/IM immediate Peak: 30–60/20 min Dur: 2–4 h | Commonly used for therapeutic sleep with prolonged latent phase; rarely used during labor ↓ FHR variability Maternal and neonatal CNS depression risk |
| Demerol (Meperidine) | Opioid agonist analgesic | 25 mg IV 50 mg IM | Onset 10–15 min Peak 30–60 min Dur: 2–4 h | Neonatal CNS depression risk if delivered within 1–4 h after administration ↓ FHR variability |
| Fentanyl | Opioid agonist analgesic | 25–50 mcg IV 100 mcg IM | Onset: 7–8 min Dur: 30–60 min | Short-acting, risk for respiratory depression in neonate and mother ↓ FHR variability Used with continuous infusion or PCA pump |
| Phenergan (Promethazine) | Phenothiazines | 12.5–25 mg IV 50 mg IM 25–50 mg PO | Dur: 4–5 h | Use in combination with opioids Antiemetic Reduces anxiety, promotes sedation Risk for hypotension |
| Vistaril (Hydroxyzine) | Antihistamine | 25–50 mg IM 50–100 mg PO NEVER IV | Dur: 4 h | Use in combination with opioids Antiemetic/anti-itch Painful injection ↓ FHR variability possible |

*Narcan: Give 0.1–0.2 mg IV Q 2–3 min until desired effect. Onset 2 min, duration 4–6 h.

**SOURCES**

McCool, W. F., Packman, J., & Zwerling, A. (2004). Obstetric anesthesia: Changes and choices. *Journal of Midwifery & Women's Health, 49,* 505.

Thompson Healthcare. (2007). *MICROMEDEX: Healthcare series.* Retrieved August 26, 2008, from http://www.micromedex.com

## LABOR: TRUE VS. FALSE, EARLY VS. ACTIVE

**True Labor**
  Regular progressive contractions
  Cervical change
  Contractions in fundus
  Position change or walking increases intensity
  Bloody show

**False Labor**
  Irregular, nonprogressive contractions
  No cervical change
  Low, crampy contractions
  No changes in intensity with position change/walking
  No other signs of labor

**Early Labor**
  Can continue normal daily activities through contractions
  Easily distracted during contractions
  Cervix dilated < 4 cm
  Contractions lasting 15–30 sec
  Contractions Q 10–30 min

**Active Labor**
  Much less distractable during contractions
  Needs support through contractions
  Incorporates coping mechanisms
  Contractions lasting ≥ 1 min
  Contractions Q 4–5 min
  Cervix dilated ≥ 5 cm
  Cervical dilation is progressing
  Pt c/o pelvic fullness/heaviness

**L**

**SOURCES**
Greulich, B., & Tarrant, B. (2007). The latent phase of labor: Diagnosis and management. *Journal of Midwifery & Women's Health, 52,* 190–198.
Varney, H., Kriebs, J. M., & Gegor, C. L. (2004). *Varney's midwifery* (4th ed.). Sudbury, MA: Jones and Bartlett.

# LAB VALUES

TABLE L–3    Lab Values

| Laboratory Test | Nonpregnant | Pregnant |
|---|---|---|
| **Hematology** | | |
| Hematocrit | 37–47% | 33–44% |
| Hemoglobin | 12–16 g/dl | 11–14 g/dl |
| Erythrocyte count | $4.8–10^6/mm^3$ | $4.0–10^6/mm^3$ |
| Leukocyte count | $6.0 (4.5–11) \times 10^3/mm^3$ | $9.2 (6–16) \times 10^3/mm^3$ |
| Neutrophils | $4.4 (1.8–7.7) \times 10^3/mm^3$ | $(3.8–10) \times 10^3/mm^3$ |
| Lymphocytes | $2.5 (1–4.8) \times 10^3/mm^3$ | $(1.3–5.2) \times 10^3/mm^3$ |
| Monocytes | $0.3 (0–0.8) \times 10^3/mm^3$ | No change |
| Eosinophils | $0.2 (0–0.45) \times 10^3/mm^3$ | No change |
| Platelet count | 130,000–400,000/ml | Slight decrease |
| Fibrinogen | 200–450 ng/dl | 400–650 ng/dl |
| Folate | | |
| Red blood cell | 150–450 ng/ml cells | 100–400 ng/ml cells |
| Ferritin | 25–200 ng/ml | 15–150 ng/ml |
| Iron | 135 mcg/dl | 90 mcg/dl |
| Iron-binding capacity | 250–460 mcg/dl | 300–600 mcg/dl |
| *Coagulation studies* | | |
| Bleeding time (Duke) | < 4 min | No change |
| Partial thromboplastin time | 24–36 sec | No change |
| Prothrombin time | 12–14 sec | No change |
| Thrombin time | 12–18 sec | No change |
| *Factors* | | |
| VIII | 60–100% | 120–200% |
| X, IX | 60–100% | 90–120% |
| VII, XII | 60–100% | No change |
| II, V, XI | 60–100% | No change |
| V | 60–100% | No change |
| **Renal** | | |
| BUN | 10–20 mg/dl | 5–12 mg/dl |
| Creatinine | < 1.5 mg/dl | < 0.8 mg/dl |
| Magnesium | 2–3 mg/dl | 1.6–2.1 mg/dl |
| Osmolarity | 285–295 mOsm/kgH$_2$O | 275–280 mOsm/kgH$_2$O |
| Sodium | 136–145 mEq/l | 130–140 mEq/l |
| Potassium | 3.5–5 mEq/l | 3.3–4.1 mEq/l |
| Carbon dioxide content | 21–30 mEq/l | 18–25 mEq/l |
| Chloride | 98–106 mEq/l | 93–100 mEq/l |
| Uric acid | 1.5–6 mg/dl | 1.2–4.5 mg/dl |
| Urinary protein | < 150 mg/day | < 250–300 mg/day |
| Creatinine clearance | 91–130 ml/min | 120–160 ml/min |
| Complement (total) | 150–250 CH50 | 200–400 CH50 |
| C3 | 55–120 mg/dl | 100–180 mg/dl |
| **Endocrine** | | |
| Glucose, fasting (plasma) | 75–115 mg/dl | 60–105 mg/dl |
| ACTH | 20–100 pg/ml | No change |
| Aldosterone (plasma) | < 8 ng/dl | < 20 ng/dl |
| Aldosterone (urinary) | 8–20 mcg/24 h | 15–40 mcg/24 h |
| Cortisol (plasma) | 5–25 mcg/dl | 15–35 mcg/dl |
| Growth hormone, fasting | < 5 ng/ml | No change |
| Insulin, fasting | 6–26 mcg/ml | 8–30 mcg/ml |
| Parathyroid hormone (Bio-intact) | 20–30 pg/ml | 10–20 pg/ml |
| Prolactin | 2–15 ng/ml | 50–400 ng/ml |
| Renin activity (plasma) | 0.9–3.3 ng/ml/h | 3–8ng/ml/h |

/ continues

TABLE L–3    Lab Values (continued)

| Laboratory Test | Nonpregnant | Pregnant |
|---|---|---|
| Thyroxin ($T_4$), total | 5–12 mcg/dl | 10–17 mcg/dl |
| Tri-iodothyronine ($T_3$) | 70–190 ng/dl | 100–220 ng/dl |
| Free $T_4$ | 1–2ng/dl | No change |
| $T_3$ resin uptake | 25–35% | 15–25% |
| Free thyroxin index | 1.75–4.95 | No change |
| TSH | 4–5 mcg/ml | |
| Calcium | | |
|   Total | 9.0–10.5 mg/dl | 8.1–9.5 mg/dl |
|   Ionized (serum) | 4.5–5.6 mg/dl | 4–5 mg/dl |
| Inorganic phosphorus | 3.0–4.5 mg/dl | No change |
| **Hepatic and Enzymes** | | |
| Bilirubin (total) | 0.3–1 mg/dl | No change |
| Cholesterol | 120–180 mg/dl | 180–280 mg/dl |
| Trigliceride | < 160 mg/dl | < 260 mg/dl |
| Amylase | 60–180 U/l | 90–350 U/l |
| Creatine phosphokinase | 10–70 U/l | 5–40 U/l |
| Lactic dehydrogenase (LDH) | 200–450 U/ml | No change |
| Lipase | 4–24 IU/dl | 2–12 IU/dl |
| Alkaline phosphatase | 30–95 mU/ml | 60–200 mU/ml |
| Alanine amino transaminase | 0–35 U/l | No change |
| Aspartate amino transaminase | 0–35 U/l | No change |
| γ–Glutamyl transpeptidase | 1–45 IU/l | No change |
| Ceruloplasmin | 27–37 mg/dl | 40–60 mg/dl |
| Copper | 70–140 ng/dl | 120–200 ng/dl |
| Protein (total) | 5.5–8 g/dl | 4.5–7 g/dl |
|   Albumin | 3.5–5.5 g/dl | 2.5–4.5 g/dl |
|   IgA | 90–325 mg/dl | No change |
|   IgM | 45–150 mg/dl | No change |
|   IgG | 800–1500 mg/dl | 700–1400 mg/dl |

Note: The exact values depend on the individual laboratory.

*Source:* Reprinted with permission from Burrow, G., Duffy, T., Copel, J. (2004). *Medical complications during pregnancy* (6th ed.). Philadelphia: Saunders.

**L**

## LESBIAN CLIENTS

### Definition
Women who engage in sexual relationships with other women

### Specific Health Concerns
Fear of prejudice by providers
Revealing sexuality
STIs
GC/CT and PID not common in women who have never had sex with men
HSV, genital warts, and trichamoniasis seem to be transmitted between female partners
Odds of having an STI increase with history of sex with men
More partners increases risk of contracting and transmitting STIs

### Pregnancy-Related Stresses
Choosing biological mother (physical health, job/career, health insurance)
Donor selection
Infertility treatment (IUI, IVF, etc.)
Gender/sex roles and expectations
Healthcare discrimination
Jealousy between partners
Legal challenges (custody)
Parenting ability
Labor fear

### Top 10 Health Issues
Breast cancer
Depression/anxiety
Heart health
Gyn cancer
Fitness
Tobacco
Alcohol
Substance use
Domestic violence
Osteoporosis

### RESOURCES
www.womenshealth.gov/faq/lesbian-health.cfm—US Department of Health and Human Services
www.lesbianhealthinfo.org—San Francisco non-profit
www.mautnerproject.org—Washington, DC non-profit

### SOURCES
Bailey, J., Farquhar, C., Owen, C., & Mangtani, P. (2004). Sexually transmitted infections in women who have sex with women. *Sexually Transmitted Infections, 80,* 244–246.
O'Hanlan, K. (2008). *Ten things lesbians should discuss with their health care providers.* Retrieved May 25, 2008, from http://www.glma.org/index.cfm?fuseaction=Page.viewPage&pageID=691

# MAGNESIUM SULFATE (MgSO₄)

### Indications

Tx of preeclampsia and eclampsia

Current data show that MgSO₄ should not be used as a tocolytic for PTL to prevent PTB

### Drug Class

Anticonvulsant

Laxative

Preg Cat B

Lact Cat L1

### Pharmacokinetics

Depresses muscle contractility through a reduction in the release of acetylcholine at the neuromuscular junction

### Half-Life

Mom—90% excreted in 24 h

Neonate—40 h

### Treatment Protocol

Loading dose: 4–6 g IV over 20 min

Maintenance: 1–2 g/h (or up to 4 g/h when necessary)

PO dosing not effective

Measure levels Q 4–6 h

Therapeutic range 6–8 mEq/l

    8–10 mEq/l—↓ DTRs

    13–15 mEq/l—respiratory paralysis

    > 15 mEq/l—cardiac anomalies/arrest

### Monitor

| | |
|---|---|
| DTRs | BUN/creatinine |
| RR | Strict fluid input and output |
| Mg²⁺ & Ca²⁺ levels | |

### Contraindications

Allergy to Mg²⁺

Poor cardiac health

Do not start therapy if calcium gluconate is not readily available

### Antidote

Calcium gluconate in 10% solution, 10 ml (1g) IV over 10 min

### Maternal Effects

| | |
|---|---|
| H/A | Urinary retention |
| N/V | Cardiac arrest |
| Weakness | Hypocalcemia |
| Visual changes | |

### Fetal Effects

| | |
|---|---|
| Hypotonia | Bony abnormalities |
| Drowsiness | Congenital rickets |

Mittendorf et al. (2002) showed increased risk of IVH in neonates with high levels of ionized magnesium at delivery

#### SOURCES

Crowther, C. A., Hiller, J. E., & Doyle, L. W. (2002). Magnesium sulphate for preventing preterm birth in threatened preterm labour. *Cochrane Database of Systematic Reviews*, (4), 001060.

Duley, L., Gulmezoglu, A. M., & Henderson-Smart, D. J. (2003). Magnesium sulphate and other anticonvulsants for women with pre-eclampsia. *Cochrane Database of Systematic Reviews*, (2), CD000025.

Mittendorf, R., Pryde, P. G., Elin, R. J., Gianopoulos, J. G., & Lee, K. S. (2002). Relationship between hypermagnesaemia in preterm labour and adverse health outcomes in babies. *Magnesium Research*, 15(3–4), 253–261.

## MECONIUM

### Definition
1st bowel movement of the fetus
Viscous
Sticky
Odorless
Tarlike

### Facts
Low-level of intestinal flora, which increases with oral nutrition
Can be tested to assess for maternal drug use during pregnancy
Meconium ileus often first symptom of CF
Primary mode of excreting bilirubin, thus there is a strong connection among
  neonatal nutrition, bowel movements, and jaundice.

### Meconium-Stained Amniotic Fluid

*Statistics*
8–15% of all pregnancies

*Etiology*
1. Expulsion of meconium by fetus in utero
2. Common at term
3. May occur as a result of fetal distress

*Management*
Record consistency of meconium (light, moderate, heavy)
Consult MD if indicated by practice agreement
Ensure that suction equipment is available and operating (routine suctioning of the
  infant on the perineum with or w/o meconium staining is not evidence based)
Current evidence suggests that routine endotracheal intubation of vigorous infants
  for meconium-staining does not decrease morbidity/mortality
*See* Table M-1.

### SOURCES

Halliday, H. L., & Sweet, D. (2000). Endotracheal intubation at birth for preventing morbidity and
  mortality in vigorous, meconium-stained infants born at term. *Cochrane Database of Systematic
  Reviews*, (4), CD000500 .

Mercer, J. S., Erickson, D. A., Graves, B., & Haley, M. M. (2007). Evidence-based practices for the
  fetal to newborn transition [Abstract]. *Journal of Midwifery & Women's Health, 52*(3), 262–272.

TABLE M-1  Current Evidence for Practices Related to Management of Infants Born with Meconium-Stained Amniotic Fluid

| Treatment | Recommendation | Reference | Study Details |
|---|---|---|---|
| Amnioinfusion | No benefit to infants found for the prevention of MAS | Fraser et al. (2005) | Multicenter RCT, women (n = 1998) in labor at term with MSAF stratified by presence of variable decelerations and randomly assigned to amnioinfusion or standard care. Amnioinfusion did not reduce risk of MAS, or perinatal death. |
| Intrapartum suctioning before delivery of shoulders | No benefit to any infants including high-risk infants; suctioning of infant before delivery is not indicated | Vain et al. (2004) | RCT, blinded, infants (n = 1176) suctioned on perineum compared with infants (n = 1225) not suctioned. No difference in Apgar scores, respiratory distress, use of oxygen, need for ventilation, MAS (4% in each group), or death. |
| Endotracheal intubation and suctioning after birth of vigorous infants | No benefit to any infants; not recommended for vigorous infants | Wiswell et al. (2000) | RCT, vigorous term infants (n = 2094) with MSAF randomly assigned to intubation and suctioning or to expectant management. Intubation and suctioning did not result in lower incidence of MAS or other respiratory disorders. |

Note: MAS = meconium aspiration syndrome; MSAF = meconium-stained amniotic fluid; RCT = randomized, controlled trial.

M

Source: Reprinted with permission from ercer, J. S., Erickson, D. A., Graves, B., & Haley, M. M. (2007). Evidence-based practices for the fetal to newborn transition [Abstract]. Journal of Midwifery & Women's Health, 52(3), 262–272.

## MENOPAUSE

### Definition

Perimenopause—the years leading to menopause with menstrual irregularities and related s/sx Usually 2–8 years with onset between 39–51 yr

Menopause—Clinical absence of menses for 12 consecutive months (in the past FSH < 40 mIU/l)

Occurs between 48–55 yr, 51 is the average age

### Pathophysiology

Cessation of ovarian production of estrogen

10–20 fold increase in FSH

3-fold increase in LH

Decreased ovarian production of androstenedione and testosterone (25% decrease)

### Signs and Symptoms

Acne

Arthralgia

Decreased libido

Decreased vaginal lubrication

Depression

Dizziness

Dry eyes

Dry/thinning hair

Dyspareunia

Dysuria

Fatigue

Forgetfulness

H/A

Hirsutism/virilization

Irregular menses/bleeding

Irritability/mood disturbances

Mastalgia

Myalgia

Nervousness/anxiety

Night sweats

Nocturia

Sleep disturbances/insomnia

Skin dryness/atrophy

Stress urinary incontinence, frequency, urgency

Vaginal atrophy

Vaginal/vulvar burning, irritation, puritis

Vasomotor instability (hot flushes)

### Differential Diagnosis

Pregnancy

Anemia

Arrhythmias

Depression

Arthritis

HTN

Diabetes

Hyper/hypothyroid

Infection

Fibroids

Polyps

Endometriosis

Ovarian cysts

Ovarian tumors

*Comorbid Conditions*
   Cardiovascular changes (*see* Cardiovascular)
   Osteoporosis (*see* Osteoporosis)

**Herbal Supplements for Menopause Symptoms**
   *See* Table M-2.

**Nonhormonal Hot Flushes Treatment**
   Antidepressants—Effexor most significantly hot flushes
   Anticonvulsants (such as Neurontin)
   Antihypertensives

**Vaginal Dryness Treatment**
   *See* Table M-3.

**SOURCES**

Decker, G. M., & Meyers, J. (2001). Commonly used herbs: Implications for clinical practice [insert]. *Clinical Journal of Oncology Nursing, 5*(2).

Dennehy, C. E. (2006). The use of herbs and dietary supplements in gynecology: An evidence based review. *Journal of Midwifery & Women's Health, 51*(6), 402.

Gaudet, T. W. (2004). CAM approaches to menopause management: Overview of the options. *Menopause Management: Women's Health Through Midlife & Beyond, 13*(Suppl. 1), 48–50.

Low Dog, T. (2004). CAM approaches to menopause management: The role for botanicals in menopause. *Menopause Management: Women's Health Through Midlife & Beyond, 13*(Suppl. 1), 51–53.

Minkin, M. J., & Wright, C. (2005). *A woman's guide to menopause and perimenopause.* New Haven, CT: Yale University Press.

North American Menopause Society. (2004). Treatment of menopause-associated vasomotor symptoms: Position statement of the North American Menopause Society. *Menopause, 11*(1), 11–33.

Reed, S., Newton, K., LaCroix, A., Grothaus, L., Grieco, V., & Ehrlich, K. (2008). Vaginal, endometrial, and reproductive hormone findings: Randomized, placebo-controlled trail of black cohosh, multibotanical herbs, and dietary soy for vagomotor symptoms: The herbal alternatives for menopause study. *Menopause, 15*(1), 51–58.

Schuiling, K. D., & Likis, F. E. (2006). *Women's gynecologic health.* Sudbury, MA: Jones and Bartlett.

Speroff, L., & Fritz, M. A. (2005). *Clinical gynecology, endocrinology, infertility* (7th ed.). Philadelphia: Lippincott Williams & Wilkins.

**M**

TABLE M-2 Herbal Supplements for Menopause Symptom Control*

| Product | Usual Dosage** | Purpose in Menopause | Comments |
|---|---|---|---|
| Black cohosh (*Cimicifuga racemosa*) | 20 mg twice daily (proprietary standardized extract) | • Vasomotor symptoms | • Multiple products and formulations available<br>• Research evidence suggests beneficial effect on menopausal symptoms, benefit similar to estrogen for hot flash relief<br>• Safety for use > 6 months not established<br>• Product labels frequently recommend much higher doses<br>• Can potentiate antihypertensives<br>• Wide variations in product ingredients, extraction processes, and purity<br>• Side effects rare, usually intestinal upset, headache, dizziness, hypotension, or painful extremities; more common with higher doses |
| Chastetree berry (*Vitex agnus castus*) | Effective dose unknown, hard to find standardized extract | • Menstrual irregularity | • More popular in Europe than the US; approved in Germany for PMS, mastalgia, and menopause symptoms<br>• Often found in combination products<br>• Research focuses on PMS symptoms, no data on relief of menopause symptoms<br>• Side effects rare, usually headache, intestinal upset |
| Dong quai (*Angelica sinensis*) | 2 capsules two to three times per day; usually in combination products | • Gynecologic conditions | • Widely used in Asia<br>• Research found no benefit for menopause symptoms<br>• Often in Chinese herb combination products (Chinese Materia Medica advises against giving it alone)<br>• A "heating" herb, can cause a red face, hot flashes, sweating, irritability, or insomnia<br>• Contains coumarin derivatives, contraindicated in those taking warfarin<br>• Can cause photosensitivity, hypotension |

/continues

TABLE M-2  Herbal Supplements for Menopause Symptom Control* (continued)

| Product | Usual Dosage** | Purpose in Menopause | Comments |
|---|---|---|---|
| Evening primrose oil (Oenothera biennis) | 3–4 gm daily in divided doses | • Hot flashes<br>• Mastalgia | • Data show no benefit in treatment versus controls<br>• Potentiates risk for seizure if taken with seizure disorder, phenothiazines, and other medications that lower the seizure threshold<br>• Side effects include diarrhea and nausea |
| Ginkgo (Ginkgo biloba) | 40–80 mg of standardized extract three times daily | • Memory changes | • Insufficient research on safety and efficacy<br>• Memory changes often related to sleep disturbances, menopausal sleep disturbances frequently related to vasomotor symptoms or other life stressors<br>• Side effects include gastrointestinal distress, hypotension; chronic use had been linked with subarachnoid hemorrhage, subdural hematoma, and increased bleeding times |
| Ginseng (Panax ginseng) | 1–2 gm root daily in divided doses | • General "tonic"<br>• Improved mood, fatigue | • Heavily adulterated<br>• Research showed no benefit on menopausal symptoms; showed benefits on well-being, general health, and depression<br>• Can cause uterine bleeding, mastalgia<br>• Contraindicated with breast cancer, and with monoamine oxidase inhibitors, stimulants, or anticoagulants; may potentiate digoxin and others (multiple drug interactions)<br>• Side effects include rash, nervousness, insomnia, hypertension |
| Kava (Piper methysticum) | 150–300 mg of root extract daily in divided doses | • Irritability<br>• Insomnia | • Banned in several countries due to hepatotoxicity, thus not recommended<br>• Contraindicated with depression<br>• Side effects include gastrointestinal discomfort, impaired reflexes and motor function, weight loss, hepatotoxicity, rash |
| Licorice root (Glycyrrhiza glabra) | 5–15 mg of root equivalent daily in divided doses | • Menopause-related symptoms | • Found in many Chinese herb mixtures<br>• No data supporting relief of hot flashes<br>• High doses can lead to primary aldosteronism cardiac arrhythmias, cardiac arrest<br>• Contraindicated if hepatic or renal disease, diabetes, hypertension, arrhythmia, hypokalemia, hypertonis, pregnancy, or on diuretics |

M

/continues

TABLE M-2  Herbal Supplements for Menopause Symptom Control* (continued)

| Product | Usual Dosage** | Purpose in Menopause | Comments |
|---|---|---|---|
| Passion flower (Passiflora incarnata) | 3–10 grains daily in divided doses | • Sedative | • Research shows mixed results in sleep improvement<br>• Menopausal sleep disturbances frequently related to vasomotor symptoms or other life stressors |
| St. John's-wort (Hypericum perforatum) | 300 mg three times daily (standardized extract) | • Vasomotor symptoms<br>• Irritability<br>• Depression | • No data supporting vasomotor relief<br>• Research findings support use for depression, there are no clinical trials for menopause<br>• Often combined with black cohosh for menopause symptom treatment<br>• Interferes with metabolism of many medications that are metabolized in the liver (C 450) (e.g., estrogen, digoxin, theophylline), reduces international normalized ratio (INR) levels, not to be used concomitantly with antidepressants, monoamine oxidase inhibitors, or immunosuppressants<br>• Side effects include photosensitivity, rash, constipation, cramping, dry mouth, fatigue, dizziness, restlessness, insomnia |
| Valerian root (Valeriana officinalis) | 300–600 mg aqueous extract 1/2–1 hour before bed (insomnia); 150–300 mg aqueous extract each morning and 300–400 mg each evening (anxiety) | • Sedative<br>• Antianxiety | • Used for insomnia in intermittent dosing, for anxiety with chronic dosing<br>• Research showed improvement in sleep and depression/mood scales<br>• Side effects include headache, uneasiness, excitability, arrhythmias, morning sedation, gastrointestinal upset, cardiac function disorders (with long-term use) |
| Wild yam (Dioscorea villosa) | Unknown | • Menopausal symptoms | • Products claim that creams are converted to progesterone; however, the human body cannot convert topical or ingested wild yam into progesterone<br>• Research showed no benefit on menopausal symptoms |

*See prescribing reference for full information on doses, side effects, contraindications, and cautions.

**Dosages vary and differ according to form (e.g., tincture, liquid extract, drops, essential oil, standardized extract).

Sources: Decker & Meyers, 2001; Gaudet, 2004; Low Dog, 2004; NAMS, 2004.

TABLE M-3  Treatment for Vaginal Dryness

| Type | Product Name | Active Ingredient | Dose |
|---|---|---|---|
| Estrogen | | | |
| Vaginal hormone creams | Estrace (Warner Chilcott) | Micronized 17-beta-estradiol | 2–4 g daily for 1–4 weeks, then 1 g daily 1–3 times per week for 1–3 weeks. Maintenance: 1 g 1–3 times a week, cyclically (3 weeks on, 1 week off). Taper dosage or discontinue at 3–6 month intervals |
| | Premarin (Wyeth) | Conjugated equine estrogen | 0.5–2 g intravaginally daily cyclically (3 weeks on, 1 week off). Reevaluate periodically. Tapering is frequently appropriate but not specified in product information |
| Vaginal tablets | Vagifem (Novo Nordisk) | Estradiol hemihydrate | 25 mcg once daily for two weeks then twice weekly |
| Ring | Estring (Pharmacia) | Micronized 17-beta-estradiol | 7.5 mcg/24 hours once every 90 days |
| | Femring (Warner Chilcott) | Estradiol acetate | 0.05 mg/day or 0.1 mg/day once every 3 months |
| Progestogen | | | |
| Gel | Crinone (Serono) | Progesterone | 4% gel–45 mg, 1 applicator every other day, give 6 doses; increase to 8% if no response |
| IUD | Mirena (Berlex) | Evonorgestrel | 20 mcg daily |

*See prescribing reference for full information on doses, side effects, contraindications, and cautions.

Source: Schuiling, K. D., & Likis, F. E. (2006). Women's gynecologic health. Sudbury, MA: Jones and Bartlett.

M

## MENOPAUSE: HORMONE THERAPY

### Indications
FDA suggests tx for moderate to severe vasomotor symptoms
Hot flashes 7–8 per d or 60 per wk
Estrogen therapy alone if hysterectomy, combination therapy for everyone else

### Contraindications to Estrogen
Breast cancer
Estrogen-dependent neoplasia
Hx of uterine or ovarian cancer
Hx of heart disease or stroke
Undiagnosed abnormal genital bleeding
Hx of thrombophlebitis or thromboembolic disorder

### Contraindication to Progesterone
Active thrombophlebitis or thromboembolic disorder
Liver problems
Breast cancer
Undiagnosed abnormal vaginal bleeding
Pregnancy

### Trial Risks
Women's Health Initiative (WHI) and Heart and Estrogen/progestin Replacement Study (HERS) studies showed increased risk of breast cancer, coronary heart disease, thromboembolism, stroke, and dementia

*WHI Conclusions*

TABLE M-4   WHI Overview of Findings

|  | Estrogen Alone in Women Without Uteruses | Estrogen and Progesterone |
|---|---|---|
| Coronary artery | Coronary artery calcium was lower in women taking estrogen | |
| Stroke | Estrogen increased risk of stroke | 31% increased risk of stroke |
| Breast cancer | CEE group had 20% lower risk of invasive breast cancer, though it was not statistically significant | 24% increased risk of breast cancer. Increased risk of mammogram abnormalities and difficulty interpreting findings |
| Venous thrombosis | Increased risk especially in first 2 years of use | 2-fold increased risk |
| Heart disease | No protective effect against heart attach | No protective effect |
| Diabetes | No significant findings | Reduced risk of new diagnosis, lower sugar and insulin levels, reduced weight and waist size |
| Bone density/osteoporosis | | 24% reduction in fractures |

*Sources:* Adapted from Women's Health Initiative. (2002). *WHI HRT update.* Retrieved August 10, 2008, from http://www.whi.org/findings/ht/update_ht2002.pdf. Women's Health Initiative. (2004). *WHI hormone program update.* Retrieved August 10, 2008, from http://www.whi.org/findings/ht/update_ht2004.pdf

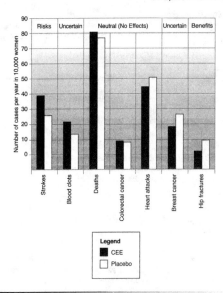

FIGURE M-3   Effects of Estrogen Alone and Placebo on Disease Rates. *Source:* Women's Health Initiative. (2002). *WHI HRT update*. Retrieved August 10, 2008, from http://www.whi.org/findings/ht/update_ht2002.pdf

M

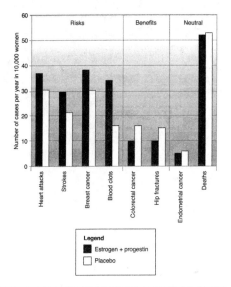

FIGURE M-4   Effects of Estrogen Plus Progesterone and Placebo on Disease Rates. *Source:* Women's Health Initiative. (2002). *WHI HRT update*. Retrieved August 10, 2008, from http://www.whi.org/findings/ht/update_ht2002.pdf

## Adverse Effects

Fluid retention—decrease salt, increase water intake, exercise, mild diuretic
Bloating—change to low-dose transdermal estrogen and lower progesterone (try micronized progesterone)
Breast tenderness—decrease or change estrogen, decrease salt, change progesterone, decrease caffeine and chocolate consumption
H/A—change to transdermal estrogen, decrease hormone levels, change to CC-EPT regimen, adequate water intake, decrease salt, caffeine, and alcohol
Mood changes—lower progesterone dose, change to CC-EPT regimen, adequate water, restrict salt, caffeine and alcohol
Nausea—take hormones with meals, change and decrease hormone levels, use transdermal estrogen

## Treatment

Start w/ 0.3 mg CEE and 0.25–0.5 mg 17-beta estradiol patch
Vasomotor symptoms usually begin to improve in 2–6 wks
Discontinuation by gradual taper

## Follow-Up

6–8 wks to adjust dose

## Hormone Therapy

*See* Table M-5.

### SOURCES

Hulley, S., Grady, D., Bush, T., Furberg, C., Herrington, D., Riggs, B., et al. (1998). Randomized trial of estrogen plus progestin for secondary prevention of coronary heart disease in postmenopausal women. Heart and Estrogen/Progestin Replacement Study (HERS) research group. *Journal of the American Medical Association, 280*(7), 605–613.

Rossouw, J. E., Anderson, G. L., Prentice, R. L., LaCroix, A. Z., Kooperberg, C., Stefanick, M. L., et al. (2002). Risks and benefits of estrogen plus progestin in healthy postmenopausal women: Principal results from the women's health initiative randomized controlled trial. *Journal of the American Medical Association, 288*(3), 321–333.

Schuiling, K. D., & Likis, F. E. (2006). *Women's gynecologic health.* Sudbury, MA: Jones and Bartlett.

Women's Health Initiative. (2002). *WHI HRT update.* Retrieved August 10, 2008, from http://www.whi.org/findings/ht/update_ht2002.pdf

Women's Health Initiative. (2004). *WHI hormone program update.* Retrieved August 10, 2008, from http://www.whi.org/findings/ht/update_ht2004.pdf

TABLE M-5  Hormone Therapy Options*

| Type | Product Name (Manufacturer) | Active Ingredient | Dosage |
|---|---|---|---|
| Estrogens, oral | Cenestin (Duramed) | Conjugated estrogens | 0.3 mg, 0.625 mg, 0.9 mg, or 1.25 mg once daily |
| | Estrace (Warner Chilcott) | Micronized estradiol | 0.5 mg, 1 mg, or 2 mg once daily |
| | Estratab (Solvay) | Esterified estrogens | 0.3 mg, 0.625 mg, or 2.5 mg once daily |
| | Menest (Monarch) | Esterified estrogens | 0.3 mg, 0.625 mg, 1.25 mg, or 2.5 mg once daily |
| | Ogen (Pharmacia) | Estropipate | 0.625 mg, 1.25 mg, or 2.5 mg once daily |
| | Ortho-est (Women First) | Estropipate | 0.625 mg or 1.25 mg once daily |
| | Premarin (Wyeth) | Conjugated equine estrogens (CEE) | 0.3 mg, 0.45 mg, 0.625 mg, 0.9 mg, 1.25 mg, or 2.5 mg once daily |
| Estrogens, transdermal | Climara (Berlex) | Estradiol | 0.025 mg, 0.0375 mg, 0.05 mg, 0.06 mg, 0.075 mg, or 0.1 mg once weekly |
| | Esclim (Women First), Vivelle, Vivelle-Dot (Novartis) | Estradiol | 0.025 mg, 0.0375 mg, 0.05 mg, 0.075 mg, or 0.1 mg twice weekly |
| | Alora (Watson) | Estradiol | 0.025 mg, 0.05 mg, 0.075 mg, or 0.1 mg twice weekly |
| | Estrogel (Solvay) | Estradiol | 1.25 g apply once daily to arm from shoulder to wrists |
| | Estraderm (Novartis) | Estradiol | 0.05 mg or 0.1 mg twice weekly |
| | Estrasorb Cream (Novavax) | Estradiol | 4.35 mg (one pouch) rubbed into each thigh every morning (total 8.7 mg daily) |

/continues

M

TABLE M-5 Hormone Therapy Options* (continued)

| Type | Product Name (Manufacturer) | Active Ingredient | Dosage |
|------|------------------------------|-------------------|--------|
| Progestogens | Provera (Pharmacia) | Medroxyprogesterone acetate (MPA) | 2.5 mg, 5 mg, or 10 mg continuously or on set cycle schedule |
| | Prometrium (Solvay) | Micronized progesterone | 100 mg or 200 mg continuously or on set cycle schedule |
| | Aygestin (Barr) | Norethindrone acetate | 5 mg or 10 mg continuously or on set cycle schedule |
| | Amen (Carnick), Cycrin (Wyeth-Ayerst) | MPA | 2.5 mg, 5 mg, or 10 mg continuously or on set cycle schedule |
| Combination estrogen + progestogen, oral preparations | Prempro (Wyeth) | CEE + MPA | 0.3 mg + 1.5 mg once daily<br>0.45 mg + 1.5 mg once daily<br>0.625 mg + 2.5 mg once daily, or<br>0.625 mg + 5 mg once daily continuously |
| | Premphase (Wyeth) | CEE (14 tabs), then CEE + MPA (14 tabs) | 0.625 mg, then 0.625 mg + 5 mg once daily sequentially |
| | Femhrt (Warner Chilcott) | Norethindrone acetate + ethinyl estradiol | 1 mg + 5 mcg once daily, continuously |
| | Prefest (Monarch) | Estradiol 3 tabs then estradiol + norgestimate 3 tabs | 1 mg, then 1 mg + 0.9 mg, once daily sequentially |
| | Activella (Novo Nordisk) | Estradiol + norethindrone acetate | 1 mg + 0.5 mg once daily |
| Combination estrogen + progestogen transdermals | Climara Pro (Berlex) | Estradiol + levonorgestrel | 0.045 mg + 0.015 mg once weekly |
| | Combipatch (Novartis) | Estradiol + norethindrone acetate | 0.05 mg + 0.14 mg per day<br>0.05 mg + 0.25 mg per day twice weekly |
| Combination estrogen + androgens | Estratest HS (Solvay) | Esterified estrogens + methyltestosterone | 0.625 mg + 1.25 mg once daily |
| | Estratest (Solvay) | Esterified estrogens + methyltestosterone | 1.25 mg + 2.5 mg once daily |

*See prescribing reference for full information on doses, side effects, contraindications, and cautions.

Source: Schuiling, K. D., & Likis, F. E. (2006). *Women's gynecologic health.* Sudbury, MA: Jones and Bartlett.

## MENSTRUAL CYCLE

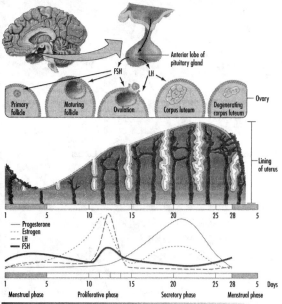

FIGURE M-1    Menstrual Cycle Overview.

M

**Gonadotropins**

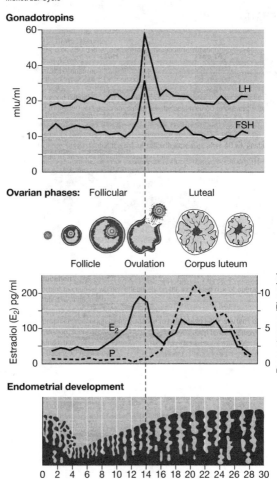

**Ovarian phases:**    Follicular                    Luteal

Follicle          Ovulation          Corpus luteum

**Endometrial development**

Days of menstrual cycle

FIGURE M-2    Menstrual Cycle.

**SOURCE**
Schuiling, K. D., & Likis, F. E. (2006). *Women's gynecologic health*. Sudbury, MA: Jones and Bartlett.

# METHADONE

### Definition
Used to prevent opioid craving

Has longer half-life than heroin

During pregnancy used to hold level stable to decrease risk of fetal withdrawal

A 2005 national survey found that nearly 4% of pregnant women between the ages of 15 and 44 reported illicit drug use in the previous month. Among pregnant women admitted to substance abuse programs, 15% identified heroin as the primary substance used. Methadone is a recommended treatment for pregnant women wishing to discontinue their use of heroin.

### Risks During Pregnancy
Reduced fetal growth

Premature birth

Lower birth rate

No known teratogenicity

### Labor Pain Management
Personal dose of methadone in addition to anesthesia and analgesia for pain

Choices other than opioid agonist/antagonists (do not give stadol or nubain)

### Neonatal Abstinence Syndrome
Never use Narcan after birth

Begins in the first week of life

Characterized by CNS irritability and GI dysfunction

May need withdrawal tx

### Breastfeeding
Studies have shown the amount of methadone in breastmilk to be small, and to have little effect on the behaviors exhibited with neonatal withdrawal syndrome. The American Academy of Pediatrics states that maternal methadone use is usually compatible with breastfeeding.

**SOURCE**

Goff, M., & O'Connor, M. (2007). Perinatal care of women maintained on methadone. *Journal of Midwifery & Women's Health, 52*(3), 23–26.

**M**

## METHERGIN

Also known as ergonovine/methylergonovine, Ergotrate, ergometrine, methylergometrine, ergotrate maleate

### Class
Ergot alkaloid
Uterine stimulant

### Indication
Postpartum hemorrhage associated with uterine atony
Uterine subinvolution

### Dose
0.2 mg IM (may be repeated Q 2–4 h intervals up to 5 doses), then 0.2 mg PO TID–QID as needed (MAX duration: 7 d)
IV dosing (same as IM) only as a lifesaving measure, d/t risk for sudden onset HTN and increased CVA risk; give slowly over 1 min with constant BP monitoring
Peak (oral): 1 h
Half-life: 3.4 h

### Monitor
Blood pressure
Heart rate
Uterine response
Uterine bleeding

### Contraindication
HTN
Preeclampsia
Eclampsia

### Side Effects
HTN
Sweating
N/V
Dizziness
H/A
Tinnitus
Angina
MI (rare)
Seizure

### Breastfeeding
Lact Cat L2 generally, Lact Cat L4 if chronic use
Anecdotal reports of impaired or delayed milk production in mothers taking oral methergine

**SOURCE**
Hale, T. W. (2008). *Medications and mothers' milk* (13th ed.). Amarillo, TX: Hale.

## MIDWIVES

TABLE M-6  Types of Midwives

| | OB/Gyn Physician | Certified Nurse Midwives | Certified Midwives | Certified Professional Midwives | Direct-Entry Midwives | Lay Midwives | Doula |
|---|---|---|---|---|---|---|---|
| Job Description | Medical professional providing comprehensive obstetric and gynecologic care including high-risk obstetrics | Multidisciplinary license in both nursing and midwifery<br><br>Provides primary health care to women of childbearing age including: prenatal care, labor and delivery care, care after birth, gynecological exams, newborn care, assistance with family planning decisions, preconception care, menopausal management, and counseling in health maintenance and disease prevention | Provides primary health care to women of childbearing age including: prenatal care, labor and delivery care, care after birth, gynecological exams, newborn care, assistance with family planning decisions, preconception care, menopausal management, and counseling in health maintenance and disease prevention | Independent midwifery practitioner who has met the standards for certification set by the North American Registry of Midwives (NARM) and is qualified to provide the midwifery model of care | Independent practitioner educated in the discipline of midwifery through self-study, apprenticeship, a midwifery school, or a college- or university-based program distinct from the discipline of nursing | Educated through informal routes such as self-study or apprenticeship rather than through a formal program.<br><br>This term does not necessarily mean a low level of education, just that the midwife either chose not to become certified or licensed, or there was no certification available for her type of education (as was the fact before the Certified Professional Midwife credential was available). | Accompanies a woman in labor taking care of her emotional needs throughout childbirth.<br><br>Offers information, assistance, and advice on topics such as breathing, relaxation, movement, and positioning.<br><br>Doulas do not perform clinical tasks, diagnose medical conditions, or give medical advice. |

/continues

M

TABLE M-6  Types of Midwives (continued)

| | OB/Gyn Physician | Certified Nurse Midwives | Certified Midwives | Certified Professional Midwives | Direct-Entry Midwives | Lay Midwives | Doula |
|---|---|---|---|---|---|---|---|
| Education | Medical school and a residency in OB/Gyn | Registered nurse and a master's level degree in midwifery | Certification according to the requirements of the American College of Nurse-Midwives | Met the standard of North American Registry of Midwives | Self-study, apprenticeship, and/or a midwifery program distinct from the discipline of nursing | Self-study or apprenticeship rather than through a formal program | Education in normal processes of childbirth via independent study, workshop style training, and experience |
| Place of Practice | Hospitals | Hospitals Birth centers Home birth | Hospitals Birth centers Home birth | Birth centers Home birth | Home birth Some birth centers | Home birth | Wherever the mother is giving birth |
| Insurance Coverage | Complete coverage | Complete coverage | Complete in certain states | Limited coverage | Limited coverage | No coverage | No coverage |
| Scope of Practice | All aspects of care including high risk | Low risk | Low risk | Out of hospital care | Out of hospital care | Out of hospital care | Strictly support and encouragement, no direct physical healthcare responsibilities |

Sources: Adapted from American College of Nurse Midwives. (2005). Become a midwife. Retrieved August 10, 2008, from http://www.midwife.org/become_midwife.cfm. DONA International. (2005). What is a doula? Retrieved August 10, 2008, from http://www.dona.org/mothers/index.php MANA. (2008). Midwives alliance of North America definitions. Retrieved August 12, 2008, from http://mana.org/definitions.html. North American Registry of Midwives. (2008). How to become a NARM certified professional midwife. Retrieved August 10, 2008, from http://www.narm.org/htb.htm.

# MOLAR PREGNANCY

Gestational trophoblastic disease (GTD)

## Statistics

1 in 1000 pregnancies in the United States and Europe
Recurs in 2% of women with previous dx
Increased risk with advance maternal age
2–8% are malignant

## Etiology

Partial—fetal tissue is often present (69,XXX or 69,XXY)
Complete—contains no fetal tissue (46,XX or 46,XY)
Resulting from either dispermy or an aberrant duplication of the paternal genomic material
Trophoblastic tissue invades the uterus

## Signs and Symptoms

Continuous or intermittent brown or bloody discharge evident by about 12 wk, usually not profuse
Uterine enlargement out of proportion to the duration of pregnancy in about half of the cases
Absence of fetal parts and fetal heart motion
Characteristic U/S appearance
Serum B-hCG level higher than expected for the stage of gestation
Preeclampsia/eclampsia developing before 24 wk
Hyperemesis gravidarum

## Diagnosis

*Complete*

U/S shows no fetal/embryonic tissue
No amniotic fluid
Central heterogeneous mass with anechoic spaces diffuse swelling of hydropic chorionic villi, theca lutein cysts ≥ 6 cm in diameter
High serum B-hCG usually > 100, 000 IU/ml

*Partial*

U/S shows fetal embryonic tissue present (may be viable), but often is IUGR
Amniotic fluid present
Focal hydatidiform swelling and/or increased echogenicity of chorionic villi, increased transverse diameter of gestational sac
Theca lutein cysts are absent

**M**

## Treatment

Refer for MD management
Counsel regarding the need for immediate evacuation and subsequent evaluation for persistent trophoblastic proliferation or malignant change
Rh neg pt needs RhoGAM

## Follow-Up

Pregnancy prevention for a minimum of 6 mos using hormonal contraception
Monitoring of serum B-hCG levels Q 2 wk
Persistence or elevation of serum B-hCG may indicate trophoblastic neoplasia (unless the woman is pregnant again)
After B-hCG levels become undetectable, evaluate level Q month for 6 mo
If level remains WNL then pregnancy can be attempted within one yr

**SOURCE**
Cunningham, G., Leveno, K. J., Bloom, S. L., Hauth, J. C., Gilstrap, L. C., & Wenstrom, K. D. (2005). *Williams obstetrics* (22nd ed.). New York: McGraw-Hill.

## MULTIPLE GESTATIONS

Identify as early in pregnancy as possible

### Signs and Symptoms
S > D

Severe N/V due to increased B-hCG

Abdominal palpation of 3 or more large parts

Auscultation of more than one (nonmaternal) distinct heart tone differing by more than 10 bpm. Higher suspicion if family hx of twins

Use of ovulation stimulators (Clomid or Pergonal)

### Risks
Fetal anomalies

Early pregnancy loss

Stillbirth

IUGR

Placenta previa

PTL

PTB

GDM

Preeclampsia

Malpresentation

Dysfunctional labor

PPH

### Types of Twins
Monozygotic: one egg, one sperm, identical

Dizygotic: two eggs, two sperms, fraternal

Monochorionic/monoamniotic: one sac, one placenta, greatest risk for cord accidents

Monochorionic/diamniotic: two sacs, one placenta

Dichorionic/diamniotic (fused placenta): two sacs, fused placenta

Dichorionic/diamniotic (separate placenta): separate sac and placenta

### Twin-to-Twin Transfusion
Cases in which there is one placenta and blood supply is shunted to one twin

Discordant growth

### Monitoring
1. NST every 2 wks 24–36 wks
2. NST weekly > 36 wks
3. Fetal growth monitored by U/S every 3–4 wks starting at 20 wks

SOURCE

Varney, H., Kriebs, J. M., & Gegor, C. L. (2004). *Varney's midwifery* (4th ed.). Sudbury, MA: Jones and Bartlett.

# NAUSEA AND VOMITING: PREGNANCY

### Differential Diagnosis

Molar pregnancy
Hyperthyroid
Multiple gestation
Pancreatitis
Cholestasis
Hepatitis
Influenza
GI upset
Hyperemesis gravidarum

### Relief Measures

Small frequent meals
Dry crackers or toast before getting out of bed and/or in the middle of the night
Do not brush teeth after eating to avoid gag reflex
Carbonated beverages (ginger ale)
Avoid smelly foods
Restrict fats
Acupressure wristbands
Rest
It will go away eventually (as HCG level drops nausea typically resolves)

### First Line Treatment

Ginger 500–1500 mg Q d, in divided doses
Vitamin $B_6$ (pyridoxine) 25 mg QID or 50 mg BID
Add Unisom (doxylamine) 12.5 mg (1/2 tab) in the morning, 12.5 mg 6–8 h later, 25 mg (1 tab) Qhs to each dose of vitamin $B_6$ if symptoms do not improve with vitamin $B_6$ alone

### Hyperemesis Gravidarum

*Signs and Symptoms*

Tachycardia
Hypotension
Dry mucous membranes
Decreased skin turgor
Wt loss or lack of appropriate Wt gain
Ketonuria
Increased urine specific gravity
Elevated HCT
Elevated BUN
Decreased serum urea level
Hyponatremia
Hypokalemia
Hypochloremia
Metabolic acidosis
Elevated liver transaminase levels

*Differential Diagnosis*

Wernicke's encephalopathy (very rare; from vitamin B deficiency)
Hepatitis
Appendicitis
Pyelonephritis
Uremia
Twisted ovarian cyst
Drug toxicity
Hyperthyroidism
CNS lesions
Vestibular disorders
Severe preeclampsia
Hydatiform mole
Psychiatric disorder

*Diagnosis*

Pregnancy test
Urinalysis and test for ketones
Serum electrolytes
TFTs and LFTs

*Treatment*

IV hydration and NPO × 24 h
Antiemetic suitable for pregnancy
Correction of electrolyte imbalances
Hyperalimentation or enteral nutrition
Organize schedule around frequent small, low-fat meals
Activity modification, if activity brings on vomiting
*See Table N-1.*

**N**

### SOURCES

Boone, S., & Shields, K. (2005). Treating pregnancy related nausea and vomiting with ginger. *Annals of Pharmacotherapy, 39*(10), 1710–1713.

Epocrates, I. (2008). *Epocrates online*. Retrieved May 27, 2008, from http://www.epocrates.com

Gabbe, S. G., Niebyl, J. R., & Simpson, J. L. (Eds.). (2002). *Obstetrics: Normal and problem pregnancies* (4th ed.). New York: Churchill Livingstone.

Hale, T. W. (2008). *Medications and mothers' milk* (13th ed.). Amarillo, TX: Hale.

Jewell, D. (2003). Nausea and vomiting in early pregnancy. *Clinical Evidence,* (9), 1561–1570.

Varney, H., Kriebs, J. M., & Gegor, C. L. (2004). *Varney's midwifery* (4th ed.). Sudbury, MA: Jones and Bartlett.

TABLE N-1 Medication for Treatment of Nausea and Vomiting

| Medication Information | Dose | Pharmacology | Contraindications | Side Effects |
|---|---|---|---|---|
| Meclazine | 12.5 mg PO TID/PRN | Antiemetic | Hypersensitivity to drug/class | Drowsiness |
| | | Antivertigo | | Dry mouth |
| | | Motion sickness | CAUTION with glaucoma, asthma, | Blurred vision |
| | | | COPD, GI obstruction | Thickened bronchial secretions |
| | | | | Confusion |
| | | | | Paradoxical CNM stimulation |
| Preg Cat B | | | | Urinary retention |
| Lact Cat L3 | | | | Constipation |
| Kytril | 1 mg PO daily | Antiemetic | Hypersensitivity to drug/class | Leukopenia |
| | | | Neonates/Premature infants | Thrombocytopenia |
| | | | | Anemia |
| | | | CAUTION recent abdominal surgery | Fetal gasping syndrome |
| | | | | Headache |
| | | | | Asthenia |
| | | | | Somnolence |
| | | | | Diarrhea |
| Preg Cat B | | | | Constipation |
| Lact Cat L3 | | | | Fever |
| | | | | Rash |
| | | | | HTN |
| | | | | Taste changes |
| | | | | Alopecia |

/continues

**TABLE N-1** Medication for Treatment of Nausea and Vomiting (continued)

| Medication Information | Dose | Pharmacology | Contraindications | Side Effects |
|---|---|---|---|---|
| Promethazine (Phenergan)<br><br>Preg Cat C<br>Lact Cat L2 | 12.5–25 mg PO/IM/PR Q 4–6 h | Antiemetic, antihistamine, phenothiazine | Hypersensitivity to drug or class, narrow-angle glaucoma<br><br>CAUTION with asthma, seizure disorder, hepatic dysfunction, bone marrow suppression | Tardive dyskinesia, extrapyramidal effects, respiratory depression, hypotension, bradycardia, tachycardia, agranulocytosis, thrombocytopenia, dry mouth, sedation, drowsiness, N/V, rash, thickened bronchial secretions |
| Ondansetron (Zofran)<br><br>Preg Cat B<br>Lact Cat L2 | 8 mg PO/IM Q 12 h | Antiemetic, serotonin receptor antagonist | Hypersensitivity to drug or class<br><br>CAUTION with hepatic dysfunction | Bronchospasm, extrapyramidal symptoms, oculogyric crisis, headache, fatigue, constipation, diarrhea, agitation, pruritus, and dizziness |
| Metoclopramide (Reglan)<br><br>Preg Cat B<br>Lact Cat L2 | 5–10 mg PO/IM Q 6–8 h | Antiemetic, antivertigo GI stimulant, Prolactin stimulant | Hypersensitivity to drug or class, pheochromocytoma, seizure disorder, GI bleeding, GI obstruction<br><br>CAUTION with cirrhosis, CHF, renal or hepatic dysfunction, Parkinson's disease, hypertension, psychosis, depression, breast cancer | Suicidal ideation, seizures, neutropenia, agranulocytosis, bronchospasm, dystonic reactions, galactorrhea, amenorrhea, hypotension, hypertension, arrhythmia, urinary frequency, insomnia, headache, confusion |

/continues

N

**TABLE N-1** Medication for Treatment of Nausea and Vomiting (continued)

| Medication Information | Dose | Pharmacology | Contraindications | Side Effects |
|---|---|---|---|---|
| Prochlorperazine (Compazine)<br><br>Preg Cat C<br>Lact Cat L3 | 5–10 mg Q 3–4 h IM/PO or 25 mg BID PR | Antiemetic, antivertigo, antipsychotic, phenothiazine | Hypersensitivity to drug or class, CNS depression, adrenergic blockade, phenothiazine blood dyscrasia<br><br>CAUTION with glaucoma, epilepsy, cardiovascular disease, bone marrow suppression | ECG abnormalities, agranulocytosis, thrombocytopenia, hemolytic anemia, hepatotoxicity, drowsiness, amenorrhea, blurred vision, rash, orthostatic hypotension, anxiety, photosensitivity |
| Chlorpromazine (Thorazine)<br><br>Preg Cat C<br>Lact Cat L3 | 25–50 mg PR Q 6–8 h or 25–50 mg IM Q 3–4 h | Tranquilizer | Hypersensitivity to drug or class, bone marrow depression, sedation, Parkinson's disease<br><br>CAUTION with hepatic failure and hypotension | Seizure, thrombocytopenia, agranulocytosis, neuroleptic malignant syndrome |
| Methylprednisolone<br><br>Preg Cat B<br>Lact Cat L2 | 16 mg TID for 3 d, then taper over 2 wk | Corticosteroid | Hypersensitivity to drug or class, systemic fungal infection<br><br>CAUTION with CHF, seizure disorder, DM, HTN, osteoporosis, tuberculin, hepatic dysfunction | Immunosuppression, HTN, peptic ulcer, CHF, adrenal insufficiency, N/V/D, insomnia, anxiety, edema, appetite change, hyperglycemia |

Sources: Epocrates, I. (2008). Epocrates online. Retrieved May 27, 2008, from http://www.epocrates.com. Hale, T. W. (2008). Medications and mothers' milk (13th ed.). Amarillo, TX: Hale Publishing.

# NEONATES: CARDIAC DEFECTS

**Vital Signs**

Respirations: 30–60 breaths/min
HR: 80–160 bpm
Temp: 36.5–37°C (97.9–98.3°F)

**Look**

General appearance: comfortable, irritable, lethargic, diaphoretic
Respiratory effort: tachypnic, nasal flaring, retractions (intercostal, diaphragmatic)
Color: mottled, cyanotic, dusky

**Listen**

You may only get one chance; do not touch the baby until your stethoscope is on the chest
Rate & rhythm: regular, tachycardic, bradycardic
Sounds: S1, S2 (single, loud, split), murmurs, systolic/diastolic, harsh/musical, loud/soft
Know where you are starting, and do not ignore changes in your exam

**Feel**

Precordium (feel with the ball of your fingers): active, hyperdynamic
Where is the PMI?
Can you feel a thrill?
Extremities: temperature, pulses (check brachial & femoral pulse)
Fontanel: sunken, bulging
Abdomen: liver enlarged, spleen enlarged (use percussion)

**Anomalies**

Acyanotic defects:
Ventricular septal defect (VSD)
Atrial septal defect (ASD)
Large patent ductus arteriosus (PDA)
Complete atrioventricular canal (CAVC)
Coarctation of the aorta
Pulmonary stenosis/atresia
Aortic stenosis
Interrupted aortic arch
Mitral stenosis
Cyanotic defects:
Tetralogy of fallot
Tricuspid atresia
Ebstein's anomaly of the tricuspid valve
Truncus arteriosus
Congestive heart failure
Transposition of the great arteries
Hypoplastic left heart syndrome

N

**SOURCE**

Thureen, P., Hall, D., Deacon, J., & Hernandez, J. (2004). *Assessment and care of the well newborn* (2nd ed.). St. Louis, MO: Saunders.

## NEONATES: PREVENTIVE MEDICATIONS

### Erythromycin

*0.5% Erythromycin Ointment*
Prophylaxis against infections caused by GC and/or CT which can cause blindness in neonates

*Instructions*
Apply to eye from inner to outer canthus
Not necessary to wash off after application
Application should be deferred until after first period of reactivity so that bonding can occur

### Vitamin K

*Purpose*
Prophylactic prevention of hemorrhagic disease of the newborn
Only prevents classic hemorrhagic disease, which occurs in the first 1–7 d, no effect on late hemorrhagic disease (2–12 wk)

*Hemorrhagic Disease of the Newborn (HDN)*
Early < 24 h
Classic 1–7 d
Late 2–12 wk

*Cochrane Review Statement*
A single dose (1.0 mg) of intramuscular vitamin K after birth is effective in the prevention of classic HDN. Either intramuscular or oral (1.0 mg) vitamin K prophylaxis improves biochemical indices of coagulation status at 1–7 days. Neither intramuscular nor oral vitamin K has been tested in randomized trials with respect to effect on late HDN. Oral vitamin K, either single or multiple dose, has not been tested in randomized trials for its effect on either classic or late HDN.

*Notes*
IM or oral administration increases coagulation on d 1–7
Oral administration has multiple dosing regimes, there is no agreed-upon dosing schedule; one example is dosing at birth, 2 wk, and 6 wk
Natural sources of vitamin K: kelp, parsley, alphalfa

**SOURCE**
Puckett, R., & Offringa, M. (2000). Prophylactic vitamin K for vitamin K deficiency bleeding in neonates. *Cochrane Database of Systematic Reviews, 4*(002776).
Varney, H., Kriebs, J. M., & Gegor, C. L. (2004). *Varney's midwifery* (4th ed.). Sudbury, MA: Jones and Bartlett.

# NEONATES: RESUSCITATION

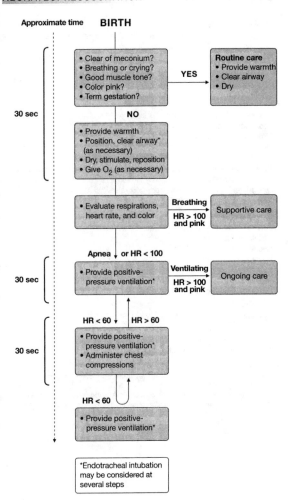

**FIGURE N-1** Neonatal Resuscitation. *Source:* Reprinted with permission from Niermeyer, S., Kattwinkel, J., Van Reempts, P., Nadkarni, V., Phillips, B., & Zideman, D., et al. (2000). International guidelines for neonatal resuscitation: An excerpt from the guidelines 2000 for cardiopulmonary resuscitation and emergency cardiovascular care: International consensus on science. *Pediatrics, 106*(3), E29.

**SOURCE**

Niermeyer, S., Kattwinkel, J., Van Reempts, P., Nadkarni, V., Phillips, B., Zideman, D., et al. (2000). International guidelines for neonatal resuscitation: An excerpt from the guidelines 2000 for cardiopulmonary resuscitation and emergency cardiovascular care: International consensus on science. Contributors and reviewers for the neonatal resuscitation guidelines. *Pediatrics, 106*(3):E29.

## NEONATES: TRANSIENT TACHYPNEA OF NEWBORN

### Definition and Statistics

Benign condition that results from delayed clearance of lung fluid in newborns

Rapid breathing (> 60 bpm), otherwise healthy

Occurs in approx. 1–2% of newborns

Breathing rate may rise as high as 100–150 breaths/min

Can start 2–6 h after birth but usually resolves in 24–48 h

May be caused, in part, by a genetic variation of surfactant protein B

### Risk Factors

C/S (especially elective with no trial of labor)

Babies who experienced asphyxia or cord prolapse

Mild surfactant deficiency

Moms who have experienced sedation, overhydration, asthma, betamimetic drugs, bleeding, or diabetes

Cord compression or vasoconstriction (due to hypoxia or cord clamping) can cause hypovolemia diminishing the swallow and cough reflex, which can lead to a poor respiratory effort and a delayed circulatory transition

Male infants are also more at risk for unknown reasons

### Differential Diagnosis

Respiratory distress syndrome

Meconium aspiration

Infection

Hypoglycemic

Hypothermia

Persistent pulmonary hypertension

Congenital heart defect

Pneumothorax

### Treatment

R/o other conditions

Give oxygen

Keep newborn warm and provide nutrition

### SOURCES

Frye, A. (2004). *Holistic midwifery A comprehensive textbook for midwives in homebirth practice.* Portland, OR: Labrys Press.

Riskin, A., Abend-Weinger, M., Riskin-Mashiah, S., Kugelman, A., & Bader, D. (2005). Cesarean section, gestational age, and transient tachypnea of the newborn: Timing is the key. *American Journal of Perinatology, 22*(7), 377–382.

Thureen, P., Hall, D., Deacon, J., & Hernandez, J. (2004). *Assessment and care of the well newborn* (2nd ed.). St. Louis, MO: Saunders.

# NONSTRESS TEST (NST)

## Definition
Assessment of the fetal heart rate in response to fetal activity as a measure of fetal well-being

## Steps for Exam
1. Patient should be in side-lying position
2. External electronic fetal monitor and tocometer placed on mother's abdomen
3. Identify FHR baseline (average for 3 min time period)
4. Monitor continuously for 20 min with the mother noting each fetal movement she feels during that time period

## Results

*Reactive*
At least 2 accelerations of the FHR within a 20 min period that are above the baseline for at least 15 sec with a minimum amplitude increase of 15 bpm

*Nonreactive*
FHR that fails to demonstrate adequate number or amplitude of FHR accelerations within any 20 min period

*Inconclusive*
Any FHR pattern that is not interpretable as reactive or nonreactive

## Notes
Before 32 wk accelerations $10 \times 10$ and before 26 wk no accelerations
Acoustic stimulation of the baby to wake it from sleeping is acceptable

## Twice Weekly Testing Suggested

| | |
|---|---|
| Bleeding in 2nd or 3rd trimester | Polyhydramnios |
| DM Type I | Macrosomia |
| GDM | Postdates (> 41 wks) |
| Chronic HTN, or HTN after 32 wk | PIH |
| Fetal arrhythmia | Rh sensitization |
| IUGR | Structural abnormalities |
| Isoimmunization | Twins |
| Elevated MSAFP (unexplained) | Variable decelerations |
| Oligohydramnios | Abnormal Quad screen (High INH A or low E3) |
| Placenta previa | IUFD hx (do NST at 32 wk or 1 wk prior to gestational age of previous demise) |

N

## Once Weekly Testing Suggested

| | |
|---|---|
| Advanced maternal age | Polyhydramnios |
| Asthma exacerbation | Poor maternal wt gain |
| Fetal bradycardia (< 100 bpm) | Substance abuse |
| Diabetes or GDM | |

## Other Fetal Assessment Tools
AFI

## Contraction Stress Test
Needs to achieve 3 contractions in 10 min
Positive if late decelerations with 50% of the contractions
Negative result is reassuring

### SOURCES
Frye, A. (1997). *Understanding diagnostic tests in the childbearing years* (6th ed.). Portland, OR: Labrys Press.
Gabbe, S. G., Niebyl, J. R., & Simpson, J. L. (Eds.). (2002). *Obstetrics: Normal and problem pregnancies* (4th ed.). New York: Churchill Livingstone.
Varney, H., Kriebs, J. M., & Gegor, C. L. (2004). *Varney's midwifery* (4th ed.). Sudbury, MA: Jones and Bartlett.

# NUTRITION DURING PREGNANCY AND LACTATION

## Pregnancy

Increase calories by 100–300 calories/d (equivalent to one extra snack/d)

### Make Sure Daily Diet Includes

6 oz of grains (1 slice bread, 1/2 cup rice, 1/2 cup pasta)
2.5 cups of vegetables
1.5–2 cups of fruit
5–5.5 oz meat/protein
3 cups milk (calcium equivalent)
400 mcg folic acid daily (see Vitamins)
Vitamin A, C, $B_6$, and $B_{12}$ daily (see Vitamins)

### Avoid

Unpasteurized milk and soft cheeses
Raw or under cooked meats, poultry, and shellfish
Prepared meats such as hotdogs and deli meats
Unwashed fruits and vegetables

## Caution with Fish

Fish is a healthy food source during pregnancy and contains important omega fatty acids that aid in brain development
Women can eat up to 12 oz of fish Q wk
Some fish contain high levels of methylmercury that can harm the development of the neurological system of a fetus

### Do Not Eat

| | |
|---|---|
| Shark | King mackerel |
| Swordfish | Tilefish |

### Maximum Intake

Farmed salmon Q month
Albacore tuna ("white" tuna) Q wk (6 oz)
Shrimp, canned light tuna, canned or wild salmon, pollock, and catfish: 1–2 meals Q wk
Check local information about locally caught fish or limit intake to once Q wk

## Vegetarian/Vegan-Specific Needs

Vitamin D—10–15 min of direct sunlight QD (hands, face, and arms exposed)
3 servings of iron-rich foods QD
One source of vitamin C, A, and folic QD
Vitamin $B_{12}$ daily (primarily found in shellfish, eggs, and dairy products so supplements probably needed)
3 servings of protein daily (1 serving = 1/2 cup beans/peas, 1/2 cup tofu, 1/4 cup nuts/seeds, 2 T peanut butter, 1 egg, 2 egg whites)

## Breastfeeding

Increase calories by 500 extra calories QD for breastfeeding

### SOURCES

American College of Nurse Midwives. (2004). Eating safely during pregnancy. *Share with Women, 49*(4).

American College of Obstetricians and Gynecologists. (2008). *Nutrition during pregnancy* (Patient Education Pamphlets No. 12345/65432). Washington, DC: Author.

Cleveland Clinic Foundation. (2008). *Nutrition during pregnancy for vegetarianism.* Retrieved August 10, 2008, from http://my.clevelandclinic.org/healthy_living/pregnancy/hic_nutrition_during_pregnancy_for_vegetarians.aspx

March of Dimes. (2007). *Mercury and fish.* Retrieved May 24, 2008, from http://search.marchofdimes.com/cgi-bin/MsmGo.exe?grab_id=6&page_id=6095104&query=fish+during+pregnancy&hiword=FISHE+FISHER+FISHERS+FISHING+FISHMAN+PREGNANCIES+PREGNANT+during+fish+pregnancy+

Penney, D. S., & Miller, K. G. (2008). Nutritional counseling for vegetarians during pregnancy and lactation. *Journal of Midwifery & Women's Health, 53,* 37–44.

Varney, H., Kriebs, J. M., & Gegor, C. L. (2004). *Varney's midwifery* (4th ed.). Sudbury, MA: Jones and Bartlett.

# OSTEOPOROSIS

## Definition
Low bone mass and microarchitectural changes in bone structure causing an increase in the possibility of bone fracture

An imbalance between osteoclasts that break down bone and osteoblasts that build up bone leading towards increased osteoclasts activity

## Bone Density Assessment
1. Dual X-ray absorptiometry (DEXA) scan—Determines bone mass of specific vulnerable bones and creates a score that is compared to the generalized scores of young healthy women
2. U/S
3. Computed tomography
4. Radiography

## Diagnosis by DEXA

*Criteria for Osteoporosis (T Score)*
Normal -1 to 0 = No tx
Osteopenia -2.5 to -1.0 = Tx if risk factor
Osteoporosis < -2.5 = Tx
Severe Osteoporosis < −2.5 + > fragility fracture = Tx

## Risk Factors
Female sex
Older age
Asian/white
Family hx
Petite stature
Low body wt < 127 lb
Amenorrhea—primary and secondary
Sedentary lifestyle
Menopause, specifically premature onset
Low calcium intake
Smoking
Excess EtOH
Excess caffeine
Low testosterone in men

*Drugs That Increase Risk*
Thyroid replacement drugs
Lithium
Glucocorticoids
Anticonvulsants
Chemotherapy
Heparin

*Disease States That Increase Risk*
Anorexia/bulimia
Cushing's syndrome
Thyrotoxicosis
RA and other neuromuscular disorders
DM type I
Thalassemia

*Calcium Requirements*
See Calcium page

## Treatment (Symptom Free/Osteopenia)
Dietary modification—increase calcium and decrease salt, animal protein, and caffeine
Exercise—weight bearing exercise such as walking or aerobics

Estrogen—hormone replacement slows bone deterioration, evaluate risks and
benefits, Calcitonin—hormone which inhibits osteoclast activity, derived from
salmon, eel, and porcine sources

## Pharmacological Treatment

TABLE 0-1   Pharmacological Tx for Osteoporosis

| Medication | FDA Approved for | Considerations |
|---|---|---|
| Alendronate (Fosamax) | Prevention—5 mg orally daily or 35 mg orally weekly | Caution if upper gastrointestinal disease, clinical association with dysphagia, esophagitis, or ulceration |
| | Treatment—10 mg orally daily or 70 mg orally weekly | Take first thing in the morning on an empty stomach with 8 oz glass of water, remain upright and take no other food or drink for at least 30 minutes |
| Risedronate (Actonel) | Prevention or treatment—5 mg orally daily or 35 mg orally weekly | Take 2 hours before antacids/calcium |
| Calcitonin (Miacalcin) | Treatment—200 IU intranasal spray daily or 100 IU IM or SC every other day | Usually administered as nasal spray. Has analgesic effect on osteoporotic fractures |
| Estrogen (i.e., Premarin, Estratab, Menest, Alora, Climara, Estraderm, Menostar, Vivelle, Vivelle Dot, Estrace, Femhrt*, Activella**, Ortho-prefest**, Prempro**, others) | Prevention—Doses and routes vary*** | Also effective in alleviating most symptoms of menopause. Comes in several forms, including pills, patch, ring, and cream |
| Raloxifene (Evista) | Prevention or treatment—60 mg orally daily | May cause hot flashes. Not recommended if taking ET or EPT |
| Teriparitide (Forteo) | Treatment—20 mcg subcutaneously daily | Reserved for use after failure of first-line agents |

*See prescribing reference for full information on doses, side effects, contraindications, and cautions.
**Also contains progesterone compounds.
***Lowest effective dose should be used. The FDA recommends considering non-estrogen
osteoporotic agents when ET/EPT use is solely for the purpose of osteoporosis prevention.

Sources: Dawson-Hughes et al., 2003; Hodgson & Watts, 2003.

## SOURCES

Dawson-Hughes, B., Gold, D. T., Rodbard, H. W., Bonner, F. J., Khosla, S., & Swift, S. (2003). Physician's guide to prevention and treatment of osteoporosis (2nd ed.). Washington, DC: National Osteoporosis Foundation.

Hodgson, S. F., & Watts, S. F. (2003). American Association of Clinical Endocrinologists medical guidelines for clinical practice for the prevention and treatment of postmenopausal osteoporosis: 2001 edition with selected updates for 2003. Endocrine Practice, 9(6), 544–564.

Kanis, J. (2002). Diagnosis of osteoporosis and assessment of fracture risk. Lancet, 359, 1929–1936.

Lindsay, R. (1993). Prevention and treatment of osteoporosis. Lancet, 341(8848), 801–805.

Schuiling, K. D., & Likis, F. E. (2006). Women's gynecologic health. Sudbury, MA: Jones and Bartlett.

Weinstein, L., & Ullery, B. (2000). Identification of at-risk women for osteoporosis screening. American Journal of Obstetrics & Gynecology, 183(3), 547–549.

# PAPANICOLAOU (PAP) SMEAR

### Indication
Used for screening of precancerous or cancerous changes in the cervix/vaginal pouch

### Statistics
Approximately 7% of Pap smears require follow-up

### Procedure
Current recommendation is the use of thin-prep w/ sample collection by extended tip spatula and cytobrush (some manufacturers offer a tool that combines these two)

### Indications
Current evidence suggests that infection w/ HPV is the leading cause of cervical cancer

Infection w/ HPV can occur in the absence of sexual intercourse through hand/mouth-to-genital contact; therefore, it is important to not discount the need for Pap smears in virginal or lesbian pts

First Pap: W/in 3 yr of onset of sexual activity or by age 21

### Colposcopy
Diagnostic tool used to assess the presence or absence of precancerous or cancerous lesions on the cervix; acetic acid is applied to cervix, cervix is viewed under magnification, and biopsies are taken of suspicious areas

### Guidelines

*ASCUS (Atypical Squamous Cells of Undetermined Significance)*

3 pathways are clinically acceptable:
1. Colposcopy, if neg for CIN then rpt 12 mo
2. Rpt in 4–6 mo, if not normal then colposcopy; if normal × 2 then return to 12 mo schedule
3. Reflexive HPV testing, if HPV positive then colposcopy/biopsy, if negative rpt 12 mo

*ASCUS, Postmenopausal*

Intravaginal estrogen therapy followed by rpt Pap w/in 1 wk of tx completion; if rpt is neg, then rpt in 4–6 mo; if that PAP is neg then routine testing can resume

If either rpt Pap after estrogen therapy is ASCUS, then colposcopy

Immediate colposcopy or HPV testing also acceptable

*ASCUS, Immunosuppressed*

Colposcopy

*ASCUS, Pregnant*

Manage as nonpregnant

*ASCH (ASC Unable to Exclude HSIL)*

HPV testing to help determine best course of management

Colposcopy, if neg then a review of Pap should be performed, management depends on all results

*AGC (Atypical Glandular Cells)*

High risk for neoplasia

Colposcopy w/ endometrial sampling if > 35 yr old or abnormal bleeding

Positive neoplasia manage per ASCCP guidelines

Negative neoplasia, rpt Pap in 4–6 mo intervals × 4, follow appropriate guidelines per result

*LSIL (Low-Grade Squamous Intraepithelial Lesions)*
1 million dx per yr
Immediate colposcopy
Usually appears as CIN I on colposcopy
57% of CIN I return to normal in 1 yr
Colposcopy neg, then HPV testing w/ rpt Pap in 6 mo to 1 yr

*LSIL Postmenopausal*
Consider intravaginal estrogen therapy if not contraindicated; additionally colposcopy or HPV testing are also reasonable therapies

*LSIL Adolescents*
Immediate colposcopy
*Or* Rpt Pap at 6 mo
*Or* HPV testing at 1 yr

*HSIL (High-Grade Squamous Intraepithelial Lesions)*
Immediate colposcopy
Further treatment depends on presence and grade of CIN and consultation of current ASSCP guidelines

*LSIL/HSIL Pregnant*
1. Immediate colposcopy w/ consideration of gestation age and predicted necessary therapy

**See http://www.asccp.org/consensus/cytological.shtml for algorithms**

**SOURCES**
American Society for Colposcopy and Cervical Pathology. (2008). *Consensus guidelines.* Retrieved August 10, 2008, from http://www.asccp.org/consensus/cytological.shtml
Wright, T., Cox, T., Massad, S., Twiggs, L., & Wilkinson, E. (2002). 2001 consensus guidelines for the management of women with cervical cytological abnormalities. *Journal of American Medical Association, 287*(16), 2120.

# PELVIC INFLAMMATORY DISEASE

### Cause
GC

CT

*Mycobacterium hominis*

*Ureaplasma urealyticum*

### Signs and Symptoms
Abnormal bleeding

Dyspareunia

Vaginal discharge

### Rule Out Other Abdominal Pain
*See* Abdominal Pain

Ectopic pregnancy

Acute appendicitis

Functional pain

### Criteria for Possible Diagnosis (Must Have All 3 of These Criteria)
Cervical or uterine motion tenderness

Hx of abdominal pain

Adnexal tenderness

### Other Warning Signs
Temp > 101°F

Mucopurulent discharge

Abundance of WBCs

Elevated sedimentation rate

Elevated C-reactive protein

Positive GC/CT

### Specific Diagnosis
Endometrial biopsy

TVU/S

MRI

Laparoscopy

### Labs

TABLE P-1  Lab Tests for Diagnosis of Pelvic Inflammatory Disease

| Lab Test | Reason |
|---|---|
| GC/CT culture | Common cause of PID |
| Pregnancy test | R/o ectopic pregnancy or undiagnosed IUP |
| Wet mount | Assess for BV and Candida, which may contribute to PID; WBCs typically present in large numbers with PID |
| CBC with sed rate | Assess for anemia, elevated WBCs; elevated sed rate may indicate infection |
| Urinalysis | R/o UTI or pyelonephritis |
| General cervical culture | Assess for organisms other than GC/CT, especially if pt has hx of BV |
| Fecal occult blood test | R/o bowel inflammation/infection/carcinoma as a possible cause of pelvic pain |

*Sources:* Desai, S. P. (2004). *Clinician's guide to laboratory medicine: A practical approach* (3rd ed.). Hudson, OH: Lexi-Comp. Varney, H., Kriebs, J. M., & Gegor, C. L. (2004). *Varney's midwifery* (4th ed.). Sudbury, MA: Jones and Bartlett.

### Treatment
Parenteral tx needed if case is severe

Levofloxacin 500 mg PO QD × 14 d

Ofloxacin 400 mg PO QD × 14 d

W/ or w/o—metronidazole 500 mg PO BID × 14 d

Ceftriazone 125 mg IM once

Doxycyline 100 mg PO BID × 7 d

PQ

### Follow-Up
S/sx should be greatly improved in 3 d, if not then pt requires hospitalization and parenteral tx

### Patient Education
Test sexual partners for STIs

Teach pt about STIs and regular screening

### Pregnancy
Hospitalize women who you think have PID d/t increased risk to fetus

### SOURCES
Centers for Disease Control and Prevention. (2006). *Sexually transmitted diseases treatment guidelines, Morbidity and Mortality Weekly Report, 55*(RR-11), 56–61.

Desai, S. P. (2004). *Clinician's guide to laboratory medicine: A practical approach* (3rd ed.). Hudson, OH: Lexi-Comp.

Hatcher, R. A., Trussell, J. Nelson, A. L., Cates, W., et al. (2007). *Contraceptive technology* (19th ed.). New York: Ardent Media Inc.

## PHYSICAL ASSESSMENT

**The Basics**
Name
Age/DOB
Race
Gender
Gravidity and parity
Last menstrual period

**Chief Complaint (CC)**
Pt's complaint should be in "quotes"

**History of Present Illness (HPI)**
More info regarding CC here
Omit this section if no CC
May write in paragraph form for this section only

*Important Aspects of Any Complaint*
Onset
Location
Duration
Character
Alleviating and aggravating factors
Radiation to other areas
Timing
Severity (on scale of 1–10)

**Past Medical History**
Established dx; include date if known
Overnight hospitalizations
Childhood illnesses
Immunizations
Blood disorders, clots, transfusions
Broken bones
Heart disease
Lung disease—asthma

**Past Surgical History**
Surgical names and dates of procedure (tonsils, wisdom teeth); also mention any
   reactions to anesthesia

**Medications**
Prescription
OTC
Herbals
Note dosage and timing; quantify PRN medications

**Allergies**
NKDA (no known drug allergies)
NKFA (no known food allergies)
If allergies, then state pt's reaction to exposure

**Family History**
Break it down by each family member or by disease state
Always get 3 generations
Ask about maternal and paternal grandparents, close aunts/uncles, parents,
   siblings, children
Important disease states: cancer, heart attack, stroke, coagulopathies

**Social History**
Home life/safety
Relationship status, number of partners, type of intercourse, domestic/partner
   abuse (physical, emotional, sexual)

Occupation/education
Diet/exercise
Caffeine/alcohol/drugs/smoking—always quantify
Recent travel
Religious beliefs

## Review of Systems (ROS)

List systems in a head-to-toe approach

Ask pt about specific symptoms that fall under each system

If positive, you need to gather more info (like CC and HPI)

If negative, use a negative or null sign before the symptom to signify that you have questioned the pt

General: fever/chills/night sweats, fatigue, appetite change, sleep difficulties, wt change

HEENT: H/A, head injuries, change in vision, hearing, taste, or smell, difficulty swallowing, eye/ear/throat pain, nasal congestion

CV: chest pain/palpitations, edema, orthopnea, edema

Respiratory: SOB, wheeze, cough (productive, color, when), sputum, TB exposure, pain, exacerbation with exertion

GI: abd pain, N/V, diarrhea/constipation, bloody or black stool, change in stool, heartburn, indigestion, bowel regularity, flatulence, hemorrhoids, colonoscopy history

GU: hematuria, dysuria, urgency, frequency, dribbling, incontinence

GYN: see GYN Exam

Musculoskeletal: joint pain, loss of coordination, motion restriction, swelling, bony deformities, reddened/hot joints

Hematology: bleeding gums, bruising, nose bleeds, anemia, transfusions

Neuromuscular: dizziness, seizures, numbness or tingling in extremities, syncope episodes

Endocrine: polyphagia/dipsia/uria, nocturia, hair loss, heat or cold intolerance, changes in facial hair, increase in hat or glove size

Dermatology: hair and nail growth, unusual moles or rashes, itching, pigment changes

Psychiatric: anxiety or panic attacks, depression or suicidal thoughts, hx of physical/emotional/sexual abuse—see Domestic Violence

## Physical Exam (PE) (Basic Normal Exam)

General: AAO × 3, pleasant, well-attired, well-nourished, also note eye contact, speech pattern, affect (anxious/withdrawn/depressed/calm, etc.)

Head: NCAT, lesions, normal distribution of hair

Eyes: conjunctiva clear, PERRLA, EOMI, fundi sharp bilaterally, hemorrhages/exudates, Snellen exam, normal color vision

*On PE and for eye-related complaints—note visual acuity w/ Snellen/Rosenbaum

Ears: pain w/ external palpation, canal clear, TM intact, normal bilateral, hearing intact and symmetrical w/ whispered word

*If hearing asymmetrical or if pt c/o hearing loss, do Rinne and Weber test and record results, e.g.: no lateralization noted

Nose: pink turbinates, edema, discharge, erythema

Throat: edema, erythema, exudates, teeth in good repair, gums without erythema, lesions

*If c/o sore throat, note whether there is palatal petechia, trismus, and/or uvular deviation; if yes, a more urgent evaluation is needed

Neck: supple, LAD, thyromegaly, 2+/2+ carotids, bruit

*If respiratory complaint, do not forget to listen over the neck for any stridor; positive stridor would require more urgent evaluation

Heart: RRR, S1/S2/S3/S4, murmur (include grade)

*You can also label this CV and include peripheral vascular system

Lungs: CTAB

*If pt c/o respiratory problem, note respiratory difficulty during hx or PE; assess for rales, wheezing, or rhonchi; if positive then peak flow reading, $O_2$ saturation, RR and rhythm, labored or nonlabored

PQ

Chest: axilla, no LAD bilaterally

Breasts: symmetrical, nodules, dimpling, nipple discharge

*If there is a nodule/mass noted, draw a picture of breast and X the area, record whether the nodule is tender, mobile, irregular

GYN: *See* GYN Exam

Abd: positive BS × 4, soft/NT, HSM, bruits, masses, CVA tenderness

*If complaint of pain, check for rebound tenderness and note any rigidity of the abdomen

Rectal, external: lesions, hemorrhoids, skin tags, bleeding

Rectal, internal: normal intact internal/external sphincter tone; lesions/masses palpated w/ digital exam; brown, soft stool in distal canal, neg hemoccult

*If hemorrhoid, then note if reducible, tender, color (flesh-color, erythematous, purple, etc.)

Lymph nodes: assess for axillary, cervical, clavicular, epitrochlear, and inguinal LAD

*If noted, describe the lymph node (size, shape, consistency, how many, location, tender/nontender, mobile, etc.)

Skin: assess moles as symmetrical, sharp borders, well demarcated, solid brown coloring without variation

Neuromuscular: AAO × 3; articulate speech, eye contact, grade and symmetry of DTRs bilaterally, CN II-XII assessment

Sensory—intact with soft touch and vibration to distal tips the extremities bilaterally; nl F–N–F test with fixed/moving finger/eyes closed; nl RAMs with smooth movements bilat; nl heel to shin bilat; nl tandem; neg Romberg; neg pronator drift; able to keep hands dorsiflexed against resistance

Muscle strength—assess upper and lower extremities bilaterally, grade 1 to 5

**SOURCE**

Seidel, H. M., Ball, J., Dains, J., & Benedict, W. (2006). *Mosby's physical assessment handbook* (6th ed.). St. Louis, MO: Mosby.

# PITOCIN/OXYTOCIN

### Classification
Endocrine-metabolic agent
Posterior pituitary hormone
Uterine stimulant

### Contraindications
Fetal distress where delivery is not imminent
Hypersensitivity
Obstetrical emergencies
Significant CPD
Unfavorable fetal position or presentation
Continued adequate uterine activity w/o cervical dilation or fetal descent
Hyperactive or hypertonic uterus
Vaginal delivery contraindicated

### Maternal Adverse Reactions
N/V
Water intoxication
Cardiac dysrhythmia
Hypertensive episode
PVCs
Afibrinogenemia
Anaphylaxis

Brain damage
CNS deficit
Coma
Postpartum hemorrhage
Uterine rupture
Death

### Fetal/Neonatal Adverse Reactions
Intrapartum bradycardia
Jaundice
Convulsions
Subarachnoid hemorrhage
Retinal hemorrhage
Hematoma
Low APGAR score at 5 min

### Induction/Augmentation

TABLE P-2   Regimens for Pitocin Induction and Augmentation

| Regimen | Starting Dose (mU/min) | Incremental Increase (mU/min) | Dose Interval (min) |
|---|---|---|---|
| Low dose | 0.5–1 | 1 | 30–40 |
|  | 1–2 | 2 | 15 |
| High dose | ~6 | ~6 | 15 |
|  | 6 | 6*, 3, 1 | 20–40 |

*Incremental increase is reduced to 3 mU/min in presence of hyperstimulation and reduced to 1 mU/min with recurrent hyperstimulation

Source: Reprinted with permission from American College of Obstetricians and Gynecologists. (1999). Induction of labor (Clinical Management Guidelines No. 10). In 2006 Compendium of selected publications (p. 562). Washington, DC: Author.

PQ

### Postpartum Hemorrhage
10–40 U of oxytocin added to running IV infusion
Max 40 U to 1000 ml IV solution
Adjust infusion rate to sustain uterine contractions and control uterine atony
10 U IM given after delivery of the placenta

#### SOURCES
American College of Obstetricians and Gynecologists. (1999). Induction of labor: Clinical management guidelines No. 10. In 2006 compendium of selected publications (p. 562). Washington, DC: Author.
Cunningham, G., Leveno, K. J., Bloom, S. L., Hauth, J. C., Gilstrap, L. C., & Wenstrom, K. D. (2005). Williams obstetrics (22nd ed.). New York: McGraw-Hill.

## PLACENTAL ABRUPTION

### Definition
Separation of the placenta from site of implantation before the delivery of the fetus

### Incidence
1 in 200 (vary per source)
80% occur before onset of labor

### Risk Factors
HTN
PIH
Advanced maternal age
Smoking
Poor nutrition
Chorioamnionitis
Blunt trauma
Hx of abruption
Sudden decrease in uterine size (ROM w/ polyhydramnios, twins)
External cephalic version
Cocaine/crack use
PPROM

### Signs and Symptoms
Bleeding (80%)
Abdominal pain
Back pain
Uterine tenderness
Frequent uterine ctx
Persistent uterine hypertonicity
Frank bleeding—coming out of vagina
Occult bleeding—trapped between placenta and myometrium

### Differential Diagnosis
Placenta previa
Labor
Uterine rupture
Coagulopathy
Genital track trauma
Fetal bleeding

### Grading
Grade 1—slight vaginal bleeding, some uterine irritability, normal BP, normal
    fibrinogen, normal FHR
Grade 2—mild to mod vaginal bleeding, irritable uterus, normal BP, elevated pulse,
    decreased fibrinogen (150–250 mg/dl), FHR shows distress
Grade 3—mod to severe bleeding, tetanic painful uterus, hypotension, fetal death,
    fibrinogen decreased (< 150 mg/dl)

### Treatment
This is an emergency!
Get to a location that can care for mother and baby
Start two large bore IVs (16 gauge), IVF 5% dextrose in Ringer's lactate
Type and cross-match at least 4 units of blood

### Labs
HCT/Hb
Fibrinogen
Platelets
Fibrin degradation products
PT
PTT or do a clot test (Fill a red-topped tube w/ blood. If a clot does not form w/in 6
    min or forms and lyses w/in 30 min a coagulation defect is probably present.)

Oxygen

Trendelenburg and warm blankets

Monitor vital signs

Continuously monitor FHR (consider fetal scalp electrode)

Foley catheter to accurately monitor maternal output

Inform woman and her partner of the emergency, possible need for C/S, blood transfusion, neonatal resuscitation

Notify appropriate staff to ready the operating room for emergency C/S

**SOURCES**

Cunningham, G., Leveno, K. J., Bloom, S. L., Hauth, J. C., Gilstrap, L. C., & Wenstrom, K. D. (2005). *Williams obstetrics* (22nd ed.). New York: McGraw-Hill.

Gabbe, S. G., Niebyl, J. R., & Simpson, J. L. (Eds.). (2002). *Obstetrics: Normal and problem pregnancies* (4th ed.). New York: Churchill Livingstone.

Tikkanen, M., Nuutila, M., Hiilesmaa, V., Paavomen, J., & Ylikorkala, O. (2006). Clinical presentation and risk factors of placental abruption. *Acta Obstetricia et Gynecologia Scandinavia, 85*(6), 700.

Varney, H., Kriebs, J. M., & Gegor, C. L. (2004). *Varney's midwifery* (4th ed.). Sudbury, MA: Jones and Bartlett Publishing.

PQ

## PLACENTAL PREVIA

### Definition
Presence of placental tissue overlying or near the internal os
Occurs in 1 in 200 to 1 in 390 pregnancies > 20 wk gestation
Previas found early in pregnancy may resolve

### Types of Previa
Complete—covers the internal cervical os
Partial—partially covers the internal cervical os
Marginal—placenta is adjacent to the internal os
Low lying—placenta is in the lower uterine segment

### Risk Factors
Increased parity
Maternal age: > in nullip, > 40 yr old
Previous C/S
Maternal smoking
High altitudes
Multiple gestation

### Bleeding
Initial bleeding episode is generally around 34 wk gestation
1/3 of affected pregnancies develop bleeding before 30 wk
1/3 of affected pregnancies between 30–36 wk
1/3 of affected pregnancies after 36 wk

### Diagnosis
Painless vaginal bleeding
TVU/S

### Differential Diagnosis
Abruption
Labor
Bloody show
Cervical polyps
Cervicitis
Rectal bleeding
UTI
Cervical irritation from manipulation or sex

### Patient Education
Complete pelvic rest
Emergency care if bleeding
Nothing in the vagina

### Treatment
Consider bethamethazone for lung maturation if < 34 wk
Manage bleeding
C/S

**SOURCE**
Varney, H., Kriebs, J. M., & Gegor, C. L. (2004). *Varney's midwifery* (4th ed.). Sudbury, MA: Jones and Bartlett.

# PLATELETS—THROMBOCYTOPENIA

**Mild Decrease: 100,000–149,000/mm3**
   Gestational thrombocytopenia

*Labs*
   Antiplatelet antibody (APA) screen
   Peripheral smear
   Recheck plt counts each trimester, at 36 wk, and in labor
   Immediate postpartum CBC on newborn or cord bloods

*Treatment*
   None needed
   Consult MD for further evaluation

**Moderate Decrease: 50,000–99,000/mm3**
   Gestational thrombocytopenia

*Labs*
   APA screen
   Peripheral smear
   Recheck plt counts each trimester, at 36 wk, and in labor
   Immediate postpartum CBC on newborn or cord bloods

*Treatment*
   None needed
   Consult MD for further evaluation and collaborative management

**Profound Decrease: < 50,000/mm3**
   Thrombocytopenia
   Gestational Thrombocytopenia
   Immune thrombocytopenia purpura (ITP)
   HELLP
   PIH
   DIC

*Labs*
   PIH labs
   APA screen
   Peripheral smear
   Recheck plt counts each trimester, at 36 wk, and in labor
   Immediate postpartum CBC on newborn or cord bloods

*Treatment*
   Medical management
   Glucocorticoids
   Consult MD for further evaluation and collaborative management
   Plt < 20,000/ mm³ or significant clinical bleeding during labor requires
      immediate tx

**PQ**

**Pathophysiology of Gestational Thrombocytopenia**
   Dilution of normal pregnancy
   Acceleration of the normal increase in plt destruction that occurs during pregnancy
      (increase in plt associated IgG)

**SOURCE**
Gabbe, S. G., Niebyl, J. R., & Simpson, J. L. (Eds.). (2002). *Obstetrics: Normal and problem
pregnancies* (4th ed.). New York: Churchill Livingstone.

## POLITICAL INVOLVEMENT

### Federal Government

*Legislative Branch*
  Congress
  House of Representatives
  Senate

*Executive Branch*
  President and vice president
  Cabinets, agencies, executive departments

*Judicial Branch*

### State Government

*Legislative Branch*
  Legislature
  State house of representatives made up of legislators
  State senate made up of senators

*Executive Branch*
  Governor
  State cabinets, agencies, executive departments

*Judicial Branch*

### How to Speak Before Committees
  Madam Chair or Mister Chairman, members of the committee
  My name is .... I am from....
  I am here today in favor of (or opposed to) bill #
  Because....
  This issue is a problem that you need to address because (why should they and
    their constituents care?)
  **Always bring a written copy of your testimony for the committee**

### Strategies for Influencing Policy
  Pick one or two concrete and specific points you want to make
  Network with other supporting organizations or individuals
  Know the opposition's position
  Present the financial/fiscal impact of your position and how it will be paid for
  Know which regulatory boards/agencies your proposal will impact and how they
    feel about the proposed change
  Outline the individuals impacted by your proposal
  Always have something in the proposal you are willing to give up in compromise
  Connect w/ the people you are talking to on a personal level
  You have information to offer—they do not know what you know
  Tell a story
  Do not be intimidated (they are people too)
  Use your passion to drive your political involvement!
  Any questions about proper procedure refer to Robert's Rules of Order, which most
    legislators have access to at any moment, or it can be found in any office or
    committee room at the state house
  State Web sites: www.*statename*.gov

## POLYCYSTIC OVARY SYNDROME (PCOS)

### Statistics
Affects 6–10% of women of reproductive age in the United States
Most common cause of infertility due to anovulation

### Diagnosis
Two of the following criteria in addition to the exclusion of all other medical
    conditions that cause irregular menses and androgen excess
Oligo-ovulation or anovulation
Hyperandrogenism: Hirsutism, acne, balding, acanthosis nigricans (darker skin
    pigmentation of neck and axilla)
Clinical

### Labs
Polycystic ovaries as defined by U/S (10 or more follicles measuring 2–9 mm
diameter and an increased central stroma > 25% the ovarian area)

### Differential Diagnosis

| | |
|---|---|
| Cushing's | Obesity |
| Hyperprolactinemia | Virilizing adrenal or ovarian neoplasm |
| Hypothyroidism | Drug-related conditions |
| Acromegaly | Hyperthecosis |
| Premature ovarian failure | 21-hydroxylase deficiency |

### Testing/Screening
Serum total testosterone
DHEA sulfate: exclude the rare possibility of androgen tumor (tumor would have
    testosterone above 200 ng/ml and DHEA-S above 7000 ng/ml)
17-hydroxyprogesterone: to rule out 21-hydroxylase deficiency (would also have
    severe hirsutism, clitoromegaly, irregular menses, familial tendency, short
    stature); < 3 ng/ml obtained during the follicular phase in pts w/ regular
    menstrual cycles excludes the dx
24 h urinary-free cortisol: if Cushing's syndrome is a consideration
TSH
Prolactin
Fasting glucose and insulin levels
Lipid profile
LH/FSH ratio
Note: d 3 FSH/LH ratio is normally 1:1, PCOS ~ 1:2, the extra LH suppresses the
    production of FSH, thus inhibiting follicle maturation

### Risks Factors
Metabolic syndrome (1/3–1/2 of all PCOS sufferers)
Type 2 DM
Cardiovascular disease

PQ

### Treatment
Lifestyle modification—increased physical activity, reduction in body wt
Metformin—inhibits output of hepatic glucose, thus increasing systemic glucose
    use; caution pts re: possible return to ovulation and risk of pregnancy
Thiazolidinediones—increase insulin sensitivity
OCPs—Yasmin, Yaz, Orthocyclen, Orthocept
See also Hyperandrogenism

#### SOURCES
Chang, R. J. (2004). A practical approach to the diagnosis of polycystic ovary syndrome. *American Journal of Obstetrics and Gynecology, 191*(3), 713–717.

Essah, P. A., Wickham, E. P., & Nestler, J. E. (2007). The metabolic syndrome in polycystic ovary syndrome. *Clinical Obstetrics and Gynecology, 50*(1), 205–225.

## POSTDATE PREGNANCY

### Definition
LMP + 294 d or 280 d after documented ovulation/fertilization
Greater than 42 wk
Greater than 10 lunar mo

### Incidence
1–3% (w/ good dating)
Early (1st trimester) and accurate dating are the best method to prevent supposed postdate pregnancies

### Controversy
Current evidence suggests that the risk of stillbirth increases after 40 wk gestation, which has lead to an increase in the induction rate

### Concerns
Postdate pregnancies are associated w/ placental insufficiency, resulting in a loss of oxygen/nutrient supply to the fetus

### Management
No standardized protocol for the management of postdate pregnancies
Common practice to initiate testing at 41 wk that includes AFI, biweekly NSTs, and a BPP
Induction is also routinely offered between 41–42 wk; however, no current protocol has been shown to significantly reduce the incidence of stillbirth

### Patient Education
It is important to counsel women effectively on the increased risk of operative birth associated w/ induction
Discuss the possible need for cervical ripening
Offer appropriate encouragement/guidance to help pt get labor started naturally
*Also see* Bishop Score
*Also see* Induction
*Also see* Dating a Pregnancy

### SOURCES

Alexander, J. M., McIntire, D. D., & Leveno, K. J. (2000). Forty weeks and beyond: Pregnancy outcomes by week of gestation. *Obstetrics & Gynecology, 96*(2), 291–294.

Divon, M. Y., & Feldman-Leidner, N. (2008). Postdates and antenatal testing. *Seminars in Perinatology, 32*(4), 295–300.

Fretts, R. C. (2005). Etiology and prevention of stillbirth. *American Journal of Obstetrics and Gynecology, 193*(6), 1923–1935.

# POSTPARTUM CHECK UP

**Basics**
Nutrition
Fluid intake

Exercise
Adjustment

**Baby**
Growth
Development
Umbilical cord
Fontanels

Sleep/wake cycles
Circumcision healing/care
Adjustment to life w/ infant

**Bonding**
Mother and baby bonding
Paternal attachment

Sibling adjustment

**Breast vs. Bottle**
Infant nutrition and growth/development

**Blues**
Maternal affect
Sense of safety and support
Maternal transition back into work

Mothering role adjustment
Reflections on her birth experience

**Breasts**
Breastfeeding
Milk production
Skin integrity

S/sx mastitis or engorgement
Supportive bras
Mother's fluid and nutrition intake

**Belly**
Abdominal exercises
Scars/stretch marks

Bowel function
Cramping or pain

**Bleeding**
When did it stop
Lochia pattern

Uterine involution
First menses after birth expectation

**Bottom**
Integrity of repair
C/S scar
Difficulty w/ urination

Kegel exercises
Hemorrhoids

**Birth Control**
Child spacing

Sexual activity

**Body Check**
Vital signs
Breast evaluation
Abdominal exam

Perineum exam
Uterine involution bimanual exam

**PQ**

**SOURCE**
Varney, H., Kriebs, J. M., & Gegor, C. L. (2004). *Varney's midwifery* (4th ed.). Sudbury, MA: Jones and Bartlett.

## POSTPARTUM INFECTIONS

**Evaluate 5 Ws for Infection**
Wind: respiratory infection
Water: UTI
Wound: lacerations
Walking: thrombophlebitis
Womb: uterus

**Perineum/Vagina**
Local pain and dysuria w/ or w/o urinary retention
Purulent discharge
Fever

**Lacerations/Episiotomy**
Wound edges erythematous, swollen
Sutures often tear through the edematous tissues, allowing the necrotic wound edges to gape, may note release of serous, serosanguinous, or purulent exudates

**Cervix**
Infection may be more common than realized d/t undiagnosed lacerations
Cervix normally harbors potentially pathogenic organisms
Deep cervical lacerations often extend directly into the tissue at the base of the broad ligament, increasing risk for lymphangitis, parametritis, and bacteremia

**Endometritis**
Uncommon after uncomplicated vaginal delivery (except when GBS pos)
Common w/ C/S

*Signs and Symptoms*
Fever range 100.4°F (38°C) to 104°F (40°C)
Malaise
Chills
Anorexia
Tachycardia
Abdominal pain extending laterally
Discharge can be foul, profuse, sometimes frothy
Subinvolution
WBC elevated beyond physiological leukocytosis

*Risk Factors*
C/S
Multiple vaginal exams
Prolonged ROM
Internal fetal monitoring
Intrapartum chorioamnionitis
GC
CT
GBS
Gardnerella infection
High BMI
Nulliparity
Multiple gestation
Prolonged labor induction
3 or more courses of betamethazone

**Salpingitis**
Inflammation of the fallopian tubes, most often involving an STI

*Causes*
GC
CT
*Staph aureus*
*E. coli* and other anaerobic and aerobic cocci and bacilli
Can cause sterility and scarring
Common among immunosuppressed women

*Signs and Symptoms*
Sometimes asymptomatic
Usually present w/ unilateral/bilateral lower abdominal pain
Fever
Chills

**Peritonitis**
Inflammation of serous membrane of the peritoneum

*Risk Factors*
C/S w/ uterine incision necrosis and dehiscence
Rupture of any organ (especially GI)

*Signs and Symptoms*
Severe pain that worsens w/ movement
Marked bowel distension leading to paralytic ileus
Nausea
Loss of appetite
Sometimes hypothermia

*Diagnosis*
Aspiration of peritoneal fluid

**Septicemia**
Pathogenic organisms in the blood

*Risk Factors*
Untreated postpartum infections
Septic abortion
Antepartum pyelonephritis

*Bacteria*
Enterobacter family
Specifically *E. coli* and less commonly from Strep A and *Staph aureus*

*Signs and Symptoms*
Decreased systemic cardiovascular resistance not fully compensated by increased
cardiac output
Lactic acidosis
Decreased tissue perfusion
End-organ dysfunction
Oligouria
Can lead to HELLP and/or DIC
Can be fatal

PQ

**Thrombophlebitis**
Inflammation of veins in conjunction w/ formation of a thrombus

*Signs and Symptoms*
Abrupt in onset
Severe pain and edema
Homan's sign
Most cases in pregnancy are confined to the deep veins of the lower extremity

*Risk Factors*
Inactivity/stasis
Smoking
Obesity
Coagulopathy
Factor V Leiden mutation
Superficial varicosities
IV catheterization

*Diagnosis*
Doppler U/S
Venography or phlebography
*See also* Antibiotics
*See also* Chorioamnionitis

**SOURCE**
Varney, H., Kriebs, J. M., & Gegor, C. L. (2004). *Varney's midwifery* (4th ed.). Sudbury, MA: Jones and Bartlett.

# PRECONCEPTION VISIT

Determine the timeline for the next pregnancy
Dependent on that timeline discuss birth control options, being sure to factor in
nonhormonally influenced menstrual cycles

## Advise Overall Increase in Wellness

Up-to-date immunizations
Improve nutrition
Increase exercise
Decrease/abstain from smoking and alcohol

## Screen For

All STIs
Blood sugar
Blood type and Rh factor
HCT/Hb
Domestic violence
Psychological readiness
Possible additions dependent on risk factors:
    Drug urine screen
    TORCH screen
    Tuberculosis

## Discuss Risks and Tests for Genetic Diagnosis w/

Woman > 35 yr old
Either partner has hx w/ birth defect
Either partner has a birth defect, genetic disorder, or family hx
Ashkenazi Jews (Tay Sachs), African, Asian, or Mediterranean descent (sickle cell,
    thalassemia)
Cystic fibrosis carrier screening
Either partner > 3 SABs
Woman has a serious medical history

## Teaching Points

Encourage starting prenatal vitamins or at least a folic acid supplement w/ a
    minimum dose of 400 mcg/d
Fertility cycle
Sperm count and life cycle
Lead poisoning
TORCH infections
Options for prenatal care

**SOURCES**

Cunningham, G., Leveno, K. J., Bloom, S. L., Hauth, J. C., Gilstrap, L. C., & Wenstrom, K. D. (2005).
    *Williams obstetrics* (22nd ed.). New York: McGraw-Hill.
Summers, L., & Price, R. A. (1993). Preconception care: An opportunity to maximize health in
    pregnancy. *Journal of Midwifery & Women's Health, 38*(4), 188–196.

**PQ**

## PREECLAMPSIA

### Incidence
8% of all pregnancies; often in women who were previously normotensive; must be distinguished from chronic HTN

### Signs and Symptoms
HTN (> 140 systolic and/or > 90 diastolic) with associated proteinuria (> 0.3 g/d)
H/A not relieved by analgesics
RUQ pain
Visual changes

### Etiology
Poorly understood
Current theories: uterine ischemia/underperfusion, endothelial activation/dysfunction, calcium deficiency, immunological activation, poor nutrition, genetic tendency

### Risk Factors
Chronic HTN
Hydatidiform mole
Previous pregnancy complicated by preeclampsia
Nulliparity
Advanced maternal age
Obesity
Multiple gestation
Diabetes or gestational diabetes
Kidney disease
Autoimmune disease (e.g., lupus)

### Diagnosis
HTN
Urine dip stick finding of +1 protein, requires confirmation with 24 h urine

### Labs
CBC—low platelets and/or hemoconcentration/anemia suggests disease
LDH—elevated levels indicate preeclampsia associated hemolysis
Peripheral blood smear—assess for microangiopathic hemolytic anemia
Serum creatinine—rising levels indicate disease
Uric acid—$\geq 6$ mg/dl indicates disease and can distinguish preeclampsia from chronic HTN, which exhibits normal uric acid levels
AST/ALT—elevation indicates disease

### Treatment
Delivery of fetus

### Treatment Medications

*Magnesium Sulfate*
Indication: prevention of seizures
Contraindications:
Allergy to magnesium products
Should not be used w/ heart block
Previous myocardial damage
Be aware of increased toxicity w/ renal impairment
*See also* Magnesium Sulfate
Oral antihypertensives

*Methyldopa*
Indications: maintain BP 130–160/80–100
Contraindications:
Current MAOI therapy
Hypersensitivity to methyldopa
Liver disease

Mechanism: alpha-adrenergic agonist, decreases sympathetic tone
Dose: 250–650 mg PO TID
Class:
Preg Cat B
Lact Cat L2

*Labetalol*
Indications: Maintain BP 130–160/80–100
Contraindications:
   COPD/bronchial asthma
   Severe bradycardia, heart block, cardiac failure
   Cardiogenic shock
Mechanism: alpha and beta-adrenergic blocker
Dose: 200 mg Q 8 h PO to a max of 600 mg Q 6 h PO
Preg Cat C
Lact Cat L2
*See also* Hypertension

**SOURCE**

MICROMEDEX: *Healthcare series* [homepage on the Internet]. Retrieved August 21, 2008, from http://www.micromedex.com

Varney, H., Kriebs, J. M., & Gegor, C. L. (2004). *Varney's midwifery* (4th ed.). Sudbury, MA: Jones and Bartlett

**PQ**

## PREMATURE RUPTURE OF MEMBRANES (PROM)

### Definition
Rupture of amniotic sac before onset of labor at greater than 37 wk gestation

### Incidence
8–10% of term pregnancies

### Management
Consider: cervical ripeness, fetal testing, length of ROM, time of day, GBS status, pt wishes, institutional policy

Expectant management contraindications: active labor, chorioamnionitis, vaginal bleeding, fetal distress

*Latency to Onset of Labor*
50% w/in 12 h
70% w/in 24 h
85% w/in 48 h
95% w/in 72 h
5000 women randomized into 4 groups
No difference in neonatal infection or C/S rates
Immediate induction w/ pit reduced latency by 12 h
Immediate induction w/ pit resulted in fewer women receiving antibiotics in labor for s/sx chorioamnionitis
Immediate induction group had fewer vag exams

### Implications for Midwifery Practice
Strictly limit vaginal exams to reduce the incidence of chorioamnionitis, especially in pts choosing expectant management

Involve pts in the decision-making process re: expectant vs. active management, providing evidence-based guidance

Neonatal: increased risk of infection*

Maternal: increased risk of postpartum infections*

*These risks are directly related to the incidence of chorioamnionitis, which, in many cases, may be prevented by limiting vaginal exams

*See also* Chorioamnionitis

*See also* Postpartum Infection

### SOURCES
Hannah, M. E., Ohlsson, A., Farine, D., Hewson, S. A., Hodnett, E. D., Myhr, T. L., et al. (1996). Induction of labor compared with expectant management for prelabor rupture of the membranes at term. TERMPROM study group. *New England Journal of Medicine, 334*(16), 1005–1010.

Marowitz, A., & Jordan, R. (2007). Midwifery management of prelabor rupture of membranes at term (Abstract). *Journal of Midwifery & Women's Health, 52*(3), 199–206.

Norwitz, E., & Schorge, J. (2001). *Obstetrics and gynecology at a glance.* Osney Mead, Oxford: Blackwell Science.

Scott, J., Gibbs, R., Karlan, B., & Haney, A. (2003). *Danforth's obstetrics and gynecology* (9th ed.). Philadelphia: Lippincott Williams and Wilkins.

# PREMENSTRUAL DYSPHORIC DISORDER (PMDD)

### Definition
Recurrent luteal phase complaints of physiological, cognitive, affective, behavioral, and somatic symptoms thought to be related to fluctuations in hormones (estrogen and progesterone) as well as neurotransmitters

### Statistics
70–90% menstruating women have some degree of symptoms
20–40% women report these symptoms are bothersome

### Signs and Symptoms
Depression
Anger outbursts
Irritability
Anxiety
Confusion
Social withdrawal
Breast tenderness
Abdominal pain
H/A
Swelling of extremities
Aches/pains

### ACOG Diagnosis
1. Complaint of at least one affective and one somatic symptom related to the last 3 menstrual cycles
2. Resolution of s/sx w/in 4 d of onset of menses
3. Symptoms clearly seen in prospective recordings; Pts should track symptom severity using an assessment tool such as the Premenstrual Assessment Form, Calendar of Premenstrual Experiences, or the Daily Record of Severity of Problems
4. Symptoms must interfere w/ daily functions

### Differential Diagnosis
Depression/anxiety
Dysthymia
Panic disorder
Bipolar disorder
Somatoform disorder
Personality disorder
Substance abuse
Anemia
Autoimmune disorders
Chronic fatigue
Diabetes
Seizure disorders
Hypothyroidism
Endometriosis
Allergies

**PQ**

**Treatment**

*Hormonal*
  COCs
  Progesterone only
  Estrogens
  Danazol
  GnRH analogs

**DIETARY TREATMENTS FOR PMDD**
  Calcium 1200–1600 mg/d
  Magnesium 400–800 mg/d
  Vitamin $B_6$ 50–100 mg/d
  Decrease vitamin E and caffeine

**HERBAL TREATMENTS FOR PMDD**
  Angus cactus fruit (Chasteberry) 4–20 mg/d
  Evening primrose oil 2–3 g/d
  Black cohosh 40 mg BID
  St.-John's-wort 300 mg TID
  Kava 100–300 mg/d
  Ginkgo 80 mg BID

**BEHAVIORAL TREATMENTS FOR PMDD**
  Cognitive behavior therapy (CBT)
  Biofeedback
  Relaxation response
  Light therapy
  Exercise—aerobics, yoga
  Support groups
  Massage
  Chiropractics
  Homeopathy

*Nonhormonal Medications*
  SSRIs
  Diuretics
  Prostaglandin inhibitors
  Antidepressants

*Surgical*
  Hysterectomy
  Oophorectomy

**Treatment Approach**
  1. Mild/moderate—nutrition, supplements, NSAIDs, COCs
  2. Persistent mild/moderate—SSRI
  3. Severe—GnRH agonists

**SOURCES**

Braverman, P. (2007). Premenstrual syndrome and premenstrual dysphoric disorder. *North American Society for Pediatric and Adolescent Gynecology, 20*, 3–12.

Girman, A., Lee, R., & Kligler, B. (2002). An integrative medicine approach to premenstrual syndrome. *American Journal of Obstetrics and Gynecology, 188*(5), S56–S63.

Salamat, S., Ismail, K., & O'Brien, S. (2007). Premenstrual syndrome. *Obstetrics, Gynecology, and Reproductive Medicine, 18*(2), 29–32.

Schuiling, K. D., & Likis, F. E. (2006). *Women's gynecologic health.* Sudbury, MA: Jones and Bartlett.

Usman, S., Indusekhar, R., & O'Brien, S. (2008). Hormonal management of premenstrual syndrome. *Best Practice and Research Clinical Obstetrics and Gynecology, 22*(2), 251–260.

# PRETERM LABOR (PTL)/PRETERM DELIVERY (PTD)

## Preterm Delivery Statistics
11–12% of births in United States
2% < 32 wk
11% < 37 wk

## Risk Factors
Intra-amniotic infection
Multiple gestation
Placental abruption
3rd trimester bleeding
2nd trimester bleeding
Prior PTD
Uterine anomalies
DES exposure
UTI
Smoking (>10 cig/d)
Illicit drug use (especially cocaine)
Maternal age > 30 yr old
African-American race
Low SES

## Prevention w/ Progesterone
IM progesterone is associated w/ reduced risk of PTD and infant birth wt < 2500 g in one trial, dosage varies

## Differential Diagnosis
PTL vs. preterm contractions
UTI vs. pyelonephritis
Gastroenteritis
Dehydration
Cervicitis, vaginitis, vaginosis
Acute surgical abdomen

## Pathophysiology

*Stress*
Fetal—IUGR, UPI
Maternal—PIH, HTN activates the HPA axis up-regulating CRH and increasing prostaglandin production, which correlates w/ PTD risk; low predictive value, not a screening tool

*Infection*
STIs
Cervicitis
Vaginitis
Asymptomatic bacteruria
Cytokines (IL, TNF) are released, increasing prostaglandin production; IL and TNF recruit collegenases and elastases that degrade membranes, causing PROM and initiating the prostaglandin cascade

*Hemorrhage*
Any bleeding increases risk 3×
Bleeding in 2nd trimesters increases risk 7×
Causes release of TNF and prostaglandins

*Mechanical*
Contents too large (multiples—twins > 50% PTD, triplets > 80% PTD, quads > 90% PTD)
Polyhydramnios
Uterine-size limit (bicornuate, Mullerian duct abnormality)
Stretch receptors release cell-protein destruction enzymes
Initiates prostaglandin cascade

PQ

**Management**

*Subjective Information*
Uterine contractions > 4/h w/ or w/o pain
Intermittent lower abdominal pain
Menstrual-like cramps w/ or w/o diarrhea
Dull backache, pelvic pressure
Vaginal bleeding 2nd or 3rd trimester
Change in vaginal discharge, amount, color, consistency
Vague complaint of "not feeling right"
Recent intercourse
Dysuria or UTI not adequately treated
PO intake inadequate by pt hx
Psychological/physical trauma
Hx of previous PTD

*Objective Information*
Vital signs, afebrile
Observed adequate hydration, PO or IV
NST-FHT appropriate for gestational age, uterine activity
Abdominal palpation for uterine tenderness, contractions
CVAT
Suprapubic tenderness
Assess for normal discomforts of pregnancy
SSE-fFN, GC/CT, wet mount, GBS, visualize cervix
Cervical exam—Length by U/S (serial digital exams not acceptable)

*Labs*
UA by clean catch
Straight catheter if necessary

*Treatment*
Tocolytics: Each has side effects, one is not better than another, two is not better
than one (terbutaline, nifedipine commonly used). Purpose—delay delivery to
allow administration of antenatal steroids, transport of mother to tertiary care
facility, prolong pregnancy to allow treatment of self-limited causes (appendicitis,
pyelonephritis)
Steroids—Betamethasone 12 mg IM Q 24 h × 2, dexamethasone 6 mg IM Q 12 h
× 4 induce maturation of lung architecture, flattening of epithelial cells, thinning
of alveolar septa, increased cytodifferentiation
*See also* Fetal Lung Maturity
*See also* Fetal Fibronectin

**SOURCES**
Cunningham, G., Leveno, K. J., Bloom, S. L., Hauth, J. C., Gilstrap, L. C., & Wenstrom, K. D. (2005).
    *Williams obstetrics* (22nd ed.). New York: McGraw-Hill.
Dodd, J. M., Flenady, V., Cincotta, R., & Crowther, C. A. (2006). Prenatal administration of
    progesterone for preventing preterm birth. *Cochrane Database of Systematic Reviews* (Online), (1),
    CD004947.
Meis, P. J., Klebanoff, M., Thom, E., Dombrowski, M. P., Sibai, B., Moawad, A. H., et al. (2003).
    Prevention of recurrent preterm delivery by 17 alpha-hydroxyprogesterone caproate. *New England
    Journal of Medicine, 348*(24), 2379–2385.
Varney, H., Kriebs, J. M., & Gegor, C. L. (2004). *Varney's midwifery* (4th ed.). Sudbury, MA: Jones and
    Bartlett.

# PRETERM PREMATURE RUPTURE OF MEMBRANES (PPROM)

**Definition**
Rupture of membranes before 37 wk

**Incidence**
2–4% singleton
7–10% in multiples

**Risk Factors**
Prior occurrence (recurrence rate 20–30%)
Vaginal bleeding
Abruption (15% in PPROM)
Cervical incompetence
Amniocentesis
Smoking
Multiples
Polyhydramnios
Connective tissue diseases
Anemia
Low SES
Unwed status
African-American race

**Diagnosis**
GA < 37 wk
Positive sterile speculum exam = ferning, pooling, nitrazine
Amnisure positive

**Management**
Risk of prematurity vs. risk of infection
Tocolysis—PPROM is a relative contraindication
Antibiotics—prolongs latency, doesn't improve outcomes
Steroids—decreases RDS in neonates

**Fetal Surveillance**
NST vs. BPP vs. fetal kick counts
Limit # of vaginal exams when SSE is sufficient

**Neonatal Complications**
RDS
IVH
Sepsis

**Maternal Complications**
Increased C/S rate
Chorioamnionitis (15–30%)
Postpartum endometritis
See also Chorioamnionitis
See also Postpartum Infection
See also Preterm Labor

**PQ**

**SOURCES**
Briggs, G., Yaffe, S., & Freeman, R. (2005). *Drugs in pregnancy and lactation* (7th ed.). Philadelphia:
    Lippincott Williams and Wilkins.
Norwitz, E., & Schorge, J. (2001). *Obstetrics and gynecology at a glance*. Osney Mead, Oxford,
    England: Blackwell Science.
Scott, J., Gibbs, R., Karlan, B., & Haney, A. (2003). *Danforth's obstetrics and gynecology* (9th ed.).
    Philadelphia: Lippincott Williams and Wilkins.

## RH STATUS AND RHOGAM

### Pertinent Medical History
Previous blood transfusions
Did babies before this one need blood transfusions?
Any stillbirth/neonatal death w/ unknown cause?
Have you received RhoGAM after past deliveries/Abs?
Rh neg blood type
Father's Rh status

### Indications for Rhogam
Mom is Rh neg
Mom is not sensitized to Rh antibodies based on screen
Infant is Rh pos
Infant has negative direct antiagglutination test (Coomb's test)

### RhoGAM Prophylaxis Information
Prophylaxis usually at 28 wk GA (protects through rest of pregnancy until
    postdates)
Duration of action = 12 wk common to administer RhoGAM w/out antibody screen,
    since sensitization is rare in the absence of trauma/amnio
RhoGam given w/in 72 h of birth
If you cannot type infant, better to just give RhoGAM than risk sensitization
If possibility of exposure, use Kleihauer-Betke test to determine appropriate dose
Rhogam dose related to amount of fetal blood that has entered mother's circulation
300 mcg dose covers 15 ml of fetal blood mixing
If suspected to be greater, adjust RhoGAM dose to 20 mcg/ml of fetal blood
If mother and FOB are Rh neg, then baby will be Rh neg (autosomal recessive
    inheritance)
Care provider must be confident of paternity if no tx is administered based on FOB
    Rh status

### Treatment

TABLE R-1    Rh (D)-Immune Globulin Dosages with Reference to Chance for
Fetomaternal Hemorrhage

| Causes of Fetomaternal Hemorrhage | Dose of Rh (D)-Immune Globulin (RhoGAM) |
|---|---|
| First trimester | |
| Abortion (spontaneous/elective) | 50 mcg |
| Ectopic pregnancy | 50 mcg |
| CVS | 50 mcg |
| Second trimester | |
| Ectopic pregnancy | 300 mcg |
| Amniocentesis | 300 mcg |
| Second/third trimester | |
| Blunt abdominal trauma | 300 mcg |
| Fetal death, stillbirth | 300 mcg |
| Fetal manipulation (external cephalic version) | 300 mcg |
| Vaginal, C/S birth | 300 mcg |
| Major hemorrhage (placental abruption, uterine rupture) | 20 mcg/ml estimated fetal whole blood *Kleihauer Betke |

Source: Varney, H., Kriebs, J. M., & Gegor, C. L. (2004). Varney's midwifery (4th ed.). Sudbury, MA:
Jones and Bartlett.

### SOURCE
Varney, H., Kriebs, J. M., & Gegor, C. L. (2004). Varney's midwifery (4th ed.). Sudbury, MA: Jones and
    Bartlett.

# SCALP SAMPLING

### Definition
Direct assessment of pH of fetal blood intrapartum

### Indications
Nonreassuring FHR patterns
Birth eminent
Intrauterine resuscitation possible

### Contraindications
Delay in delivering baby
Intact membranes
No cervical dilation
Inability to achieve maternal comfort/cooperation
Maternal infection such as HSV, HIV, hepatitis
Few maternal and fetal complications
Cervix dilated at least 2–3 cm
Membranes ruptured

### Influencing Factors
Fetal caput
Maternal posture
Analgesia
Hyperventilation
Uterine contractions
Medications
Few maternal and fetal complications
Cervix dilated at least 2–3 cm
Membranes ruptured

### Procedure
Position mother on her side in a supported lithotomy position
Place amnioscope on fetal head
Secure good light source for full visualization of fetal head
Clean fetal skin and apply a drop of silicone gel to place of incision
Puncture fetal skin w/ a 2 mm blade
Collect blood in a heparinized capillary tube
Quickly transport blood to blood gas machine for analysis
Repeat as many times as needed to assure accurate assessment

### Follow-Up
Assess maternal and fetal well-being
Educate mother and partner about risks and benefits as well as F/U management
Evaluate fetal head for hemorrhage and abscesses

TABLE S-1    Scalp pH, Diagnosis, and Management

| Scalp pH | Diagnosis | Management |
|---|---|---|
| Less than 7.20 | Acidosis | Immediate delivery |
| 7.20–7.25 | Equivocal | Repeat every 30 min |
| Greater than 7.25 | Normal | Manage expectantly; rpt Q h if FHR still abnormal |

S

SOURCES
AWHONN. (2003). *Fetal heart monitoring: Principles and practices* (3rd ed.) Dubuque, IA: Kendall/Hunt.
Elimian, A., Figueroa, R., & Tejani, N. (1997). Intrapartum assessment of fetal well-being: A comparison of scalp stimulation with scalp blood pH sampling. *Obstetrics and Gynecology, 89,* 373–376.
Varney, H., Kriebs, J. M., & Gegor, C. L. (2004). *Varney's midwifery* (4th ed.). Sudbury, MA: Jones and Bartlett.

## SCREENING GUIDELINES

**TABLE S-2**  Preventive Services Recommendations

The U.S. Preventive Services Task Force (USPSTF) recommends that clinicians discuss these preventive services with eligible patients and offer them as a priority. All these services have received an "A" (strongly recommended) or a "B" (recommended) grade from the Task Force. For definitions of all grades used by the USPSTF, see the original document.

| Recommendation | Adults | | Special Populations | |
| --- | --- | --- | --- | --- |
| | Men | Women | Pregnant Women | Children |
| Abdominal aortic aneurysm, screening[1] | ✓ | | | |
| Alcohol misuse screening and behavioral counseling interventions | ✓ | ✓ | ✓ | |
| Aspirin for the primary prevention of cardiovascular events[2] | ✓ | ✓ | | |
| Bacteriuria, screening for asymptomatic | | | ✓ | |
| Breast cancer, chemoprevention[3] | | ✓ | | |
| Breast cancer, screening[4] | | ✓ | | |
| Breast and ovarian cancer susceptibility, genetic risk assessment and BRCA mutation testing[5] | | ✓ | | |
| Breastfeeding, behavioral interventions to promote[6] | | ✓ | ✓ | |
| Cervical cancer, screening[7] | | ✓ | | |
| Chlamydial infection, screening[8] | | ✓ | ✓ | |
| Colorectal cancer, screening[9] | ✓ | ✓ | | |
| Dental caries in preschool children, prevention[10] | | | | ✓ |
| Depression, screening[11] | ✓ | ✓ | | |
| Diabetes mellitus in adults, screening for type 2[12] | ✓ | ✓ | | |
| Diet, behavioral counseling in primary care to promote a healthy[13] | ✓ | ✓ | | |

TABLE S-2  Preventive Services Recommendations (continued)

| Recommendation | Adults | | Special Populations | |
| | Men | Women | Pregnant Women | Children |
| --- | --- | --- | --- | --- |
| Gonorrhea, screening[14] | | ✓ | ✓ | |
| Gonorrhea, prophylactic medication[15] | | | | ✓ |
| Hepatitis B virus infection, screening[16] | | | ✓ | |
| High blood pressure, screening | ✓ | ✓ | | |
| HIV, screening[17] | ✓ | ✓ | ✓ | ✓ |
| Iron deficiency anemia, prevention[18] | | | | ✓ |
| Iron deficiency anemia, screening[19] | | | ✓ | |
| Lipid disorders, screening[20] | ✓ | ✓ | | |
| Obesity in adults, screening[21] | ✓ | ✓ | | |
| Osteoporosis in postmenopausal women, screening[22] | | ✓ | | |
| Rh (D) incompatibility, screening[23] | | | ✓ | |
| Sickle cell disease, screening[24] | | | | ✓ |
| Syphilis infection, screening[25] | ✓ | ✓ | ✓ | |
| Tobacco use and tobacco-caused disease, counseling[26] | ✓ | ✓ | ✓ | |
| Visual impairment in children younger than age 5 years, screening[27] | | | | ✓ |

[1]One-time screening by ultrasonography in men aged 65 to 75 who have ever smoked.
[2]Adults at increased risk for coronary heart disease.
[3]Discuss with women at high risk for breast cancer and at low risk for adverse effects of chemoprevention.

/ continues

S

TABLE S-2  Preventive Services Recommendations (continued)

4Mammography every 1-2 years for women 40 and older.

5Refer women whose family history is associated with an increased risk for deleterious mutations in BRCA1 or BRCA2 genes for genetic counseling and evaluation for BRCA testing.

6Structured education and behavioral counseling programs.

7Women aged 21-65 who have been sexually active and have a cervix.

8Sexually active women 24 and younger and other asymptomatic women at increased risk for infection. Asymptomatic pregnant women 24 and younger and others at increased risk.

9Men and women 50 and older.

10Prescribe oral fluoride supplementation at currently recommended doses to preschool children older than 6 months whose primary water source is deficient in fluoride.

11In clinical practices with systems to assure accurate diagnoses, effective treatment, and follow-up.

12Adults with hypertension or hyperlipidemia.

13Adults with hyperlipidemia and other known risk factors for cardiovascular and diet-related chronic disease.

14Sexually active women, including pregnant women 25 and younger, or at increased risk for infection.

15Prophylactic ocular topical medication for all newborns against gonococcal ophthalmia neonatorum.

16Pregnant women at first prenatal visit.

17All adolescents and adults at increased risk for HIV infection and all pregnant women.

18Routine screening for asymptomatic children aged 6 to 12 months who are at increased risk for iron deficiency anemia.

19Routine screening in asymptomatic pregnant women.

20Men 35 and older and women 45 and older. Younger adults with other risk factors for coronary disease. Screening for lipid disorders to include measurement of total cholesterol and high-density lipoprotein cholesterol.

21Intensive counseling and behavioral interventions to promote sustained weight loss for obese adults.

22Women 65 and older and women 60 and older at increased risk for osteoporotic fractures.

23Blood typing and antibody testing at first pregnancy-related visit. Repeated antibody testing for unsensitized Rh (D)-negative women at 24-28 weeks gestation unless biological father is known to be Rh (D) negative.

24Newborns.

25Persons at increased risk and all pregnant women.

26Tobacco cessation interventions for those who use tobacco. Augmented pregnancy-tailored counseling to pregnant women who smoke.

27To detect amblyopia, strabismus, and defects in visual acuity.

Source: U.S. Preventive Services Task Force. (2008). The guide to clinical preventative services, 2008. AHRQ publication no. 08-05122. Rockville, MD: Agency for Healthcare Research and Quality. Retrieved March 26, 2009, from http://www.ahrq.gov/clinic/pocketgd08/pocketgd08.pdf

# SEIZURES

### Incidence

Second most common neurological disorder (2% of the US population)
1 in 10 have a seizure at some point in their life
Temporal lobe epilepsy most common

### Definition

Brief disturbance in the electrical activity of the brain
Often w/ bursts of activity in one or more regions

### Etiology

Epileptogenic focus w/ paroxysmal discharges of brain electrical activity
  sometimes accompanied by a prodromal phase or aura

### Diagnosis

MRI
CT
EEG is the gold standard
May require 24 h monitoring to dx

### Types

*Generalized*

Affects both hemispheres

Absence (petit mal):

  Lasts 2–5 sec

  Seizure symptoms include stare, eye flutter, and automatisms

  Postseizure symptoms include amnesia for seizure events, but daily activities
    can be immediately resumed

Tonic-clonic (grand mal):

  Lasts 1–2 min

  Seizure symptoms include vocalizations, falling, tonicity and clonicity, occasional
    cyanosis

  Postseizure symptoms include amnesia for seizure events, confusion,
    exhaustion, sleep

*Partial Seizures*

Affects one hemisphere

Most common type

Simple partial:

  Lasts –90 sec

  Seizure symptoms include sudden jerking, sensory phenomena, w/o loss of
    consciousness

  Postseizure the sufferer may experience transient weakness or loss of sensation

Complete partial:

  Lasts 1–2 min

  Seizure symptoms include a preseizure aura, automatisms, detachment from
    surroundings, wandering

  Postseizure symptoms include amnesia for the seizure event, mild to moderate
    confusion, sleepiness

### Treatment

Antiseizure/anticonvulsant medications (may need to be altered for pregnancy and
  breastfeeding)
Hormonal birth control efficacy is affected by many antiseizure medications

S

**SOURCE**

Epilepsy Foundation. (2005). *Seizures and syndromes.* Retrieved August 28, 2008, from http://www.
  epilepsyfoundation.org/about/types/types/index.cfm

## SEXUAL ASSAULT

Hotline: 1-800-656-HOPE (4673)

### History

Identifying information

Date, time, and location of assault

Circumstances

Details of sexual contact (penile, digital, oral, anal, object in vagina, ejaculation/ urination by the assailant)

Restraints used (weapon, drugs, alcohol, physical restraint)

Activities of pt after the assault (change of clothing, bathing, douching, dental hygiene, urination, defecation)

GYN hx (LMP, contraceptive use, pregnancy hx, last voluntary sexual encounter, recent GYN infections or pelvic surgery)

### Physical Exam

Assess woman for physical injuries and collect evidence for forensic evaluation

Some jurisdictions require evidence be collected w/in 72–120 h

Pelvic exam: identify signs of recent sexual activity, engorgement of clitoris (lasts 1–2 h), condition of hymen, perineal trauma, lubricate speculum w/ sterile water so DNA evidence is not compromised

### Labs

| | |
|---|---|
| GC | Syphilis |
| CT | Herpes |
| Pregnancy (r/o before EC) | Hepatitis |
| HIV | |

### Documentation

Body maps

Photographic wound record

Document w/ the phrase "reported sexual assault" or "sexual assault by history"

Be specific and state facts as reported by the pt

Include pt's affect while sharing hx

Rape kit: clothing, hair, fingernail scrapings, body secretions collection, full statement, photographs

### Statistics

1–5% of sexual assaults result in pregnancy

Risk of STI from single encounter 5–10%

Risk of hep B or HIV from single encounter < 1%

### Treatment

Emergency contraception

Hep B vaccine

Prophylaxis for GC, CT, trichonomiasis, and BV

HIV prophylaxis discussed on a case-by-case basis

Repeat testing for HIV and syphilis at 6, 12, and 24 wk after assault

### Psychological

Rape trauma syndrome

| Short Term | Long Term |
|---|---|
| Denial | Phobias |
| Shock | Sexual problems |
| Disbelief | Difficulty functioning |
| Disruption | 50% experience depression during the first year |
| Guilt | 20–40% report sexual dysfunction up to 6 yr later |
| Shame | |
| Blame | |
| Hostility | |

#### SOURCE
Schuiling, K. D., & Likis, F. E. (2006). *Women's gynecologic health.* Sudbury, MA: Jones and Bartlett.

# SEXUAL DYSFUNCTION

## Women Report
27–32% lack of interest in sex
22–28% unable to achieve orgasm
17–27% sex is not pleasurable
18–27% experience pain during sex

## Classification
Sexual desire disorders: hypoactive sexual desire, sexual aversion
Sexual arousal disorder
Orgasmic disorder
Sexual pain disorder: dyspareunia, vaginismus, other disorders

## Patient Education
Review normal sexual response w/ pt
Use a diagram to explain genital anatomy and physiology
Address issue that *most* women cannot achieve orgasm w/out direct stimulation
    of the clitoris
Medications that cause or exacerbate female sexual dysfunction: anorectics,
    anticholinergics, anticonvulsants, antidepressants, antiestrogens,
    antihistamines, antihypertensives, antipsychotics, antiulcer drugs, barbiturates,
    benzodiazepines, GnRH agonists, narcotics, oral contraceptives

## Ten Suggestions for Patient
Encourage foreplay
Advocate speaking up about personal sexual desires and needs
Encourage the use of sex toys
Say no if the sexual activity is not desired or needs to change
Investigate whether sex is really the issue
Encourage nonpenetrative sex
Define necessary conditions for sex (dishes done, kids gone, lights on/off)
Write down your ideal encounter in as much detail as possible
Activate your sexuality by taking fantasy breaks during the day (10 min to dream
    about sex)
Encourage masturbation

## Resources
American Association of Sex Educators, Counselors, and Therapists (AASECT),
    www.aasect.org

### SOURCES
Hanfling, S. (2008). Sexual health: Talking with women (patients) about their sexual concerns. Paper
    presented at the 53rd Annual Meeting of the American College of Nurse-Midwives, Boston, MA.
Laumann, E., Paik, A., & Rosen, R. (1999). Sexual dysfunction in the United States: Prevalence and
    predictors. *Journal of the American Medical Association, 281*, 537–544.
Schuiling, K. D., & Likis, F. E. (2006). *Women's gynecologic health.* Sudbury, MA: Jones and Bartlett.

S

# SEXUALLY TRANSMITTED INFECTION (STI) OVERVIEW

TABLE S-3   Sexually Transmitted Infections

| STI | S/sx Women | S/sx Men | Testing | First-line Treatment |
|---|---|---|---|---|
| Chlamydia | Usually asymptomatic<br>Pain with urination<br>Pain with intercourse<br>Spotting with intercourse | Pain with urination<br>Urethral discharge | Urethral swab (men)<br>Cervical swab (women)<br>Urine sample (men and women) | Azithromycin 1 g PO × 1 |
| Genital warts | Skin-colored, raised, painless, irregular growths on vulva and/or rectum | Skin-colored, raised, painless, irregular growths on penis, scrotum, or rectum | Visual inspection | TCA or BCA applied to wart directly |
| Gonorrhea | Usually asymptomatic | Pain with urination<br>Urethral discharge | Urethral swab (men)<br>Cervical swab (women)<br>Urine sample (men and women) | Ceftriaxone 125 mg IM × 1 |
| Hepatitis B and C | Variable | Variable | Serum testing | Refer to specialist |
| Herpes | Painful ulcers on vulva | Painful ulcers on penis | Ulcer swab, DNA testing | Acyclovir, dosing variable |
| HIV | Variable | Variable | Serum or sputum testing | Refer to specialist |
| Syphilis | Palmar and solar rash<br>Painless ulcers | Palmar and solar rash<br>Painless ulcers | Serum testing | Penicillin IM (variations on dosing) |
| Trichamonas | Usually asymptomatic<br>Green/yellow frothy discharge<br>Malodorous discharge | Usually asymptomatic<br>Pain with urination<br>Penile discharge | Saline wet smear<br>Pap testing | Metronidazole 2 g PO × 1 |

# SHOULDER DYSTOCIA

## Definition

Impingement or impaction of the anterior shoulder or both shoulders above the pelvic brim

## Risk Factors

Hx of previous dystocia or large infants      Postdates
Fetal macrosomia                              CPD
Diabetes

## Clues in Labor

Prolonged active phase and/or 2nd stage       Caput
Turtle sign

## Be Prepared

Foot stool in room for suprapubic pressure    Be attentive to signs of a dystocia
Know EFW by Leopold's or U/S

## Do's and Don'ts

Don't panic
Call for help (OB and Pediatrics)
Request preparations be made for PPH
Designate one person to record times
Note time of delivery of head, shoulder, and body
Inform mother of the situation
Caution her about discomfort, and request her undivided attention
She must *only* push when you tell her
No fundal massage or pressure
Do not attempt to twist the baby's head into position
If baby has not delivered after repositioning of mother and/or baby, then stop
    and reassess (–45 sec): bladder status (catheterize if necessary), need for
    episiotomy, vaginal exam to r/o other issues (short cord, gross fetal deformities)

## HELPERR

Call for **H**elp
**E**valuate for episiotomy
**L**egs into McRoberts position
Suprapubic **P**ressure
**E**nter maneuvers
**R**emove posterior arm
**R**oll the patient to hands and knees

## Maneuvers

McRoberts—sharp flexion of maternal thighs against the abdomen
Suprapubic pressure—steady downward pressure just above the symphysis pubis,
    inform assistant of needed direction of pressure based on shoulder position
Assess shoulder position and rotate them to the oblique position if they are
    transverse or anteroposterior; do this by placing all of your fingers on the baby's
    chest/back and exerting equal force to achieve rotation
Rubin—achieved by placing fingers of one hand on the posterior aspect of the
    anterior fetal shoulder and adducting it towards the fetal chest
Wood's corkscrew—combine with Rubin maneuver by adding fingers of other hand
    to the anterior aspect of the posterior shoulder to assist with rotating fetus into
    the oblique position
Reverse Wood's corkscrew—attempt to rotate shoulders in opposite direction if
    unable to deliver fetus after previous maneuver
Gaskin—hands and knees, easiest if no epidural was placed

## Postdelivery

Anticipate hemorrhage
Document all times and maneuvers clearly and accurately

**S**

## SOURCES

Baxley, G. B., & Gobbo, R. W. (2004). Shoulder dystocia. *American Family Physician, 89*, 1707–1714.
Varney, H., Kriebs, J. M., & Gegor, C. L. (2004). *Varney's midwifery* (4th ed.). Sudbury, MA: Jones and Bartlett.

## SMOKING

### Health Effects

*Cancer*

Cause of 80% of lung cancer deaths in women

Causes bladder, oral cavity, pharynx, larynx, esophagus, cervix, kidney, lung, pancreas, and stomach cancer

### Cardiovascular

2–4× higher risk of CAD

Double the risk of stroke

10× risk of peripheral vascular disease

Respiratory

10× increased risk of dying from COPD

*Women*

1. Increased risk for infertility, PTD, stillbirth, LBW, and sudden infant death syndrome
2. Postmenopausal women have lower bone density and increased risk of hip fracture

### Secondhand Smoke

Of the 250 known toxic chemicals in cigarettes, 50 of those chemicals are known to cause cancer

No risk-free level of exposure

Not smoking inside does not eliminate exposure

Ventilation systems and air filters do not eliminate all hazardous particles

### Children, Increased Risk For

Sudden infant death syndrome

Acute respiratory infections

Ear infections

Severe asthma

Slowed lung growth

Premature death

### Pregnancy, Increased Risk For

LBW (approx 200 g less)

Placental abruption

Placenta previa

PTD

PROM/PPROM

**Smoking Cessation**

*Keys to Success*

1. Get ready:
   - Set a quit date
   - Get rid of all cigarettes and ash trays
   - Notify people around you
2. Get support:
   - Tell your family and friends
   - Talk to a healthcare provider
   - Join a counseling group
   - Join a free program
3. Learn new skills:
   - Distract yourself from the urge to smoke w/ activities such as walking, talking to a friend, drinking tea
   - Find alternative ways to reduce stress—baths, exercise, books
   - Drink a lot of water or fluids
4. Get non-Rx medication:
   - Nicotine gum
   - Nicotine lozenge
   - Nicotine patch
5. Get Rx medication:
   - Bupropion SR (Zyban)
   - Nicotine inhaler
   - Nicotine nasal spray
   - Nicotine patch
   - Varenicline
   - Clonidine
   - Nortriptyline
   - Chantix
6. Be prepared for relapses and difficult situations
   - Most relapses happen in first 3 mo
   - Do not be disappointed if you relapse
   - Avoid alcohol
   - Avoid other smokers
   - Expect an average of 10 lb wt gain
   - Expect mood swings
   - Web site resources for quitting:
     www.smokefree.gov
     http://1800quitnow.cancer.gov

**SOURCES**

Centers for Disease Control and Prevention. (2006). *Secondhand smoke.* Retrieved May 26, 2008, from http://www.cdc.gov/tobacco/data_statistics/Factsheets/SecondhandSmoke.htm

Centers for Disease Control and Prevention. (2007). *You can quit smoking: Five keys for quitting smoking.* Retrieved May 26, 2008, from http://www.cdc.gov/tobacco/quit_smoking/you_can_quit/five_keys.htm

Centers for Disease Control and Prevention. (2008). *Health effects of cigarette smoking.* Retrieved May 26, 2008, from http://www.cdc.gov/tobacco/data_statistics/Factsheets/health_effects.htm

Centers for Disease Control and Prevention. (2008). *Tobacco use and pregnancy.* Retrieved May 26, 2008, from http://www.cdc.gov/reproductivehealth/TobaccoUsePregnancy/

U.S. Department of Health and Human Services. (2007). *The health consequences of involuntary exposure to tobacco smoke: A report of the surgeon general, U.S. Department of Health and Human Services.* Retrieved May 27, 2008, from http://www.surgeongeneral.gov/library/secondhandsmoke/factsheets/factsheet6.html

U.S. Department of Health and Human Services. (2008). *Treating tobacco use and dependency 2008 update.* Retrieved May 26, 2008, from http://www.surgeongeneral.gov/tobacco/treating_tobacco_use08.pdf

S

## STATISTICS

### Sensitivity
Proportion of persons w/ the condition who correctly test positive for the disease

### Specificity
Proportion of persons w/out the condition who correctly test negative for the disease

### Positive Predictive Value (PPV)
Likelihood that a positive test indicates disease

### Evidence
Level I: clinical trials, randomized controlled trials (RCTs)

Level II: Controlled trials w/out randomization

Observational

Level II-2: cohort and case control studies, observes the natural course of events of exposure and outcome; investigator has no role in assignment of study exposures

Level II-3: cross-sectional studies, assess the status of individuals w/ respect to the presence or absence of exposure and outcome as well as uncontrolled investigational studies that report results of treatment or interventions but lack a control group for comparison

Level III: descriptive studies, expert opinion, case study, provide limited information about exposure and outcome

Type I error: the error of rejecting a true null hypothesis

Type II error: the error of failing to reject a false null hypothesis

### SOURCE
American College of Obstetricians and Gynecologists. (1999). Reading the medical literature. In *2006 compendium of selected publications* (pp. 329–336). Washington, DC: Author.

# SUTURING

### Degree of Perineal Tear

Classified first to fourth degree based on depth

First degree—involves just the vaginal mucosa, perineal muscle is intact

Second degree—the vaginal mucosa and perineal muscle are involved, external anal sphincter is intact; tear > 1.25 cm deep in the vaginal floor

Third degree—the vaginal mucosa, entire perineal muscle, and external anal sphincter are involved

Fourth degree—the vaginal mucosa, perineal muscle, anal sphincter, and rectal mucosa are involved

### Stitches

Blanket (continuous locked)—repair of vaginal mucosa

Continuous unlocked—closure of subcutaneous layer

Deep interrupted—deep muscle repair

Continuous mattress—subcuticular closure

Crown stitch—bulbocavernosus muscle repair (3rd- and 4th-degree lacerations)

### Tissue

Vaginal mucosa—locked blanket running stitch using a 3-0 chromic synthetic suture w/ a standardized taper needle

Subcutaneous tissue—uninterrupted unlocked basting stitches using a 3-0 chromic synthetic suture w/ a standardized taper needle

Subcuticular tissue—running mattress stitch with suture used in the repair of the subcutaneous tissue (typically 3-0 chromic synthetic or gut with tapered needle)

Rectal sphincter—interrupted stitches w/ a 2-0 absorbable synthetic suture w/ a large taper needle

Perineal body/deep muscle—continuous running stitch from the vaginal mucosa by using the Hobb's maneuver to bring the stitch into the perineal plane using a 3-0 synthetic w/ a taper needle

### Suture

3-0: vaginal mucosa, subcutaneous tissue, perineal body, deep muscle

2-0: rectal sphincter

TABLE S-4    Sutures

| Type | Characteristics | Tensile Strength Length | Absorption Complete | Information |
|------|-----------------|------------------------|---------------------|-------------|
| Plain gut | Pig or cow small intestine | 7–10 d | 70 d | Epidermal use, natural materials |
| Chromic | Intestine treated w/ chromium salt | 10–14 d | 90 d | Natural knots may fray |
| Vicryl | Braded multifilament with polyglactin 910 | 65% strength at 14 d | 56–70 d | Precise knots |
| Monocryl | Monofilament coated with poliglecaprone 25 | 50–60% strength at 7 d, lost at 21 d | 91–119 d | Good pliability |
| Polysorb | Lactomer copolymer | 80% strength at 14 d, 30% at 21 d | 56–70 d | Decreased friction |

*Source:* Adapted from Lai, S. (2008). *Sutures and needles.* Retrieved August 28, 2008, from http://www.emedicine.com/ent/TOPIC38.HTM

**SOURCES**

Frye, A. (1995). *Healing passage: A midwife's guide to the care and repair of the tissue involved in birth.* Portland, OR: Labrys Press.

Lai, S. (2008). *Sutures and needles.* Retrieved August 28, 2008, from http://www.emedicine.com/ent/TOPIC38.HTM

# SYPHILIS

## Cause
*Treponema pallidum*

## Statistics
2nd or 3rd leading cause of genital ulcers

## Stages
Primary—indurated and painless ulcer or chancre present 9–90 d after exposure

Secondary—generalized nonitchy rash on the palms and soles, orogenital mucosal lesions, and lymphadenopathy develops w/in 4–10 wk after s/sx of primary infection

Tertiary—cardiac, ophthalmic, auditory, and gummatous lesions

Latent—no clinical symptoms but test positive

Early latent—acquired in last 2 yr

Latent—acquired > 2 yr ago

Unknown—duration unknown

## Neurosyphilis
Diagnosed clinically by symptoms as well as cerebrospinal fluid testing

## Serologic Testing
Nontreponemal tests—Venereal Disease Research Laboratory (VDRL) and rapid plasma reagin (RPR)

Trepanemal tests—fluorescent treponemal antibody absorbtion and particle agglutination

VDRL and RPR have high false-positive rates, rpt test for confirmation

All tests have a low specificity, so dx needs to be confirmed by multiple tests

Sexual transmission only occurs when mucocutaneous syphilitic lesions are present, which is uncommon after 1st yr of infection; always check current tx guidelines before initiating therapy

## Treatment
Benzathine penicillin G 50,000 U/kg IM up to adult dose of 2.4 million U in a single dose (pregnant and nonpregnant)

PCN allergic pts must be desensitized

## Patient Education
Suggest HIV testing for all pts w/ syphilis

Test children and partners if at risk

F/U serologically at 6 and 12 mo

Looking for a 4-fold decline in titer values w/in 6 mo

## Pregnancy
Untreated may cause IUGR, nonimmune hydrops fetalis, 30% chance of still birth, 60% chance of congenital infection, 40% change of mental retardation, PTD

Infection readily crosses placenta, and transmission can occur during any stage of disease or fetal development

Tx reduces risk of fetal infection from 100% to 1–2%

Congenital syphilis—asymptomatic at birth, develop rash, jaundice, hepatosplenomegaly, ascites, meningitis, and snuffles as 1st s/sx

### SOURCES
Centers for Disease Control and Prevention. (2006). Sexually transmitted diseases treatment guidelines, 2006. *Morbidity and Mortality Weekly Report, 55*(RR-11), 22–35.

Edwards, R. (2000). Syphilis in women. *Primary Care Updates for OB/GYNS, 7*(5), 186–191.

Goh, B. T. (2005). Syphilis in adults. *Sexually Transmitted Infections, 81,* 448–452.

Vaules, M., Ramin, K., & Ramsey, P. (2000). Syphilis in pregnancy: A review. *Primary Care Updates for OB/GYNS, 7*(1), 26–30.

# TANNER STAGING

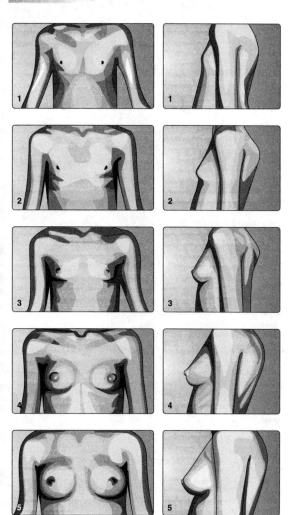

FIGURE T-1   Tanner Stages for Breast Development

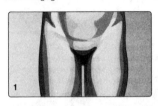
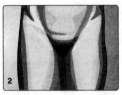
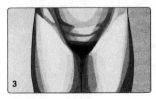
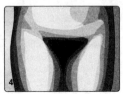

FIGURE T-2  Tanner Stages for Genital Development

### Tanner Stage 1 (Prepubertal)

Age: 10–14 yr old
Ht increase rate: 5–6 cm/yr
Breast—nipple elevation only
Pubic hair—villus hair only, no coarse pigmented hair

### Tanner Stage 2

Ht increase rate: 7–8 cm/yr
Breast—buds palpable and areolae enlarge
Pubic hair—minimal coarse pigmented hair mainly on labia
White: stage 2 changes appear 1 yr earlier
Black: stage 2 changes appear 2 yr earlier

### Tanner Stage 3

Age: 12–14 yr old
Ht increase rate: 8 cm/yr
Breast—elevation of breast contour; areolae enlarge
Pubic hair—dark, coarse, curly hair spreads over mons pubis
Other changes—axillary hair develops, acne vulgaris develops

### Tanner Stage 4

Ht increase rate: 7 cm/yr
Breast—areolae forms secondary mound on the breast
Pubic hair—hair of adult quality, no spread to junction of medial thigh with perineum

### Tanner Stage 5

No further height increases after age 16 yr old
Breast—adult breast contour, areola recesses to general contour of breast
Pubic hair—adult distribution of hair; pubic hair spreads to medial thigh; pubic hair
does not extend up linea alba

**SOURCES**

Marshall, W. A., & Tanner, J. M. (1970). Variations in the pattern of pubertal changes in boys. *Archives of Disease in Childhood, 45*(239), 13–23.

Schuiling, K. D., & Likis, F. E. (2006). *Women's gynecologic health.* Sudbury, MA: Jones and Bartlett.

## THERAPEUTIC REST

### Rationale
Prodromal and/or prolonged latent phase is a tough time for women, and sometimes they just need to rest

### Outpatient Treatment
Hydroxyzine (Vistaril) 50–100 mg (PO/IM)
  Antianxiety and sedative properties
  Maternal sedation is achieved without significant maternal or newborn side effects
Diphenhydramine (Benadryl) 50 mg (PO)
  Hypnotic and may help with rest
Zolpidem (Ambien) 5–10 mg (PO)
  Hypnotic that may help with rest

### Inpatient Treatment
Morphine—10–15 mg IM
  20 min to onset
  3–4 h duration
  Risk of neonatal respiratory depression if given in active phase just prior to delivery

### Morphine Can Be Combined With
Vistiril 50 mg IM
Phenergan 50 mg IM

### Effectiveness
Approximately 85% of women treated with this regimen [referring to morphine treatment] will wake up in the active phase of labor, 10% will not be in labor (suggesting a diagnosis of false labor), and 5% will have a persistent dysfunctional pattern
Tx is particularly useful in women who are tired, uncomfortable, and in early latent phase

**SOURCES**

Greulich, B., & Tarrant, B. (2007). The latent phase of labor: Diagnosis and management. *Journal of Midwifery and Women's Health, 52*, 190–198.

Koontz, W. L., & Bishop, E. (1982). Management of the latent phase of labor. *Clinical Obstetrics and Gynecology, 25*(1), 111–114.

T

# THYROID

TABLE T-1  Thyroid Disorders

|  | TSH | Free T4 |
| --- | --- | --- |
| Primary hypothyroidism | Increased | Decreased |
| Secondary hypothyroidism | Decreased | Decreased |
| Mild thyroid failure | Increased | Normal |
| Hyperthyroidism | Decreased | Increased |
| Subclinical hypothyroidism | Decreased | Normal |

Source: Adapted from Arcangelo, V. P., & Peterson, A. M. (2006). Pharmacotherapeutics for advanced practice (2nd ed.). New York: Lippincott Williams & Wilkins.

## Thyroid Stimulating Hormone (TSH)

TSH is released from the anterior pituitary and induces thyroid hormone (TH) to be released from the thyroid gland

TH then feeds back to the pituitary gland to inhibit the continued release of TSH, thereby regulating the level of free TH; only free TH is bioavailable

*Tissue Effects*

Increased metabolic rate

Increased heart rate and contractility

Affects the growth and maintenance of skin, hair, and nails

*Neurological Effects*

Alertness

Sleep pattern

Reflexes

## Hypothyroidism (High TSH)

*Signs and Symptoms*

Fatigue

Constipation

Menorrhagia

Wt gain

Hair loss

Cold intolerance

Hoarseness

Depression

Dry skin

Infertility

Difficulty with memory and concentration

Bradycardia

Delayed deep tendon reflexes

Hyperlipidemia

Goiter

Hypothermia

Periorbital swelling

Jaundice

Ataxia

Edema

Myalgias

## Hashimoto's Autoimmune Thyroiditis

*When to Treat*

Increased TSH and decreased $T_4$

TSH > 10 mU/l and $T_4$ WNL

Goiter present

If TSH 5–10 mU/l, retest in 3–4 mo

*Treat*

Levothyroxine—start low at 50 mcg QD; can go up to 100–125 mcg

Normal dose for complete replacement 1.6 mcg/kg

Generous dose can lead to fewer dosage changes = less blood testing = happier pts

*Goal*

12.5–25.0 mcg less than full TH replacement with goal of TSH = 1.0–2.0 mU/l

Recommend take 1/2 daily dosage × 1–2 wk then increase

Should feel better within 1–2 wk of starting tx

2–3 wk to steady state

Check TSH 6 wk after start

*If Pt Continues to Complain of S/Sx After TSH WNL r/o Other Causes*

Anemia

Depression

Hypercalcemia
Hypercaloric diet
Lack of exercise

*Monitoring*
Recheck Q 6 mo × 2 yr then Q yr or with any surgery

*Drug Holiday*
Every 1–2 yr of therapy stop TH abruptly, and check TSH over 6–12 wk
If TSH increases, pt needs lifelong replacement

*Pregnancy*
$T_4$ is 1.5 × higher than nonpregnant
TSH is low especially in 1st trimester

## Hyperthyroidism (Low TSH)

*Signs and Symptoms*

| | |
|---|---|
| Dyspnea | Goiter |
| Heat intolerance | Brisk reflexes |
| Palpitations | Tachycardia |
| Infertility | Tremor |
| Insomnia | Lid lag |
| Irritability | Exopthalamos |
| Nervousness | Wt loss |
| Sweatiness | Amneorrhea or oligomenorrhea |
| Frequent bowel movements | |

*Causes*
Autoimmune (Grave's disease)
Thyroid nodules
Abuse of thyroid medication

*Clinical*
Decreased TSH (< 0.04 mU/l)
Increased $T_3$ and $T_4$
Decreased HCT
Increased AST and ALT
Increased Alkaline phosphatase
Increased WBC
Increased serum calcium (flag for thyroid nodule)

*Thyroid Nodules and Goiter*
Benign: solitary nodule vs. multinodular goiter
May be euthyroid, hypothyroid, or hyperthyroid
Thyroid cancer (often euthyroid)

*Treatment*
Radioiodine—safe, curative; tx of choice
Antithyroid medications: propylthiouracil (PTU), methimazole
Beta-blockers (propranolol, etc.) are useful for short-term management

*Antithyroid Drugs in Pregnancy and Lactation*
Thyroid hormone requirements change during pregnancy
$T_4$ is 1.5 × higher, and TSH is low especially in the 1st trimester
Methimazole is contraindicated in pregnancy, use PTU

## Postpartum Thyroiditis

*Initial Hyperthyroid Phase*
Usually within 3 mo
S/sx: agitation, fatigue, poor sleep

*Later Hypothyroid Phase*
Usually 3–9 mo
S/sx: fatigue, wt gain, depression
Thyroid function usually WNL at 12 mo

T

**SOURCE**
Arcangelo, V. P., & Peterson, A. M. (Eds.). (2006). *Pharmacotherapeutics for advanced practice: A practical approach* (2nd ed.). Philadelphia, PA: Lippincott Williams and Wilkins.

## TOCOLYTICS

### Goal

Used to prevent preterm birth by 48 h in order to allow time for a course of glucocorticoids to enhance fetal lung maturity

Many of the medications work by decreasing intracellular calcium, which decreases muscle contractility

### Definition of PTL

Before 37 wk

2 cm and 80%

Change in dilation > 1 cm

Cervical length < 30 mm

Positive fFN

### FDA-Approved Treatment

Ritodrine hydrochloride (Yutopar; IV only) for labor between 20 and 36 wk gestation and fetus weighing between 500 and 2499 g

### General Findings

Maintenance oral tocolytic therapy does not decrease uterine activity, reduce the rate of recurrent PTL or PTB, or improve perinatal outcome

Overall improvement in perinatal outcome may be achieved with a comprehensive program of PTD prevention without the use of maintenance oral tocolytic therapy

### MgSO$_4$

MgSO$_4$ has been used for seizure prophylaxis and to treat seizures in preeclamptic and eclamptic pts for almost 100 years

Its first use as a tocolytic was in the 1960s, but it was used in laboratory experiments rather than in clinical tests

This drug is often chosen as the first-line therapy for preterm labor

### Medications

*See* Table T-2.

*See also* Preterm Labor

*See also* Magnesium Sulfate

#### SOURCES

Crowther, C. A., Hiller, J. E., & Doyle, L. W. (2002). Magnesium sulphate for preventing preterm birth in threatened preterm labour. *Cochrane Database of Systematic Reviews*, (4), 001060.

Epocrates, I. (2008). *Epocrates online*. Retrieved May 27, 2008, from www.epocrates.com

Gyetvai, K., Hannah, M. E., Hodnett, E. D., & Ohlsson, A. (1999). Tocolytics for preterm labor: A systematic review. *Obstetrics & Gynecology, 94*(5 Pt 2), 869–877.

Pryde, P. G., Besinger, R. E., Gianopoulos, J. G., & Mittendorf, R. (2001). Adverse and beneficial effects of tocolytic therapy. *Seminars in Perinatology, 25*(5), 316–340.

Rideout, S. L. (2005). Tocolytics for pre-term labor. What nurses need to know. *AWHONN Lifelines/ Association of Women's Health, Obstetric and Neonatal Nurses, 9*(1), 56–61.

Rust, O. A., Bofill, J. A., Arriola, R. M., Andrew, M. E., & Morrison, J. C. (1996). The clinical efficacy of oral tocolytic therapy. *American Journal of Obstetrics and Gynecology, 175*(4 Pt 1), 838–842.

**TABLE T-2** Tocolytic Medications

| Drugs | Magnesium sulfate | Terbutaline, ritodine | Nifedipine, nicardipine | Indomethicin |
|---|---|---|---|---|
| Class | Anticonvulsant, laxative | Beta adrenergic agonist | Ca channel blocker | NSAID/prostaglandin inhibitor |
| Loading Dose | 4–6 g IV over 20 m | Multiple options IV/IM/SC/PO | 10 mg PO | 50 mg PO |
| Maintenance | 1–4 g/h (requires monitoring of MgSO$_4$ levels) | | 10–20 mg Q 4–6 h | 25–50 mg PO Q 6 h |
| Peak | | 10 min | 30–60 min | 4–5 h |
| Half-Life | 90% excreted in 24 h | Ritodine: 2 h<br>Terbutaline: 3–4 h | 1–2 h | 15 h |
| Pregnancy Category | B | B | C | B |
| Maternal Effects | HA, N/V, weakness, visual changes, urine retention, cardiac arrest, hypocalcemia | Tachycardia, anxiety, hyperglycemia, hypokalemia, BP changes, fluid retention, pulmonary edema, respiratory depression | N/V, HA, flushing, vasodilation, hepatotoxicity, transient tachycardia | N/V, HA, diarrhea, peptic ulcer, thrombocytopenia |
| Fetal Effects | Hypotonia, drowsiness, bony abnormalities, congenital rickets | Tachycardia, hypoglycemia, hyperinsulinemia, hydrops | Decreased uteroplacental blood flow | Oligohydramnios, decreased renal function, premature closure of ductus arteriosus |

*Source:* Adapted from Epocrates, I. (2008). *Epocrates online.* Retrieved May 27, 2008, from http://www.epocrates.com

T

## TRANSGENDER

### Vocabulary

*Gender*—psychosocial construct that culture uses to identify male, female, neither, and both

*Queer*—the sexual orientation called *queer* is most often individually defined though in general usually means that their sexual attraction is blind to sex and/or gender

*Sex*—physiological makeup of a person including genetics, hormones, morphology, biochemistry, and anatomy

*Sex reassignment surgery* (also known as gender reassignment surgery)—surgical procedures that modify the biological body to align with the individual's gender identity (e.g., mastectomy, breast implants, metoidioplasty, vaginoplasty, phalloplasty)

*Transgender*—the umbrella term used to describe people with gender identities and expressions that are not traditionally associated with their biological sex

*Transgender man*—female sex who gender identifies as a male

*Transgender woman*—male sex who gender identifies as female

*Transition*—the process through which transgender individuals move in aligning their gender identity; particularly physical, legal, and psychological

*Transsexual*—individuals who believe that their physical bodies do not represent their true sex. Transsexuals usually desire sex reassignment surgery but may choose varying degrees of surgical transition

### Resources for Treatment Guidelines

Callen Lorde Community Health Center, 356 West 18th St., New York, NY 10011. 212-271-7200. www.callen-lorde.org/index.html

Tom Waddell Health Center Transgender Protocol, 50 Lech Walesa (Ivy) St., San Francisco, CA. 415-355-7400

The World Professional Association for Transgender Health, *Standards of Care* (6th version). 612-624-9397. www.wpath.org

### SOURCES

Dean, L., Meyer, I. H., Robinson, K., Sell, R. L., Sember, R., Silenzio, V. M. B., et al. (2000). Lesbian, gay, bisexual, and transgender health: Findings and concerns. *Journal of the Gay and Lesbian Medical Association, 4*(3), 101–151.

Dutton, L., Koenig, K., & Fennie, K. (2008). Gynecological care of the female-to-male transgender man. *Journal of Midwifery & Women's Health, 53,* 331–337.

Harry Benjamin International Gender Dysphoria Association. (2001). *Standards of care for gender identity disorders* (6th version). Retrieved April 23, 2006, from www.hbigda.org/soc.htm

Oriel, K. A. (2000). Medical care of transsexual patients. *Journal of the Gay and Lesbian Medical Association, 4*(4), 185–194.

# TRICHOMONIASIS VAGINALIS

## Cause
*Trichomonas vaginalis*

## Statistics
8 million new cases/yr in North America
Incubation period 4–28 d

## Signs and Symptoms

*Women*
25–50% asymptomatic
Diffuse yellow-green odiferous discharge with vulvar irritation
Symptoms usually develop within 6 mo of infection
'Strawberry cervix' seen on colposcopy 90% of the time

*Men*
Asymptomatic usually but occasionally experience urethral discharge, urge to
urinate, or pain and burning with urination

## Diagnosis
Saline wet prep of vaginal secretions that shows motile protozoans; 60–70%
sensitivity
OSOM Trich rapid test—an immunochromatographic capillary flow dipstick
technology; 83% sensitivity and 97% specificity, results in 10 min
Affirm VP III—a nucleic acid probe test; 83% sensitivity, 97% specificity, results in
45 min
Vaginal cultures are the most specific and sensitive

## Treatment (Pregnant and Nonpregnant)
Metronidazole 2 g PO × 1 (Preg Cat B, Lact Cat L3)
Tinidazole 2 g PO × 1 (Preg Cat C, Lact Cat L4)
Metronidazole 500 mg PO BID × 7 d (Preg Cat B, Lact Cat L3)
Tx the partner also

## Follow-Up
None needed if pt becomes asymptomatic
If symptoms do not resolve, move to longer duration of tx

## Patient Education
Transmission and protection
No ETOH with metronidazole for 24 h and tinidazole for 72 h after last dose
No sex until both partners are treated and cured

## Pregnancy and Lactation
Increased risk of PROM, PTD, LBW, and postpartum endometritis
Defer treatment until after 37 wk if asymptomatic
Do not breastfeed for 12–24 h after metronidazole tx and for 3 d after tinidazole tx

### SOURCES
Centers for Disease Control and Prevention. (2004). *Trichomonas infection.* Retrieved May 25, 2008,
from http://www.cdc.gov/ncidod/dpd/parasites/trichomonas/factsht_trichomonas.htm
Centers for Disease Control and Prevention. (2006). *Sexually transmitted diseases treatment
guidelines, 2006.* Morbidity and Mortality Weekly Report, 55(RR-11), 52–54.
Hale, T. W. (2008). *Medications and mothers' milk* (13th ed.). Amarillo, TX: Hale.

T

# TUBERCULOSIS

## Cause

*Mycobacterium tuberculosis*, transmitted through droplet inhalation

Creates a primary lesion in the lungs that in most people gets encapsulated, and they have no further symptoms

Spreads in the lungs and can move into lymphatic nodes and throughout the body

## Risk Factors

Overcrowded environment
Immigration from TB epidemic areas
Nosocomial exposure
Prior TB infection
HIV
Diabetes
Steroid therapy
Immunosuppressive therapy
Head and neck cancer
Renal disease
Malabsorption syndromes
Gastrectomy
Malnutrition
Alcoholism
Substance abuse

## Signs and Symptoms

Fever
Night sweats
Wt loss
Chronic cough
Productive cough
Pleurisy with effusion
Spontaneous atelectasis
Crepitant rales

## Screening with PPD (Mantaux)

0.1 ml of purified protein derivative tuberculin containing 5 tuberculin units administered intradermally in forearm

Read in 48–72 h, > 10 mm of induration is positive for pt with no known risk factors for TB and a healthy immune system

Induration > 5 mm is positive for an immunocompromised pt

BCG vaccination used in many countries and will result in a positive PPD

## Diagnosis

CXR (in pregnant women use abdominal shield)
Sputum culture

## Treatment

*Latent TB*

Isoniazid prophylaxis 300 mg PO daily × 9 mo

*Pregnant*

Isoniazid, rifampin, ethambutol for 9-mo therapy, include vitamin $B_6$ therapy
Breastfeeding is not contraindicated
Tx family also

## Comply with State Reporting Regulations

### SOURCE

Varney, H., Kriebs, J. M., & Gegor, C. L. (2004). *Varney's midwifery* (4th ed.). Sudbury, MA: Jones and Bartlett.

# ULTRASOUND

## Indications

Gestational age with uncertain conception dates
Fetal growth evaluation
Vaginal bleeding
Assess fetal presentation if not easily palpated externally
Suspected multiple gestation
During procedures: amniocentesis, version, fetoscopy, cordocentesis, CVS, IVF, cervical cerclage placement
Size/dates discrepancy
Pelvic mass assessment
Suspected hydatidiform mole
Suspected ectopic pregnancy
Suspected fetal death
Suspected uterine abnormality
Localization of IUD
Surveillance of ovarian follicle development
Biophysical profile
Manual removal of placenta
Measure AFI
Suspected abruptio placentae
Estimate fetal weight
Abnormal AFP
Follow-up evaluation for fetal anomaly
Placental location
Fetal condition in late registrants for care

## Components of Exam

*1st Trimester*
Gestational sac location (r/o ectopic pregnancy)
Embryo identification (r/o molar pregnancy)
Crown-rump length (accurate EDD estimate)
Assessment of fetal cardiac activity
Fetal number
Evaluation of the uterus: size, shape, location, adnexa

*2nd and 3rd Trimesters*
Fetal number/presentation
Documentation of cardiac activity
Doppler flow studies
Placental location
BPP
AFI
Gestational age
Survey for fetal anatomy

## Effects

Studies have demonstrated no adverse bioeffects on the human embryo or fetus

## SOURCE

Varney, H., Kriebs, J. M., & Gegor, C. L. (2004). *Varney's midwifery* (4th ed.). Sudbury, MA: Jones and Bartlett.

## UMBILICAL CORD

2 arteries
1 vein
Venous blood has a higher pH than arterial blood
Cord pH = 7.25–7.40
Base excess:
  Measurement of the overall buffering ability of the blood
  > 12 indicates significant compromise
  A base excess of 0 is optimal

TABLE U-1   Acid-Base and Blood Gas Values in Umbilical Cord Vessels

|  | Umbilical Artery | Umbilical Vein |
|---|---|---|
| pH | 7.33 ± 0.07[*] | 7.38 ± 0.06 |
| Carbon dioxide pressure (mmHg) | 45 ± 10 | 38 ± 8 |
| Bicarbonate (mEq • l$^{-1}$) | 23 ± 5 | 23 ± 5 |
| Base excess (mEq • l$^{-1}$) | −3 ± 3 | +0.5 ± 4 |
| Oxygen content (mM • l$^{-1}$) | — | 6.7 ± 0.6 |
| Oxygen pressure (mmHg) | 35 ± 15 | 41 ± 20 |
| Hemoglobin (g • dl$^{-1}$) | 13 | 13 |

Note: n = [3] 50.
[*]Mean ± 2 SD.

*Source:* Reprinted with permission from Ecker, J. L., & Parer, J. T. (1999). Obstetrical evaluation of fetal acid-base balance. *Critical Reviews in Clinical Laboratory Science, 36*(5), 407.

TABLE U-2   Relationship Between Fetal Blood pH and Fetal Heart Rate Patterns in Preceding 20 Minutes

| FHR Deceleration Pattern | Fetal Blood pH* |
|---|---|
| Early, mid variable, or absent | 7.30 ± 0.04 |
| Moderate variable | 7.26 ± 0.04 |
| Mild or moderate late | 7.22 ± 0.06 |
| Severe late or variable | 7.14 ± 0.07 |

*Approximate mean ± standard deviation.

*Source:* Reprinted with permission from Ecker, J. L., & Parer, J. T. (1999). Obstetrical evaluation of fetal acid-base balance. *Critical Reviews in Clinical Laboratory Science, 36*(5), 407.

**SOURCE**

Ecker, J. L., & Parer, J. T. (1999). Obstetrical evaluation of fetal acid-base balance. *Critical Reviews in Clinical Laboratory Science, 36*(5), 407.

# URINALYSIS

**TABLE U-4** Urinalysis

| Observations | Normal | Abnormal | Interpretation |
|---|---|---|---|
| Color | Clear, pale yellow | Cloudy | Pyuria, lipiduria |
| | | Brown | Bile pigments, myoglobin |
| | | Brownish-black | Bile pigments, melanin, methemoglobin |
| | | Green or blue | Pseudomonal UTI, biliverdin |
| | | Orange | Bile pigments |
| | | Red | Hematuria, hemoglobinuria, myoglobinuria, porphyria |
| | | Dark yellow | Concentrated urine |
| RBCs | Negative | Positive | UTI, pyelonephritis, exercise-induced hematuria |
| Leukocyte esterase | Negative | Positive | UTI, pyelonephritis |
| Nitrites | Negative | Positive | Bacturia |
| Protein | Negative | Trace (5–10 mg/dl) | Typically insignificant finding |
| | | 1+ (30 mg/dl) | Dehydration, exercise, fever, emotional stress |
| | | 2+ (100 mg/dl) | Dehydration, exercise, vaginal secretions, UTI, Gestational HTN, preeclampsia if associated with elevated BP in pregnancy |
| | | 3+ (300 mg/dl) | UTI, vaginal secretions, Gestational HTN, preeclampsia in pregnancy |
| Glucose | Negative | Positive | DM, Cushing's syndrome, high sugar intake |
| Ketones | Negative | Positive | Uncontrolled DM, starvation, high protein diet, dehydration from N/V/D |
| Bilirubin | Negative | Positive | Hemolysis, liver disease |
| Urine pH | Normal range is 4.5 to 8.0, usually urine is acidic (5.5 to 6.5) | Dependent on symptoms | Useful in determining cause of calculi. Alkaline suggests MgNH₄PO₄ containing calculi. Acidic suggests uric acid calculi |
| Urine specific gravity | 1.003–1.030 | < 1.010 | Hydrated |
| | | > 1.020 | Dehydration |

Source: Adapted from Simerville, J. A., Maxted, W. C., & Pahira, J. J. (2005). Urinalysis: A comprehensive review. *American Family Physician, 71*(6), 1153–1162.

U

## URINARY TRACT INFECTION (UTI)

### Signs and Symptoms
Dysuria
Frequency
Urgency
Suprapubic heaviness/discomfort/pressure

### History/Exam
Dysuria
CVAT
Urine dip
Fever
Chills

### Important to r/o Pylonephritis
Acute onset chills
Fever
Flank pain/CVAT
H/A
Malaise
Hematuria

### Risk Factors
Increased sexual activity
Diaphragm/spermicide use
Failure to void after sex
Anal to vaginal penetration
Pregnancy
Postponing urination or incomplete voiding
Diabetes

### Diagnosis
Urine dip: leukocytes, nitrites, possibly protein, possibly blood
Microscopic analysis: > 5 WBCs, > 5 RBCs, positive bacteria
C&S: bacterial colony > 100,000

### Organisms
*E. coli*
*Staphylococcus saprophyticus*

### Treatment
*See* Table U-3.

### Refer
Pyelonephritis
Multiple recurrent infections
Infections with unusual organisms

### Follow-Up
Test of cure 1–2 wk after finishing antibiotics (optional)

### Recurrent UTI
Follow closely with urine cultures Q 1–2 mo

#### SOURCES
Epocrates, I. (2008). *Epocrates online*. Retrieved May 27, 2008, from http://www.epocrates.com
Hale, T. W. (2008). *Medications and mothers' milk* (13th ed.). Amarillo, TX: Hale.
Varney, H., Kriebs, J. M., & Gegor, C. L. (2004). *Varney's midwifery* (4th ed.). Sudbury, MA: Jones and Bartlett.

**TABLE U-3** Treatment for Urinary Tract Infections

| Medication | Dose | Pharmacology | Side Effects |
|---|---|---|---|
| Nitrofurantoin (Macrobid) <br><br> Preg Cat B <br> Lact Cat L2 | 100 mg BID × 7 d | Bactericidal <br> Antimicrobial <br> Urine excreted <br> CYP 450 active <br> Liver processed | N/V <br> Allergic reaction <br> Dizziness <br> Hemolytic anemia <br> Flatulence <br> Vertigo <br> Anorexia |
| Amoxicillin <br><br> Preg Cat B <br> Lact Cat L1 | 500 mg Q 8 h × 7 d | Bactericidal <br> Antimicrobial <br> Urine excreted <br> CYP 450 active <br> Liver processed | N/V <br> Diarrhea <br> Rash <br> Urticaria <br> Eosinophilia <br> Black hairy tongue <br> Candidiasis |
| Keflex (Cefalexin) <br><br> Preg Cat B <br> Lact Cat L1 | 500 mg PO BID × 7 d | Bactericidal <br> Antimicrobial <br> Urine excreted <br> CYP 450 active | Diarrhea <br> Rash <br> N/V <br> Abdominal pain <br> Steven-Johnson syndrome <br> Otitis <br> Dizziness <br> HA |
| Bactrim (trimethoprim/ sulfamethoxazole) <br><br> Preg Cat C <br> Lact Cat L3 | 80/160 mg BID × 3 d | Combination antimicrobicide <br> Urine excreted <br> CYP 450 active <br> Liver processed | N/V <br> Allergic reaction (sulfa) <br> Urticaria <br> Photosensitivity <br> Diarrhea <br> Dizziness <br> Lethargy |
| Pyridium (Phenazopyridine HCl) (analgesic only) <br><br> Preg Cat B <br> Lact Cat L3 | 100 mg PO TID × 2 d | Urine excreted <br> CYP 450 active <br> Liver processed | GI upset <br> HA <br> Rash <br> Orange urine <br> Hemolytic anemia <br> Pruritus <br> Dyspepsia <br> Anaphylaxis |

*Sources:* Adapted from Epocrates, I. (2008). *Epocrates online.* Retrieved May 27, 2008, from http://www.epocrates.com. Hale, T. W. (2008). *Medications and mothers' milk* (13th ed.). Amarillo, TX: Hale.

U

TABLE V-1  Vaccination of Pregnant Women

| | Vaccine | Should Be Considered If Indicated | Contraindicated | Special Consideration |
|---|---|---|---|---|
| | Hepatitis A | | | Low theoretical risk—inactivated vaccine |
| | Hepatitis B | ✔ | | |
| | Human papillomavirus (HPV) | | | No data available. Even if mid series, delay further dosing until after pregnancy |
| | Influenza (inactivated) | ✔ | | |
| | Influenza (LAIV)* | | X | |
| | Measles* | | X | |
| Routine | Meningococcal (MCV4) | | | No data available on its use in pregnancy |
| | Mumps* | | X | |
| | Pneumococcal | | | No data available |
| | Polio (IPV) | | | Theoretical risk |
| | Rubella | | X | |
| | Tetanus-diphtheria | ✔ | | |
| | Tetanus-diphtheria-pertussis (Tdap) | | | Not contraindicated but little data available. Prefer 2nd or 3rd trimester administration if needed |
| | Varicella | | X | Pregnancy should be avoided for 1 mo after vaccination |

/ continues

TABLE V-1 Vaccination of Pregnant Women (continued)

| Vaccine | Should Be Considered If Indicated | Contraindicated | Special Consideration |
|---|---|---|---|
| Anthrax | | | No studies. Weigh risks and benefits. |
| BCG* | | X | |
| Japanese encephalitis | | | Theoretical risk. Weigh risks and benefits. |
| Meningococcal (MPSV4) | ✔ | | |
| Rabies | ✔ | | Postexposure prophylaxis indicated |
| Typhoid (parenteral and oral*) | | | No data |
| Vaccinia* (smallpox) | | X | Fetal risk; only vaccinate for direct exposure. Weigh risks and benefits. |
| Yellow fever* | | | Only when traveling to an endemic area |
| Zoster* | | X | |

(The rows "Typhoid (parenteral and oral*)", "Vaccinia* (smallpox)", "Yellow fever*", and "Zoster*" are grouped under the label **Travel**.)

*Live attenuated vaccine

Source: Adapted from Centers for Disease Control and Prevention. (2007). Guidelines for vaccinating pregnant women. Retrieved May 26, 2008, from http://www.cdc.gov/vaccines/pubs/preg-guide.htm

**SOURCE**
Centers for Disease Control and Prevention. (2007). Guidelines for vaccinating pregnant women.
Retrieved May 26, 2008, from http://www.cdc.gov/vaccines/pubs/preg-guide.htm

V–Z

# VAGINAL BIRTH AFTER CESAREAN BIRTH (VBAC)

Every woman who has had a previous cesarean birth must consider the risks and benefits of deciding between trial of labor or elective repeat cesarean birth. This decision must be made with careful consideration of the contributing factors—see tables below

The predominant concern with VBAC is the risk of uterine rupture, which is calculated at approximately 1% of cases

## Decreasing Risk of Uterine Rupture

Do not use prostaglandins for induction

Only women with a low transverse incision in the uterus

Adherence to labor curves

TABLE V-2   Factors Associated with Probability of Successful VBAC

| Factor | Probability of Successful VBAC (%) |
|---|---|
| Indication for prior cesarean birth | |
| CPD | 65% |
| Breech | 89% |
| Fetal distress | 77% |
| Cervical dilation at prior cesarean | |
| Less than 5 centimeters | 67% |
| 6–9 centimeters | 73% |
| Second stage | 13% |
| Cervical dilation on admission | |
| Greater than 4 centimeters | 86% |
| Cervical effacement on admission | |
| Less than 25% effaced | 52% |
| 25% to 75% effaced | 70% |
| Greater than 75% effaced | 81% |
| Prior vaginal birth | |

Vaginal birth following cesarean birth is more predictive of success than vaginal birth prior to the cesarean birth

*Source:* Reprinted with permission from King, T. (2004). Vaginal birth after previous cesarean section. *Journal of Midwifery & Women's Health, 49*(1), 68–75.

TABLE V-3   Risk Stratification on the Basis of Obstetric History and Labor Characteristics

| Low Risk | Medium Risk | High Risk |
|---|---|---|
| 1 prior low transverse cesarean birth | Mechanical or Pitocin induction of labor | Repetitive nonreassuring FHR abnormalities not responsive to clinical intervention |
| Spontaneous onset of labor | Pitocin augmentation | Bleeding suggestive of abruption |
| No need for augmentation | 2 or more previous low transverse cesarean births | 2 hours without cervical change in the active phase of adequate labor |
| No repetitive FHR abnormalities | < 18 months between prior cesarean birth and current delivery | |
| Previous successful VBAC | | |

*Source:* Reprinted with permission from King, T. (2004). Vaginal birth after previous cesarean section. *Journal of Midwifery & Women's Health, 49*(1), 68–75.

## SOURCE

King, T. (2004). Vaginal birth after previous cesarean section. *Journal of Midwifery & Women's Health, 49*(1), 68–75.

# VERSION

## Goal

Turn the fetus so that a more favorable part of the fetus is presenting at the cervix

Performed in cases of breech or transverse presentation or with second twin after the birth of the first twin

The objective is to increase the likelihood of vaginal birth and decrease the need for C/S

## Types

External: both hands on mother's abdomen

Internal: fingers or hand are inserted into the uterus with other hand placed externally on maternal abdomen

## Contraindications

Low AFI

Contracted uterus

Unstable fetal condition

Placenta previa

Fetal intolerance of the procedure

## Tocolytics Are Often Used to Relax the Uterus Before Attempting Version

Done at 36 wk to term when fetus is mature enough to be delivered if a complication arises

The earlier it is done the more room a baby has to turn

Average success of external cephalic version = 58%

### SOURCES

American College of Obstetricians and Gynecologists. (1999). External cephalic version. In *2006 compendium of selected publications* (p. 562). Washington, DC: Author.

Frye, A. (2004). *Holistic midwifery: A comprehensive textbook for midwives in homebirth practice.* Portland, Oregon: Labrys Press.

V–Z

# VIRAL INFECTIONS (ANTENATAL)

*See* Table V-4.

TABLE V-4  TORCH: Toxoplasmosis, Other Infections (Varicella, Parvovirus, Syphilis), Rubella, Cytomegalovirus, Herpes

|  | Toxoplasmosis | Rubella | Cytomegalovirus | Varicella | Parvovirus B19 (Fifth Disease) | Syphilis |
|---|---|---|---|---|---|---|
| Cases | 1 in 1000 pregnant women infected each year (Varney, 2004) | Most people in the United States are immunized | Affects 50–85% of the adults in United States by age 40 Primary infection of pregnant women 1–3% (Varney, 2004) | 95% of adults have hx of infection Of 5% w/o hx, 75% exhibit serologic immunity (Varney, 2004) | 50% population over age 12 yr are immune (Frye, 2007) | See Syphilis |
| Transmission | Cat feces Raw or undercooked meat (most frequently pork) |  | Close intimate contact with body fluids | Direct contact and respiratory droplets Varicella zoster immune globulin (VZIG) at exposure | Contact with respiratory secretions Blood exposure | Sexually transmitted |
| At Risk | Cat owners Undercooked meat Gardeners | International travel Nonimmunized | Child care providers Pregnant women should not care for children who are chronic congenital CMV carriers | Incubation 10–21 d Communicable 2 d before lesions appear until 10 d after all lesions are crusted over | Those working or living with elementary and middle school children | Sex with infected partners |

/ continues

TABLE V-4 TORCH: Toxoplasmosis, Other Infections (Varicella, Parvovirus, Syphilis), Rubella, Cytomegalovirus, Herpes (continued)

| | Toxoplasmosis | Rubella | Cytomegalovirus | Varicella | Parvovirus B19 (Fifth Disease) | Syphilis |
|---|---|---|---|---|---|---|
| S/sx | Mostly asymptomatic<br>Fatigue<br>Malaise<br>Muscle pain<br>Fever<br>Sore throat<br>Enlarged posterior cervical lymph nodes<br>If mono comes back neg, test for toxoplasmosis | Low-grade fever<br>Drowsiness<br>Sore throat<br>Rash (spread from face over body and fades rapidly)<br>Swollen neck glands<br>Duration 3–5 d | Suspect if s/sx of mono or hepatitis w/ negative test results for both | Fever<br>Chills<br>Myalgia<br>Arthralgia<br>Vesicles (pruritic, start at head and spread down)<br>Associated w/ respiratory infection | Slapped cheek<br>Flushing fever<br>Malaise<br>Myalgias<br>HA<br>Maculopapular lacelike pruritic rash on trunk that moves outward | Painless chancre at site of infection<br>Adenopathy<br>Palmar and solar rash<br>Patchy alopecia<br>Fever<br>Sore throat<br>Hoarseness<br>Malaise<br>HA<br>Anorexia |
| Dx/Testing | IgM<br>IgG<br>Repeat in 3 wk (many IgM false positives) | IgG<br>IgM<br>Rubella antibody titer | ELISA<br>IgG Q 2 wk<br>IgM | Seriological testing | IgM<br>IgG | RPR<br>VDRL |
| Tx | Sulfonamides<br>Pyrimethadine<br>Spiramycin | | | Acyclovir<br>VZIG | Monitor fetus<br>U/S | Penicillin G 2.4 million units IM |

/ continues

V–Z

TABLE V-4  TORCH: Toxoplasmosis, Other Infections (Varicella, Parvovirus, Syphilis), Rubella, Cytomegalovirus, Herpes (continued)

| | Toxoplasmosis | Rubella | Cytomegalovirus | Varicella | Parvovirus B19 (Fifth Disease) | Syphilis |
|---|---|---|---|---|---|---|
| Risks Fetus | Severe congenital malformations<br>Most severe cases are those contracted late in 1st trimester<br>Seizures<br>Motor and cognitive deficits<br>Mental retardation | Greatest risks in 1st trimester: 50% chance of baby with fetal rubella syndrome (cataracts, cardiac defects, deafness, IUGR)<br>Miscarriage<br>Stillbirth<br>Fetal anomalies | Of exposed, 30% of fetuses are infected, and 15% of those will have symptoms<br>Enlargement of liver and spleen with jaundice<br>Hearing loss<br>Vision impairment<br>Mental retardation | 20–40% of fetuses exposed will be affected<br>Congenital varicella syndrome<br>Most risk in first 20 wk and 2–6 d before delivery | 20–30% placental transfer<br>Aplastic anemia<br>Nonimmune hydrops<br>Death | 40% fetal loss with untreated syphilis, another 40% give birth to babies with congenital syphilis |

Sources: Adapted from Frye, A. (1997). *Understanding diagnostic tests in the childbearing years* (6th ed.). Portland, OR: Labrys Press. Kriebs, J. M. (2008). Breaking the cycle of infection: TORCH and other infections in women's health. *Journal of Midwifery & Women's Health, 53*(3), 173–174. Varney, H., Kriebs, J. M., & Gegor, C. L. (2004). *Varney's midwifery* (4th ed.). Sudbury, MA: Jones and Bartlett.

# VITAMINS

Fat-soluble vitamins are D, E, A, and K

TABLE V–5 Vitamin Guide

| | RDA Pregnant or Lactating | RDA Nonpregnant, Nonlactating Women 14–70 Yr Old | Max Daily Dose | Source | Function |
|---|---|---|---|---|---|
| Calcium | 1000–1300 mg/d | 1000 mg/d | 2500 mg/d | Milk, cheese, yogurt, corn tortillas (calcium-set), tofu, kale, broccoli | Blood clotting, muscle contraction, nerve transmission, bone formation |
| Folic acid | 600 mcg/dl | 0.4 mg (400 mcg/dl) | 1000 mcg/dl | Enriched cereals, green leafy vegetables, enriched whole grain bread, fortified foods | Coenzyme in nucleic acid metabolism, prevents megaloblastic anemia |
| Iodine | Pregnancy 220 mcg/d Lactating 290 mcg/d | 150 mcg | 1000–1100 mcg/d | Processed food, iodized salt | Component of thyroid hormones |
| Iron | Pregnancy 27 mg/d Lactation 9–10 mg/d | 18 mg/d | 45 mg/d | Fortified dairy products and cereals, fish liver oil, egg yolk | Component of hemoglobin |
| Vitamin A | Pregnancy 750–770 mcg/dl Lactation 1200–1300 mcg/dl | 700 mcg | 3000 mcg/d | Liver, dairy, egg yolk, fish, carrots, green vegetables, pumpkin, sweet potato | Vision, gene expression, reproduction, embryonic development, immune function |
| Vitamin $B_{12}$ | 2.6–2.8 mcg/d | 2.4 mcg | None | Fortified cereal, meat, fish, shellfish, poultry, dairy | Coenzyme in nucleic acid metabolism, prevents megaloblastic anemia |
| Vitamin $B_6$ | 1.9–2.0 mg/d | 1.3 mg | 100 mg/d | Fortified cereal, whole grain bread, organ meat, meat, poultry, legumes | Coenzyme in metabolism of amino acids and glycogen |

/ continues

V–Z

**TABLE V–5** Vitamin Guide (continued)

| | RDA Pregnant or Lactating | RDA Nonpregnant, Nonlactating Women 14–70 Yr Old | Max Daily Dose | Source | Function |
|---|---|---|---|---|---|
| Vitamin C | Pregnancy 80–85 mg/d Lactation 115–120 mg/d | 75 mg | 2000 mg/d | Citrus fruit, tomatoes, potatoes, broccoli, brussel sprouts, spinach | Cofactors in reactions involving copper or iron metalloenzymes |
| Vitamin D | 5 mcg/d | 5 mcg/d | 50 mcg/d | Fortified dairy and cereal, fish liver oil, egg yolk | Maintains serum calcium and phosphorus level for bone maintenance |
| Vitamin E | 15–19 mg | 15 mg | 1000 mg/d | Vegetable oil, unprocessed grains, nuts, fruit, vegetables, meat, wheat germ | Nonspecific chain-breaking antioxidant |
| Vitamin K | 75–90 mcg/d | 90 mcg | None | Green leafy vegetables, brussel sprouts, cabbage, plant oils, margarine | Coenzyme during creation of clotting factors |
| Zinc | 11–13 mg/d | 8 mg/d | 34–40 mg/d | Fortified cereals, red meat, some seafood | Component of enzymes and proteins, regulation of gene expression |
| Fiber | 28–29 g/d | 25–26 g/d | None | Grains (oats, wheat, rice), fruit | Improves bowel function, reduces risk of coronary artery disease |

*Sources:* Adapted from Institute of Medicine Food and Nutrition Board. (2008). *Dietary reference intakes: Elements.* Retrieved August 12, 2008, from http://www.iom.edu/Object.File/Master/7/294/0.pdf. Institute of Medicine Food and Nutrition Board. (2008). *Dietary reference intakes: Macronutrients.* Retrieved August 12, 2008, from http://www.iom.edu/Object.File/Master/7/300/Webtablemacro.pdf. Institute of Medicine Food and Nutrition Board. (2008). *Dietary reference intakes: Vitamins.* Retrieved August 12, 2008, from http://www.iom.edu/Object.File/Master/7/296/webtablevitamins.pdf

# VULVODYNIA

### Definition
Vulvar discomfort
Occurs in the absence of any other dx

### Diagnosis
*Test For*
HPV
Yeast
Urine crystals
Pudendal nerve neuropathy

### Signs and Symptoms
Burning
Rawness
Stinging
Tingling
May affect vulva, inner thighs, buttocks

### Vulvar Vestibulitis
Localized pain with touch at 3, 6, 9, 12 o'clock of vulva
Characterized by pain, tingling, and/or burning

### Treatment
Hygiene
Decrease oxylate ingestion (coffee, tea, chocolate)
Treat underlying cause
TCA (amatryptyline) low dose
Gabapentin < 1200 mg/d

### Resources
www.vulvarpainfoundation.org
www.nva.org
www.vulvodynia.com

### SOURCES
Glazer, H., & Rodke, G. (2002). In Kahn, B. (Ed.), *The vulvodynia survival guide: How to overcome painful vaginal symptoms and enjoy an active lifestyle.* Oakland, CA: New Harbinger Publications.
Stewart, E. (2000). *The V book: A doctor's guide to complete vulvovaginal health.* New York: Bantam Books.
Stone-Godena, T. (2006). Vulvar pain syndrome: Vestibulodynia. *Journal of Midwifery & Women's Health, 51*(6), 502–509.

# ABBREVIATIONS

17-OHP = 17-hydroxyprogesterone

AA = African American

AAO = awake, alert, and oriented

AAP = American Academy of Pediatrics

Ab = abortion

aCL = anticardiolipin antibody

ACNM = American College of Nurse-Midwives

ACOG = American College of Obstetricians and Gynecologists

ADA = American Diabetes Association

AFI = amniotic fluid index

AFLP = acute fatty liver of pregnancy

AFP = alpha fetoprotein

AFV = amniotic fluid volume

AGC = atypical glandular cells

AIDS = acquired immunodeficiency syndrome

ALT (SGPT) = alanine aminotransferase test

APA = antiphospholipid antibody

aPL = antiphospholipid antibody

approx = approximately

APS = antiphospholipid syndrome

ARDS = acute respiratory distress syndrome

AROM = artificial rupture of membranes

ASCH = atypical squamous cells, unable to exclude HSIL

ASCUS = atypical squamous cells of undetermined significance

ASD = atrial septal defect

AST (SGOT) = aspartate aminotransferase test

BBT = basal body temperature

BCA = bichloroacetic acid

BCG = bacillus of Calmette and Guerin, TB vaccine

B-hCG = beta human chorionic gonadotropin

BID = two times per day

BMI = body mass index

BP = blood pressure

bpm = beats per minute

BPP = biophysical profile

BRAT = bread/bananas, rice, apple sauce, tea

BS = bowel sounds

BSE = breast self-exam

BUN = blood urea nitrogen

BV = bacterial vaginosis

c/o = complaint of

C/S = cesarean section

C&S = cultures and sensitivities

CAD = coronary artery disease

Cat = category

cath = catheterize

CAVC = complete atrioventricular canal

CBC = complete blood count

CBE = clinical breast exam

CBT = cognitive behavior therapy

CC = chief complaint

CC-EPT = continuous combined estrogen–progestin therapy

CDC = Centers for Disease Control and Prevention

CEE = conjugated equine estrogens

CF = cystic fibrosis

CHD = coronary heart disease

CIN = cervical intraepithelia neoplasia

CM = certified midwife

CMT = cervical motion tenderness

CMV = cytomegalovirus

CNM = certified nurse–midwife

CNS = central nervous system

COC = combined oral contraceptive pills

colpo = colposcopy

COPD = chronic obstructive pulmonary disease

CP = cerebral palsy

CPD = cephalopelvic disproportion

CPR = cardiopulmonary resuscitation

CPS = Canadian Paediatric Society

CRH = corticotropin-releasing hormone

CT = *Chlamydia trachomatis*

CTAB = clear to ascultation, bilaterally

CTFR = cystic fibrosis transmembrane conductance regulator gene

ctx = contraction

CVA = cerebrovascular accident

CVAT = costovertebral angle tenderness

CVD = cardiovascular disease

CVS = chorionic villi sampling

CXR = chest X-ray

d = day(s)

d/c = discontinue

d/t = due to

D&C = dilation and curettage

DDx = differential diagnosis

Def = definition

DES = diethylstilbestrol

DEXA = dual energy X-ray absorption
DHEA = dehydroepiandrosterone
DHES = dehydropinadrosterone sulfate
DIC = disseminated intracoagulopathy
dl = deciliter
DM = diabetes mellitus
DMPA = depot medroxyprogesterone acetate
DOB = date of birth
DTR = deep tendon reflex
DUB = dysfunctional uterine bleeding
DVT = deep vein thrombosis
dx = diagnosis
E3 = estriol
EC = emergency contraception
EDD = estimated date of delivery
EE = ethinyl estradiol
EFM = electronic fetal monitoring
EFW = estimated fetal weight
EOMI = extra ocular movements intact
EONS = early onset neonatal GBS infection
ERT = estrogen replacement therapy
EtOH = ethanol/alcohol
F/U = follow-up
fFN = fetal fibronectin
FHR = fetal heart rate
FHT = fetal heart tone
FKC = fetal kick counts
F–N–F = finger–nose–finger test
FOB = father of baby
FSE = fetal scalp electrode
FSH = follicle-stimulating hormone
g = gram(s)
GA = gestational age
GBS = group B streptococcus
GC = *Gonorrhea*
GCT = glucose challenge test
GDM = gestational diabetes mellitus
GI = gastrointestinal
GIFT = gamete intrafallopian tubal transfer
GnRH = gonadotropin-releasing hormone
GTD = gestational trophoblastic disease
GTT = glucose tolerance test
GU = genitourinary
GYN = gynecological

h = hour(s)

H/A = headache

Hb = hemoglobin

hCG = human chorionic gonadotropin

HCT = hematocrit

HDL = high-density lipoprotein

HDN = hemorrhagic disease of the newborn

HEENT = head, ears, eyes, nose, throat

HIV= human immunodeficiency virus

H/o = history of

HPA = hypothalamic-pituitary axis

HPI = history of present illness

HPV = human papilloma virus

HRT = hormone replacement therapy

HS = hour of sleep

HSG = hysterosalpingogram

HSIL = high-grade squamous intraepithelial lesions

HSM = hepatosplenomegaly

HSV = herpes simplex virus

ht = height

HTN = hypertension

HUS = hemolytic-uremic syndrome

hx = history

IA = intermittent auscultation

IBS = inflammatory bowel disease

IDDM = insulin-dependent diabetes

IL = interleukin

IM = intramuscular

in = inches

INH-A = inhibin A

IP = intrapartum

ITP = idiopathic thrombocytopenia

IU = international units

IUD = intrauterine device

IUFD = intrauterine fetal demise

IUGR = intrauterine growth restriction

IUI = intrauterine insemination

IUP = intrauterine pregnancy

IUPC = intrauterine pressure catheter

IV = intravenous

IVF = in vitro fertilization

IVH = intraventricular hemorrhage

l = liter

L/S = lecithin/sphinogomyelin

LA = lupus anticoagulant

LAD = lymphadenopathy

lb = pound

LBW = low birth weight

LDL = low-density lipoprotein

LFT = liver function test

LGA = large for gestational age

LH = luetinizing hormone

LMP = last menstrual period

LR = light reflex

LRI = lower respiratory tract infection

LSIL = low-grade squamous intraepithelial lesions

MAOI = monoamine oxidase inhibitor

mcg = microgram

MCHC = mean corpuscular hemoglobin concentration

MCV = mean corpuscular volume

mEq = milliequivalent

mg = milligram

MI = myocardial infarction

min = minute

ml = milliliter

mm = millimeters

$mm^3$ = millimeters cubed

mo = month(s)

MOA = mechanism of action

MoM = multiple of the median

MRI = magnetic resonance imaging

MSAFP = maternal serum alpha fetoprotein

multip = multiparous

MVU = Montevideo units

N/V = nausea, vomiting

NCAT = normocephalic atraumatic

neg = negative

NIH = National Institutes of Health

NPO = nothing by mouth

NSAID = nonsteroidal anti-inflammatory drug

NST = nonstress test

NSVD = normal spontaneous vaginal delivery

NT = nontender

NTD = neural tube defect

nulip = nuliparous

OCP = oral contraception pill

OP = occiput posterior

OTC = over the counter

PAPP-A = pregnancy-associated plasma protein A

PCOS = polycystic ovarian syndrome

PCT = postcoital testing

PDA = patent ductus arteriosus

PE = physical exam

PERRLA = pupils equal, round, reactive to light and accommodation

PET = positive emission tomography

pg = picogram

PGE 1 = prostaglandin

PID = pelvic inflammatory disease

PIH = pregnancy-induced hypertension

pit = pitocin

plt = platelet

PMDD = premenstrual dysphoric disorder

PMI = point of maximal impulse

PMS = premenstrual syndrome

PO = by mouth

POC = products of conception

POCP = progestin-only contraceptive pill

pos = positive

PPD (Mantoux test) = purified protein derivative

PPH = postpartum hemorrhage

PPROM = preterm, premature rupture of membranes

PPV = positive predictive value

PR = by rectum

primip = primiparous

PRN = as needed

PROM = premature rupture of membranes

pt = patient

PT = prothrombin time

PTB = preterm birth

PTD = preterm delivery

PTL = preterm labor

PTSD = post-traumatic stress disorder

PTT = partial thromboplastin time

PTU = propylthiouracil

PV = per vagina

Q or q = every

QD = one time per day

Qhs = at bedtime

QID = four times per day

QOD = every other day

RA = rheumatoid arthritis

RAM = rapid alternating movement

RBC = red blood cell(s)

RCT = randomized control trial

RDS = respiratory distress syndrome

RDW = red blood cell distribution width

RhoGam = Rh (D) immunoglobulin

R/o = rule out

ROM = rupture of membranes

ROS = review of systems

rpt = repeat

RR = respiratory rate

RRR = regular rate and rhythm

RTC = return to clinic

RUQ = right upper quadrant

Rx = prescription

s/sx = signs and symptoms

S > D = size greater than dates

SAB = spontaneous abortion

SBE = self breast exam

sec = seconds

sed rate = erythrocyte sedimentation rate

SES = socioeconomic status

SHBG = sex hormone-binding globulin

SHSG = sonohysterosalpingogram

SIADH = syndrome of inappropriate anti-diuretic hormone release

SLE = systemic lupus erythematosus

SOB = shortness of breath

SROM = spontaneous rupture of membranes

SSE = sterile speculum exam

SSRI = selective serotonin reuptake inhibitor

STI = sexually transmitted infection

sx = symptom(s)

T = tablespoon

TB = tuberculosis

TCA = tricyclic antidepressant or trichloroacetic acid

TCB = transcutaneous bilirubinometry

TFT = thyroid function test

TG = triglycerides

TIBC = total iron binding capacity

TID = three times per day

TM = tympanic membrane

TNF = tissue necrosis factor

TOC = test of cure

TSH = thyroid stimulation hormone

tsp = teaspoon

TSS = toxic shock syndrome

TTP = thrombotic thrombocytopenia purpura

TVU/S = transvaginal ultrasound

tx = treatment

U = unit

UPI = uterine-placental insufficiency

URI = upper respiratory tract infection

U/S = ultrasound

US = United States

USPSTF = United States Preventive Services Task Force

UTI = urinary tract infection

VBAC = vaginal birth after cesarean section

VS = vital signs

VSD = ventricular septal defect

w/ = with

w/o = without

WA = well adjusted

WBC = white blood cell(s)

WHO = World Health Organization

WHO 3/4 = WHO medical eligibility criteria for contraceptive use;
    Category 3 = Use of method not usually recommended unless other more
    appropriate methods are not available or not acceptable.
    Category 4 = Method not to be used.

WN = well nourished

WNL = within normal limits

wt = weight

x = times

yr = year(s)

# REFERENCES

Abrams, P., Cardozo, L., Fall, M., Griffiths, D., Rosier, P., Ulf, U., et al. (2002). The standardization of terminology of lower urinary tract function: Report from the standardization sub-committee of the International Continence Society. *Neurourology and Urodynamics, 21*, 167–178.

Alexander, G., Himes, J., Kaufman, R., Mor, J., & Kogan, M. (1996). A United States national reference for fetal growth. *Obstetrics & Gynecology, 87*(2), 163–168.

Alexander, J. M., McIntire, D. D., & Leveno, K. J. (2000). Forty weeks and beyond: Pregnancy outcomes by week of gestation. *Obstetrics & Gynecology, 96*(2), 291–294.

Alfirevic, Z., & Mousa, H. (2007). Treatment for primary postpartum haemorrhage. *Cochrane Database of Systematic Reviews,* (3).

Aliyu, M. H., Jolly, P. E., Ehiri, J. E., & Salihu, H. M. (2005). High parity and adverse birth outcomes: Exploring the maze. *Birth, 32*(1), 45–59.

Allen, R. H., Kumar, D., Fitzmaurice, G., Lifford, K. L., & Goldberg, A. B. (2006). Pain management of first-trimester surgical abortion: Effects of selection of local anesthesia with and without lorazepam or intravenous sedation. *Contraception, 74*(5), 407–413.

American Academy of Pediatrics Subcommittee on Hyperbilirubinemia. (2004). Management of hyperbilirubinemia in the newborn infant 35 or more weeks of gestation. *Pediatrics, 114*(1), 297–316.

American College of Nurse-Midwives. (2001). Endometrial biopsy: Clinical bulletin No. 5. *Journal of Midwifery & Women's Health, 46*(5), 321.

American College of Nurse-Midwives. (2002). Abnormal and dysfunctional uterine bleeding: Clinical bulletin No. 6. *Journal of Midwifery & Women's Health, 47*(3), 207–213.

American College of Nurse-Midwives. (2003). Early-onset group B strep infection in newborns: Prevention and prophylaxis: Clinical Bulletin No. 2. *Journal of Midwifery & Women's Health, 48*(5), 375.

American College of Nurse-Midwives. (2004). Eating safely during pregnancy. *Journal of Midwifery & Women's Health, 49*(4), 373.

American College of Nurse-Midwives. (2005). *Become a midwife.* Retrieved August 10, 2008, from http://www.midwife.org/become_midwife.cfm

American College of Nurse-Midwives. (2005). *Position statement: Homebirth.* Washington, DC: Author.

American College of Nurse-Midwives. (2007). Intermittent auscultation for intrapartum fetal heart rate surveillance: Clinical bulletin No. 9. *Journal of Midwifery & Women's Health, 52*(3), 314.

American College of Obstetricians and Gynecologists. (1996). Assessment of fetal lung maturity: Educational bulletin No 230. In *2006 compendium of selected publications* (p. 267). Washington, DC: American College of Obstetricians and Gynecologists.

American College of Obstetricians and Gynecologists. (1996). Use and abuse of the Apgar score. In American Academy of Pediatrics (Ed.), *2006 compendium of selected publications* (p. 257). Washington, DC: American College of Obstetricians and Gynecologists.

American College of Obstetricians and Gynecologists. (1998). Medical management of tubal pregnancy: Practice bulletin No. 3. In *2008 compendium of selected publications* (p. 1023). Washington, DC: American College of Obstetricians and Gynecologists.

American College of Obstetricians and Gynecologists. (1999). Antepartum fetal surveillance. In *2006 compendium of selected publications* (p. 337). Washington, DC: American College of Obstetricians and Gynecologists.

American College of Obstetricians and Gynecologists. (1999). External cephalic version. In *2006 compendium of selected publications* (p. 562). Washington, DC: American College of Obstetricians and Gynecologists.

American College of Obstetricians and Gynecologists. (1999). Induction of labor: Clinical management guidelines No. 10. In *2006 compendium of selected publications* (p. 562). Washington, DC: American College of Obstetricians and Gynecologists.

American College of Obstetricians and Gynecologists. (1999). Reading the medical literature. In *2006 compendium of selected publications* (pp. 329–336). Washington, DC: American College of Obstetricians and Gynecologists.

American College of Obstetricians and Gynecologists. (1999). Teratology. In *2006 compendium of selected publications* (p. 311). Washington, DC: American College of Obstetricians and Gynecologists.

American College of Obstetricians and Gynecologists. (2000). Breastfeeding: Maternal and infant aspects. In *2006 compendium of selected publications* (p. 274). Washington, DC: American College of Obstetricians and Gynecologists.

American College of Obstetricians and Gynecologists. (2001). Prenatal diagnosis of fetal chromosomal abnormalities. In *2006 compendium of selected publications* (p. 867). Washington, DC: American College of Obstetricians and Gynecologists.

American College of Obstetricians and Gynecologists. (2002). Obstetric analgesia and anesthesia. In *2006 compendium of selected publications* (p. 765). Washington, DC: American College of Obstetricians and Gynecologists.

American College of Obstetricians and Gynecologists. (2003). Breast cancer screening. In *2006 compendium of selected publications* (p. 386). Washington, DC: American College of Obstetricians and Gynecologists.

American College of Obstetricians and Gynecologists. (2003). Neural tube defects: Clinical management guidelines for obstetricians and gynecologists. In *2006 compendium of selected publications* (p. 754). Washington, DC: American College of Obstetricians and Gynecologists.

American College of Obstetricians and Gynecologists. (2005). Human papillomavirus ACOG practice bulletin No. 61. In American College of Obstetricians and Gynecologists (Ed.). *ACOG 2008 compendium* (pp. 1231–1243). Washington, DC: American College of Obstetricians and Gynecologists.

American College of Obstetricians and Gynecologists. (2005). Update on carrier screening for cystic fibrosis ACOG committee opinion No. 325. In American College of Obstetricians and Gynecologists (Ed.). *ACOG 2008 compendium of selected publications: Committee opinions and policy statements* (Vol. 1, pp. 236–239). Washington, DC: American College of Obstetricians and Gynecologists.

American College of Obstetricians and Gynecologists. (2006). *Amnioinfusion does not prevent meconium aspiration syndrome: Committee opinion* No. 346. Washington, DC: Author.

American College of Obstetricians and Gynecologists. (2007). Endometrial ablation. ACOG practice bulletin No. 81. In American College of Obstetricians and Gynecologists (Ed.). *ACOG 2008 compendium of selected publications: Practice bulletins* (Vol. II, pp. 1356–1385). Washington, DC: American College of Obstetricians and Gynecologists.

American College of Obstetricians and Gynecologists. (2007). Hemoglobinopathies in pregnancy (Practice Bulletin No. 78). *Obstetrics & Gynecology, 109*(1), 229–238.

American College of Obstetricians and Gynecologists. (2007). Screening for fetal chromosomal abnormalities (Practice Bulletin No. 77). *Obstetrics & Gynecology, 109*(1), 217–228.

American College of Obstetricians and Gynecologists. (2007). Use of psychiatric medications during pregnancy and lactation (ACOG Practice Bulletin No. 87).

*ACOG 2008 compendium of selected publications: Practice bulletins* (Vol. II, pp. 978–997). Washington, DC: American College of Obstetricians and Gynecologists.

American College of Obstetricians and Gynecologists. (2008). *ICD-9 abridged, diagnostic coding in obstetrics and gynecology.* Atlanta, GA: American College of Obstetricians and Gynecologists.

American College of Obstetricians and Gynecologists. (2008). *Nutrition during pregnancy* (Patient education pamphlets No. 12345/65432). Washington, DC: American College of Obstetricians and Gynecologists.

American College of Obstetricians and Gynecologists, American Academy of Pediatrics, & Gynecologists and Committee on Obstetric Practice. (2006). The Apgar score. *Pediatrics, 117,* 1444.

American Diabetes Association. (2004). Gestational diabetes mellitus position statement. *Diabetes Care, 27*(Suppl. 1), S88–S90.

American Pregnancy Association. (2007). *Homepage.* Retrieved May 27, 2008, from http://www.americanpregnancy.org

American Society for Colposcopy and Cervical Pathology. (2007). 2006 consensus guidelines for the management of women with abnormal cervical cancer screening tests. *Journal of Lower Genital Tract Disease, 11*(4), 346–355.

American Society for Colposcopy and Cervical Pathology. (2007). 2006 consensus guidelines for the management of women with cervical intraepithelial neoplasia or adenocarcinoma in situ. *Journal of Lower Genital Tract Disease, 11*(4), 223–239.

American Society for Colposcopy and Cervical Pathology. (2008). *Consensus guidelines.* Retrieved August 10, 2008, from http://www.asccp.org/consensus/cytological.shtml

Anderson, D., Novak, P., Keith, J., & Elliott, M. (2007). *Dorland's medical dictionary* (30th ed.). Retrieved April 24, 2008, from http://www.dorlands.com

Arcangelo, V. P., & Peterson, A. M. (Eds.). (2006). *Pharmacotherapeutics for advanced practice: A practical approach* (2nd ed.). Philadelphia: Lippincott Williams and Wilkins.

Association of Women's Health, Obstetric and Neonatal Nurses (AWHONN). (2003). *Fetal heart monitoring: Principles and practices* (3rd ed.). Dubuque, IA: Kendall/Hunt.

Bailey, J., Farquhar, C., Owen, C., & Mangtani, P. (2004). Sexually transmitted infections in women who have sex with women. *Sexually Transmitted Infections, 80,* 244–246.

Ballard, J. L., Auer, C. E., & Khoury, J. C. (2002). Ankyloglossia: Assessment, incidence, and effect of frenuloplasty on the breastfeeding dyad. *Pediatrics, 110*(5), e63.

Barton, J., & Sibai, B. (2004). Diagnosis and management of hemolysis, elevated liver enzymes, and low platelets syndrome. *Clinics of Perinatology, 31*(4), 807–833.

Baxter, J., & Weinstein, L. (2004). HELLP syndrome: The state of the art. *Obstetrics and Gynecology Survey, 59*(12), 838–845.

Betzold, C. M. (2007). An update on the recognition and management of lactational breast inflammation (Abstract). *Journal of Midwifery & Women's Health, 52*(6) 595–605.

Boone, S., & Shields, K. (2005). Treating pregnancy related nausea and vomiting with ginger. *Annals of Pharmacotherapy, 39*(10), 1710–1713.

Braverman, P. (2007). Premenstrual syndrome and premenstrual dysphoric disorder. *North American Society for Pediatric and Adolescent Gynecology, 20,* 3–12.

Bricker, L., & Luckas, M. (2000). Amniotomy alone for induction of labour. *Cochrane Database of Systematic Reviews*, (4), 002862.

Bridges, M. (2006). *Midwifery management of stillbirth, part 1: Epidemiology, pathophysiology, and diagnostic evaluation*. New Haven, CT. Unpublished master's dissertation, Yale University School of Nursing.

Briggs, G., Yaffe, S., & Freeman, R. (2005). *Drugs in pregnancy and lactation* (7th ed.). Philadelphia: Lippincott Williams and Wilkins.

Brucker, M. (2001). Management of the third stage of labor: An evidence based approach. *Journal of Midwifery & Women's Health, 46*(6), 381.

Burrow, G., Duffy, T., & Copel, J. (2004). *Medical complications during pregnancy* (6th ed.). Philadelphia: Elsevier Saunders.

Cady, B., Stelle, G. D., Morrow, M., Gardner, B., Smith, B., Lee, N., et al. (1998). Evaluation of common breast problems: Guidance for primary care providers. *CA Cancer Journal for Clinicians, 48*(1), 49–63.

Cararach, V., Palacio, M., Martinez, S., Deulofeu, P., Sanchez, M., Cobo, T., et al. (2006). Nifedipine versus ritodrine for suppression of preterm labor. Comparison of their efficacy and secondary effects. *European Journal of Obstetrics, Gynecology, & Reproductive Biology, 127*(2), 204–208.

Centers for Disease Control and Prevention. (2004). *Trichomonas infection*. Retrieved May 25, 2008, from http://www.cdc.gov/ncidod/dpd/parasites/ trichomonas/factsht_trichomonas.htm

Centers for Disease Control and Prevention. (2005). *Pediatric and pregnancy nutrition surveillance system health indicators*. Retrieved May 29, 2008, from http://www.cdc.gov/pednss/what_is/pnss_health_indicators.htm#Maternal%20 Health%20Indicators

Centers for Disease Control and Prevention. (2006). Sexually transmitted diseases treatment guidelines. *Morbidity and Mortality Weekly Report, 55*(RR-11), 1–94.

Centers for Disease Control and Prevention. (2007). *Breast cancer*. Retrieved March 5, 2008, from http://www.cancer.gov/cancertopics/types/breast

Centers for Disease Control and Prevention. (2007). *Body mass index: BMI for adults*. Retrieved May 27, 2008, from http://www.cdc.gov/nccdphp/dnpa/bmi/ adult_BMI/about_adult_BMI.htm

Centers for Disease Control and Prevention. (2007). *Genital HPV*. Retrieved May 26, 2008, from http://www.cdc.gov/std/hpv/default.htm

Centers for Disease Control and Prevention. (2007). *Guidelines for vaccinating pregnant women*. Retrieved May 26, 2008, from http://www.cdc.gov/vaccines/ pubs/preg-guide.htm

Centers for Disease Control and Prevention. *Powerful bones, powerful girls*. (2007). Retrieved May 27, 2008, from http://www.cdc.gov/powerfulbones/ parents/index.html

Centers for Disease Control and Prevention. (2008). *HPV vaccine information for young women*. Retrieved May 26, 2008, from http://www.cdc.gov/std/Hpv/ STDFact-HPV-vaccine.htm#hpvvac1

Centers for Disease Control and Prevention, United States Department of Health and Human Services. (2006). *Secondhand smoke*. Retrieved May 26, 2008, from http://www.cdc.gov/tobacco/data_statistics/Factsheets/ SecondhandSmoke.htm

Centers for Disease Control and Prevention, United States Department of Health and Human Services. (2007). *You can quit smoking: Five keys for quitting smoking*. Retrieved May 26, 2008, from http://www.cdc.gov/tobacco/quit_ smoking/you_can_quit/five_keys.htm

Centers for Disease Control and Prevention, United States Department of Health and Human Services. (2008). *Health effects of cigarette smoking.* Retrieved May 26, 2008, from http://www.cdc.gov/tobacco/data_statistics/Factsheets/health_effects.htm

Centers for Disease Control and Prevention, United States Department of Health and Human Services. (2008). *Tobacco use and pregnancy.* Retrieved May 26, 2008, from http://www.cdc.gov/reproductivehealth/TobaccoUsePregnancy

Chang, R. J. (2004). A practical approach to the diagnosis of polycystic ovary syndrome. *American Journal of Obstetrics and Gynecology, 191*(3), 713–717.

Christensen, F. C., & Rayburn, W. F. (1999). Fetal movement counts. *Obstetrics & Gynecology Clinics of North America, 26*(4), 607–621.

Clinical bulletin no. 6: Abnormal and dysfunctional uterine bleeding (Abstract). (2002). *Journal of Midwifery & Women's Health, 47*(3), 207–213.

Cleveland Clinic Foundation. (2008). *Nutrition during pregnancy for vegetarians.* Retrieved August 10, 2008, from http://my.clevelandclinic.org/healthy_living/pregnancy/hic_nutrition_during_pregnancy_for_vegetarians.aspx

Cohen, S. M. (2006). Jaundice in the full-term newborn. *Pediatric Nursing, 32*(3), 202–208.

Cox, J. L., Holden, J. M., & Sagovsky, R. (1987). Detection of postnatal depression: Development of the 10-item Edinburgh postnatal depression scale. *British Journal of Psychiatry, 150,* 782–786.

Creasy, R. K., & Resnik, R. (2004). *Maternal-fetal medicine* (5th ed.). Philadelphia: Saunders.

Crowther, C. A., Hiller, J. E., & Doyle, L. W. (2002). Magnesium sulphate for preventing preterm birth in threatened preterm labour. *Cochrane Database of Systematic Reviews,* (4), 001060.

Cunningham, F. G. (2002). Postoperative complications. In L. C. Gilstrap, F. G. Cunningham, & J. P. vanDorsten (Eds.), *Operative Obstetrics* (2nd ed.). New York: McGraw-Hill.

Cunningham, G., Leveno, K. J., Bloom, S. L., Hauth, J. C., Gilstrap, L. C., & Wenstrom, K. D. (2005). *Williams obstetrics* (22nd ed.). New York: McGraw-Hill.

DAC Consultants. (2001). *Herpes diagnosis.* Retrieved May 25, 2008, from http://www.herpesdiagnosis.com

Dawson-Hughes, B., Gold, D. T., Rodbard, H. W., Bonner, F. J., Khosla, S., & Swift, S. (2003). *Physician's guide to prevention and treatment of osteoporosis* (2nd ed.). Washington, DC: National Osteoporosis Foundation.

Dean, L., Meyer, I. H., Robinson, K., Sell, R. L., Sember, R., Silenzio, V. M. B., et al. (2000). Lesbian, gay, bisexual, and transgender health: Findings and concerns. *Journal of the Gay and Lesbian Medical Association, 4*(3), 101–151.

Decker, G. M., & Meyers, J. (2001). Commonly used herbs: Implications for clinical practice [insert]. *Clinical Journal of Oncology Nursing, 5*(2).

Dennehy, C. E. (2006). The use of herbs and dietary supplements in gynecology: An evidence based review. *Journal of Midwifery & Women's Health, 51*(6), 402.

Dennis, C. L., & Creedy, D. (2004). Psychosocial and psychological interventions for preventing postpartum depression. (Comment). *Cochrane Database of Systematic Reviews,* (4), 001134.

Department of Reproductive Health and Research, World Health Organization. (2003). *Managing complications in pregnancy and childbirth: A guide for midwives and doctors.* Geneva, Switzerland: Author.

Desai, S. P. (2004). *Clinician's guide to laboratory medicine: A practical approach* (3rd ed.). Hudson, OH: Lexi-Comp.

Devane, D., Lalor, J., Daly, S., & McGuire, W. (2005). Cardiotocography versus intermittent auscultation of fetal heart on admission to labour ward for assessment of fetal wellbeing (protocol). *Cochrane Database of Systematic Reviews,* (1).

Dickey, R. P. (2005). *Managing contraceptive pill patients* (12th ed.). Dallas, TX: EMIS Medical.

Divon, M. Y., & Feldman-Leidner, N. (2008). Postdates and antenatal testing. *Seminars in Perinatology, 32*(4) 295–300.

Dodd, J. M., Flenady, V., Cincotta, R., & Crowther, C. A. (2006). Prenatal administration of progesterone for preventing preterm birth. *Cochrane Database of Systematic Reviews, (1),* CD004947.

DONA International. (2005). *What is a doula?* Retrieved August 10, 2008, from http://www.dona.org/mothers/index.php

Duley, L., Gulmezoglu, A. M., & Henderson-Smart, D. J. (2003). Magnesium sulphate and other anticonvulsants for women with pre-eclampsia. *Cochrane Database of Systematic Reviews, (2),* CD000025.

Dunne, E., Unger, E., Sternberg, M., McGuillan, G., Swan, D., Patel, S., et al. (2007). Prevalence of HPV infection among females in the United States. *Journal of the American Medical Association, 297*(8), 813–819.

Dutton, L. (2006). *Antenatal care outline.* Unpublished manuscript.

Dutton, L., Koenig, K., & Fennie, K. (2008). Gynecological care of the female-to-male transgender man. *Journal of Midwifery & Women's Health, 53,* 331–337.

Eberhard-Gran, M., Eskild, A., Tambs, K., Opjordsmoen, S., & Samuelsen, S. O. (2001). Review of validation studies of the Edinburgh postnatal depression scale. *Acta Psychiatrica Scandinavia, 104*(4), 243–249.

Eberl, M., Fox, C., Edge, S., Carter, C., & Mahoney, M. (2006). BI-RADS classification for management of abnormal mammograms. *Journal of the American Board of Family Medicine, 19*(2), 161–164.

Ecker, J. L., & Parer, J. T. (1999). Obstetrical evaluation of fetal acid-base balance. *Critical Reviews in Clinical Laboratory Science, 36*(5), 407.

Edwards, R. (2000). Syphilis in women. *Primary Care Updates for OB/GYNS, 7*(5), 186–191.

Elimian, A., Figueroa, R., & Tejani, N. (1997). Intrapartum assessment of fetal well-being: A comparison of scalp stimulation with scalp blood pH sampling. *Obstetrics and Gynecology, 89,* 373–376.

Epilepsy Foundation. (2005). *Seizures and syndromes.* Retrieved August 28, 2008, from http://www.epilepsyfoundation.org/about/types/types/index.cfm

Epocrates, I. (2008). *Epocrates online.* Retrieved May 27, 2008, from http://www.epocrates.com

Essah, P. A., Wickham, E. P., & Nestler, J. E. (2007). The metabolic syndrome in polycystic ovary syndrome. *Clinical Obstetrics and Gynecology, 50*(1), 205–225.

Fahey, J. O. (2008). Clinical management of intra-amniotic infection and chorioamnionitis: A review of the literature (Abstract). *Journal of Midwifery & Women's Health, 53*(3) 227–235.

Fantl, J. A., Newman, D. K., Colling, J., et al. (1996). *Urinary incontinence in adults: Acute and chronic management* (AHCPR Publication No. 96-0682). Rockville, MD: U.S. Department of Health and Human Services, Public Health Service, Agency for Health Care Policy and Research.

Farquhar, C. (2007). Endometriosis. *British Medical Journal, 334*(7587), 249–253.

Feinstein, N. (2000). Fetal heart rate auscultation: Current and future practices. *Journal of Obstetric, Gynecologic, & Neonatal Nursing, 29*(3), 306–315.

French, L. M., & Smaill, F. M. (2004). Antibiotic regimens for endometriosis after delivery. *Cochrane Database of Systematoc Reviews, 4,* CD001067.

Fretts, R. C. (2005). Etiology and prevention of stillbirth. *American Journal of Obstetrics and Gynecology, 193*(6), 1923–1935.

Friedman, E. (1978). *Labor: Clinical evaluation and management* (2nd ed.). New York: Appleton-Century-Crofts.

Frye, A. (1995). *Healing passage: A midwife's guide to the care and repair of the tissue involved in birth.* Portland, OR: Labrys Press.

Frye, A. (1997). *Understanding diagnostic tests in the childbearing years* (6th ed.). Portland, OR: Labrys Press.

Frye, A. (2004). *Holistic midwifery: A comprehensive textbook for midwives in homebirth practice.* Portland, OR: Labrys Press.

Gabbe, S. G., Niebyl, J. R., & Simpson, J. L. (Eds.). (2002). *Obstetrics: Normal and problem pregnancies* (4th ed.). New York: Churchill Livingstone.

Gates, E. A. (2004). Communicating risk in prenatal genetic testing. *Journal of Midwifery Women's Health, 49*(3), 220.

Gaudet, T. W. (2004). CAM approaches to menopause management: Overview of the options. *Menopause Management: Women's Health Through Midlife & Beyond, 13*(Suppl. 1), 48–50.

Gavin, N. I., Gaynes, B. N., Lohr, K. N., Meltzer-Brody, S., Gartlehner, G., & Swinson, T. (2005). Perinatal depression: A systematic review of prevalence and incidence. *Obstetrics and Gynecology, 106*(5 Pt 1), 1071–1083.

Gaynes, B. N., Gavin, N., Meltzer-Brody, S., Lohr, K. N., Swinson, T., Gartlehner, G., et al. (2005). Perinatal depression: Prevalence, screening accuracy, and screening outcomes. *Evidence Report/Technology Assessment, 119,* 1–8.

Giacalone, P. L., Vignal, J., Daures, J. P., Boulot, P., Hedon, B., & Laffargue, F. (2000). A randomised evaluation of two techniques of management of the third stage of labour in women at low risk of postpartum hemorrhage. *British Journal of Obstetrics and Gynaecology, 107,* 396–400.

Gilbert, D. N., Moellering, R. C., Eliopoulos, G. M., & Sande, M. A. (2007). Table 1: Clinical approach to initial choice in antimicrobial therapy. In *The Sanford Guide to Antimicrobial Therapy.* Hyde Park, VT: Antimicrobial Therapy.

Girman, A., Lee, R., & Kligler, B. (2002). An integrative medicine approach to premenstrual syndrome. *American Journal of Obstetrics and Gynecology, 188*(5), S56–S63.

Glazer, H., & Rodke, G. (2002). In B. Kahn (Ed.), *The vulvodynia survival guide: How to overcome painful vaginal symptoms and enjoy an active lifestyle.* Oakland, CA: New Harbinger.

Goff, M., & O'Connor, M. (2007). Perinatal care of women maintained on methadone. *Journal of Midwifery & Women's Health, 52*(3), 23–26.

Goh, B. T. (2005). Syphilis in adults. *Sexually transmitted infections, 81,* 448–452.

Gomez, R., Romero, R., Medina, L., Nien, J. K., Chaiworapongsa, T., Carstens, M., et al. (2005). Cervicovaginal fibronectin improves the prediction of preterm delivery based on sonographic cervical length in patients with preterm uterine contractions and intact membranes. *American Journal of Obstetrics and Gynecology, 192*(2), 350–359.

Goodarzi, M. O., & Korenman, S. G. (2003). The importance of insulin resistance in polycystic ovary syndrome. *Fertility and Sterility, 80*(2), 255–258.

Goodman, N. F., Bledsoe, M. B., Futterweit, W., Goldzeiher, J. W., Petak, S. M., Smith, K. D., et al. (2001). American Association of Clinical Endocrinologists medical guidelines for clinical practice for the diagnosis and treatment of hyperandrogenic disorders. *Endocrine Practice, 7*(2), 120–134.

Goodwin, L. (2000). Intermittent auscultation of the fetal heart rate: A review of general principles. *Journal of Perinatal and Neonatal Nursing, 14*(3), 53–61.

Graves, B. W., & Barger, M. K. (2001). A "conservative" approach to iron supplementation during pregnancy. *Journal of Midwifery & Women's Health, 46*(3), 159.

Greulich, B., & Tarrant, B. (2007). The latent phase of labor: Diagnosis and management. *Journal of Midwifery & Women's Health, 52*, 190–198.

Griffiths, D. M. (2004). Do tongue ties affect breastfeeding? *Journal of Human Lactation, 20*(4), 409–414.

Gyetvai, K., Hannah, M. E., Hodnett, E. D., & Ohlsson, A. (1999). Tocolytics for preterm labor: A systematic review. *Obstetrics & Gynecology, 94*(5 Pt 2), 869–877.

Hackley, B., Kriebs, J. M., & Rousseau, M. E. (2007). *Primary care of women.* Sudbury, MA: Jones and Bartlett.

Hale, T. W. (2006). *Medications and mothers' milk* (12th ed.). Amarillo, TX: Hale.

Hale, T. W. (2008). *Medications and mothers' milk* (13th ed.). Amarillo, TX: Hale.

Halliday, H. L., & Sweet, D. (2000). Endotracheal intubation at birth for preventing morbidity and mortality in vigorous, meconium-stained infants born at term. *Cochrane Database of Systematic Reviews,* (4), CD000500.

Hanfling, S. (2008). *Sexual health: Talking with women (patients) about their sexual concerns.* Boston: American College of Nurse Midwives.

Hannah, M. E., Ohlsson, A., Farine, D., Hewson, S. A., Hodnett, E. D., Myhr, T. L., et al. (1996). Induction of labor compared with expectant management for prelabor rupture of the membranes at term. TERMPROM study group. *New England Journal of Medicine, 334*(16), 1005–1010.

Harry Benjamin International Gender Dysphoria Association. (2001). *Standards of care for gender identity disorders (6th ed.).* Unpublished manuscript. Retrieved April 23, 2006, from htpp://www.hbigda.org/soc.htm

Hart, A. C., Hopkins, C. A., & Ford, B. (Eds.). (2006). *ICD-9-CM professional* (6th ed.). Salt Lake City, UT: Ingenix.

Hatcher, R. A. (2007). *Contraceptive technology* (19th ed.). San Francisco: Ardent Media.

Healthwise WebMD. (2007). *Semen analysis.* Retrieved May 27, 2008, from http://www.webmd.com/hw/infertility_reproduction/hw5612.asp?src=RSS_BLOGGER

Higdon, J. V., & Frei, B. (2006). Coffee and health: A review of recent human research. *Critical Reviews in Food Science and Nutrition, 46*, 101.

Hodgson, S. F., & Watts, S. F. (2003). American Association of Clinical Endocrinologists medical guidelines for clinical practice for the prevention and treatment of postmenopausal osteoporosis: 2001 edition with selected updates for 2003. *Endocrine Practice, 9*(6), 544–564.

Hofmeyr, G. (2005). Amnioinfusion for potential and suspected umbilical cord compression during labour. *Cochrane Database of Systematic Reviews, 2*(CD001182).

Hollander, M., Paarlberg, M., & Huisjes, A. (2007). Gestational diabetes: A review of the current literature and guidelines. *Obstetrical and Gynecology Survey, 62*(2), 125.

Horner, N. K., & Lampe, J. W. (2000). Potential mechanisms of diet therapy for fibrocystic breast conditions show inadequate evidence of effectiveness. *Journal of the American Dietetic Association, 100*(11), 1368–1380.

Howard, L. M., Hoffbrand, S., Henshaw, C., Boath, L., & Bradley, E. (2005). Antidepressant prevention of postnatal depression. *Cochrane Database of Systematic Reviews,* (2), 004363.

Hughes, L. E. (1991). Classification of benign breast disorders: The ANDI classification based on physiological processes within the normal breast. *British Medical Bulletin, 47*(2), 251–257.

Hulley, S., Grady, D., Bush, T., Furberg, C., Herrington, D., Riggs, B., et al. (1998). Randomized trial of estrogen plus progestin for secondary prevention of coronary heart disease in postmenopausal women. Heart and Estrogen/ Progestin Replacement Study (HERS) research group. *Journal of the American Medical Association, 280*(7), 605–613.

Hutton, E., & Hassan, E. (2007). Late vs. early clamping of the umbilical cord in full-term neonates. *Journal of the American Medical Association, 297*(11), 1241–1252.

Iams, J. D., Newman, R. B., Thom, E. A., Goldenberg, R. L., Mueller-Heubach, E., Moawad, A., et al. (2002). Frequency of uterine contractions and the risk of spontaneous preterm delivery. *New England Journal of Medicine, 346*(4), 250–255.

Ilse, S., & Hammer Burns, L. (1992). *Miscarriage: A shattered dream.* Maple Plain, MN: Wintergreen Press.

Institute of Medicine. (1990). *Nutrition during pregnancy: Part 1 weight gain, part 2 nutrient supplements.* Washington, DC: National Academy Press.

Institute of Medicine. (2008). *Dietary reference intakes: Elements.* Retrieved August 12, 2008, from http://www.iom.edu/Object.File/Master/7/294/0.pdf

Institute of Medicine. (2008). *Dietary reference intakes: Macronutrients.* Retrieved August 12, 2008, from http://www.iom.edu/Object.File/Master/7/300/ Webtablemacro.pdf

Institute of Medicine. (2008). *Dietary reference intakes: Vitamins.* Retrieved August 12, 2008, from http://www.iom.edu/Object.File/Master/7/296/ webtablevitamins.pdf

Jacobson, P., & Turner, L. (2008). Management of the second stage of labor in women with epidural analgesia. *Journal of Midwifery & Women's Health, 53*(1), 82–85.

Jewell, D. (2003). Nausea and vomiting in early pregnancy. *Clinical Evidence, 9,* 1561–1570.

Joint National Committee. (2003). *Seventh report of the joint national committee on prevention, detection, evaluation, and treatment of high blood pressure.* Bethesda, MD: National Heart Lung and Blood Institute.

Jolivet, R. (2002). Early-onset neonatal group B streptococcal infection: 2002 guidelines for prevention (Abstract). *Journal of Midwifery & Women's Health, 47*(6), 435–446.

Kaaja, R. J., & Greer, I. A. (2005). Manifestations of chronic disease during pregnancy. *Journal of the American Medicine Association, 294*(21), 2751–2757.

Kanis, J. (2002). Diagnosis of osteoporosis and assessment of fracture risk. *Lancet, 359,* 1929–1936.

Kent, J. C. (2007). How breastfeeding works (Abstract). *Journal of Midwifery & Women's Health, 52*(6), 564–570.

Schuiling, K. D., Sipe, T. A., & Fullerton, J. (2005). Findings from the analysis of the American College of Nurse-Midwives membership surveys (Abstract). *Journal of Midwifery & Women's Health, 50*(1), 8–15.

King, T. (2004). Vaginal birth after previous cesarean section. *Journal of Midwifery & Women's Health, 49*(1), 68–75.

King, J., Flenady, V., Cole, S., & Thornton, S. (2005). Cyclo-oxygenase (COX) inhibitors for treating preterm labour. *Cochrane Database of Systematic Reviews,* (2), 001992.

Knoche, A., Selzer, C., & Smolley, K. (2008). Methods of stimulating the onset of labor: An exploration of maternal satisfaction (Abstract). *Journal of Midwifery & Women's Health, 53*(4), 381–387.

Knutson, D., & Steiner, E. (2007). Screening for breast cancer: Current recommendations and future directions. *American Family Physician, 75*(11), 1660–1666.

Koontz, W. L., & Bishop, E. (1982). Management of the latent phase of labor. *Clinical Obstetrics and Gynecology, 25*(1), 111–114.

Kriebs, J. M. (2008). Breaking the cycle of infection: TORCH and other infections in women's health. *Journal of Midwifery & Women's Health, 53*(3), 173–174.

Kriebs, J. M., & Fahey, J. O. (2006). Ectopic pregnancy. *Journal of Midwifery & Women's Health, 51*, 431.

Lai, S. (2008). *Sutures and needles.* Retrieved August 28, 2008, from http://www.emedicine.com/ent/TOPIC38.HTM

Laumann, E., Paik, A., & Rosen, R. (1999). Sexual dysfunction in the United States: Prevalence and predictors. *Journal of the American Medical Association, 281*, 537–544.

Lindsay, R. (1993). Prevention and treatment of osteoporosis. *Lancet, 341*(8848), 801–805.

Little, C. M., & Lewis, J. A. (2005). Genetic resources for midwifery practice. *Journal of Midwifery & Women's Health, 50*(3), 246.

Lockwood, C. L., & Lemons, J. A. (Eds.). (2007). *Guidelines for perinatal care* (6th ed.). Washington, DC: American College of Obstetricians and Gynecologists.

Loder, E., & Martin, V. (2004). *Headaches.* Philadelphia: American College of Physicians.

Low Dog, T. (2004). CAM approaches to menopause management: The role for botanicals in menopause. *Menopause Management: Women's Health Through Midlife & Beyond, 13*(Suppl. 1), 51–53.

Lucero, J., Harlow, B. L., Barbieri, R. L., Sluss, P., & Cramer, D. W. (2001). Early follicular phase hormone levels in relation to patterns of alcohol, tobacco, and coffee use. *Fertility and Sterility, 76*(4), 723–729.

Lumley, J., Austin, M. P., & Mitchell, C. (2004). Intervening to reduce depression after birth: A systematic review of the randomized trials. *International Journal of Technology Assessment in Health Care, 20*(2), 128–144.

Lusk, M. J., & Konecny, P. (2008). Cervicitis: A review. *Current Opinions in Infectious Diseases, 21*, 49–55.

MacArthur, C., Winter, H. R., Bick, D. E., Lilford, R. J., Lancashire, R. J., Knowles, H., et al. (2003). Redesigning postnatal care: A randomised controlled trial of protocol-based midwifery-led care focused on individual women's physical and psychological health needs. *Health Technology Assessment, 7*(37), 1–98.

MANA. (2008). *Midwives alliance of North America definitions.* Retrieved August 12, 2008, from http://mana.org/definitions.html

Manning, F. (1999). Fetal biophysical profile. *Obstetrics and Gynecology Clinics of North America, 26*(4), 557–577.

March of Dimes. (2007). *Mercury and fish.* Retrieved May 24, 2008, from http://search.marchofdimes.com/cgi-bin/MsmGo.exe?grab_id=6&page_id=6095104&query=fish+during+pregnancy&hiword=FISHE+FISHER+FISHERS+FISHING+FISHMAN+PREGNANCIES+PREGNANT+during+fish+pregnancy+

Marowitz, A., & Jordan, R. (2007). Midwifery management of prelabor rupture of membranes at term (Abstract). *Journal of Midwifery & Women's Health, 52*(3), 199–206.

Marshall, W. A., & Tanner, J. M. (1970). Variations in the pattern of pubertal changes in boys. *Archives of Disease in Childhood, 45*(239), 13–23.

Martin, J. A., Hamilton, B. E., Sutton, P. D., Ventura, S. J., Menacker, F., Kirmeyer, S., et al. (2007). Births: Final data for 2005. *National Vital Statistics, 56*(6), 1–103.

Martin, J. A., Kochanek, K. D., Strobino, D. M., Guyer, B., & MacDorman, M. F. (2005). Annual summary of vital statistics—2003. *Pediatrics, 115,* 619–634.

Mayo Clinic. (2005). *Caffeine content of common beverages.* Retrieved May 27, 2008, from http://www.mayoclinic.com/health/caffeine/AN01211

McCool, W. F., Packman, J., & Zwerling, A. (2004). Obstetric anesthesia: Changes and choices. *Journal of Midwifery & Women's Health, 49,* 505.

McFarlane, J., Greenberg, L., Weltge, A., & Watson, M. Identification of abuse in emergency departments: Effectiveness of a two question screening tool. *Journal of Emergency Nursing, 21*(5), 391–394.

Medical Information Systems, Inc. (1998). *Pediatric normal values.* Stamford, CT: Author.

Meis, P. J., Klebanoff, M., Thom, E., Dombrowski, M. P., Sibai, B., Moawad, A. H., et al. (2003). Prevention of recurrent preterm delivery by 17 alpha-hydroxyprogesterone caproate. *New England Journal of Medicine, 348*(24), 2379–2385.

Mercer, J. S. (2001). Current best evidence: A review of the literature on umbilical cord clamping. *Journal of Midwifery & Women's Health, 46*(6), 402.

Mercer, J. S., Erickson, D. A., Graves, B., & Haley, M. M. (2007). Evidence-based practices for the fetal to newborn transition (Abstract). *Journal of Midwifery & Women's Health, 52*(3) 262–272.

Mercer, J. S., Nelson, C. C., & Skovgaard, R. L. (2000). Umbilical cord clamping: Beliefs and practices of American nurse midwives. *Journal of Midwifery & Women's Health, 45*(1), 58.

Mersy, D. J. (2003). Recognition of alcohol and substance abuse (Comment). *American Family Physician, 67*(7), 1529–1532.

Miller, S., & Alpert, P. (2006). Assessment and differential diagnosis of abdominal pain. *Nurse Practitioner, 31*(7), 38–47.

Minkin, M. J., & Wright, C. (2005). *A woman's guide to menopause and perimenopause.* New Haven, CT: Yale University Press.

Mittendorf, R., Pryde, P. G., Elin, R. J., Gianopoulos, J. G., & Lee, K. S. (2002). Relationship between hypermagnesaemia in preterm labour and adverse health outcomes in babies. *Magnesium Research, 15*(3–4), 253–261.

Mohrbacher, N., Stock, J., & La Leche League International. (2003). *The breastfeeding answer book* (3rd ed.). Schaumburg, IL: La Leche League International.

Mulholland, C., Njoroge, T., Mersereau, P., & Williams, J. (2007). Comparison of guidelines available in the United States for diagnosis and management of diabetes before, during, and after pregnancy. *Journal of Women's Health, 16*(6), 790.

National Abortion Federation. (2002). *Protocol recommendations for use of methotrexate and misoprostol in early abortion* (Protocol). Washington, DC: Author. Retrieved May 8, 2008, from http://www.prochoice.org/pubs_research/publications/downloads/professional_education/medical_abortion/protocol_recs_meth_miso.pdf

National Abortion Federation. (2007). *2007 clinical policy guidelines* (Clinical guidelines). Washington, DC: Author. Retrieved May 8, 2008, from http://www.guidelines.gov

National Abortion Federation. (2008). *Facts about mifepristone (RU-486)* (Factsheet). Washington, DC: Author. Retrieved May 8, 2008, from http://www.prochoice.org/pubs_research/publications/downloads/about_abortion/facts_about_mifepristone.pdf

National Abortion Federation. (2008). *Management of side effects and complications in medical abortion: A guide for triage and on-call staff* (Clinical guidelines). Washington, DC: Author. Retrieved May 8, 2008, from http://www.prochoice.org/pubs_research/publications/downloads/professional_education/medical_abortion/phone_triage_guide.pdf

National Abortion Federation. (2008). *NAF protocol for mifepristone/misoprostol in early abortion.* Retrieved May 8, 2008, from http://www.prochoice.org/pubs_research/publications/downloads/professional_education/medical_abortion/protocol_mife_rniso.pdf

National Cancer Institute. (2008). *Breast cancer.* Retrieved March 3, 2008, from http://www.cancer.gov/cancertopics/types/breast

National Cancer Institute. (February 2008). *Breast cancer risk assessment tool.* Retrieved February 23, 2008, from http://www.cancer.gov/bcrisktool

National Institute of Allergy and Infectious Diseases. (2005). *Is it a cold or the flu?* (Consumer Information). Washington, DC: U.S. Department of Health and Human Services.

National Institute of Diabetes, Digestive, and Kidney Diseases. (2004). *Hemorrhoids* (Patient Information No. 07-3021). Bethesda, MD: NIH.

NIH National Resource Center. (2005). *Calcium supplements: What to look for* (Patient handout). Bethesda, MD: National Institute of Health.

National Heart, Lung, and Blood Institute. (2001). *ATP III guidelines at-a-glance quick desk reference.* Retrieved April 2, 2008, from http://www.nhlbi.nih.gov/guidelines/cholesterol/atglance.pdf

National Heart, Lung, and Blood Institute. (2002). *Guidelines for the diagnosis and management of asthma* (No. 02-5075). Bethesda, MD: NIH.

National Heart, Lung, and Blood Institute. (2003). Seventh report of the joint national committee on prevention, detection, evaluation, and treatment of high blood pressure (JNC 7). Retrieved April 4, 2008, from http://www.nhlbi.nih.gov/guidelines/hypertension/phycard.pdf

National Heart, Lung, and Blood Institute. (2008). *Body mass index table.* Retrieved May 10, 2008, from http://www.nhlbi.nih.gov/guidelines/obesity/bmi_tbl.pdf

Nazeer, S. (2007). *Unaided visual inspection of the cervix "clinical downstaging" picture atlas.* Retrieved April 15, 2008, from http://www.gfmer.ch/Books/Cervical_cancer_modules/Unaided_visual_inspection_atlas.htm

Newton, E. (2005). Preterm labor, preterm premature rupture of membranes, and chorioamnionitis. *Clinics of Perinatology, 32*(3), 571.

Niermeyer, S., Kattwinkel, J., Van Reempts, P., Nadkarni, V., Phillips, B., Zideman, D., et al. (2000). International guidelines for neonatal resuscitation: An excerpt from the guidelines 2000 for cardiopulmonary resuscitation and emergency cardiovascular care: International consensus on science. Contributors and reviewers for the neonatal resuscitation guidelines. *Pediatrics, 106*(3), E29.

North American Menopause Society. (2004). Treatment of menopause-associated vasomotor symptoms: Position statement of the North American Menopause Society. *Menopause, 11*(1), 11–33.

North American Registry of Midwives. (2008). *How to become a NARM certified professional midwife.* Retrieved August 10, 2008, from http://www.narm.org/htb.htm

NorthPoint Domain. (2008). *UFE info.* Retrieved January 2, 2008, from http://www.ufeinfo.com

Norwitz, E., Bahtiyar, M., & Sibai, B. (2004). Defining standards of care in maternal fetal medicine. *American Journal of Obstetrics and Gynecology, 191*(4), 1491–1496.

Norwitz, E., & Schorge, J. (2001). *Obstetrics and gynecology at a glance.* Osney Mead, Oxford, England: Blackwell Science.

NovaSure, I. (2007). *NovaSure.* Retrieved May 27, 2008, from http://www. novasure.com

O'Brien, J., & Barton, J. (2005). Controversies with the diagnosis and management of HELLP syndrome. *Clinical Obstetrics and Gynecology, 48*(2), 460–477.

Office of Dietary Supplements National Institutes of Health. (2005). *Dietary supplement fact sheet: Calcium.* Retrieved June 29, 2008, from http://ods. od.nih.gov/factsheets/calcium.asp

Office of Dietary Supplements National Institutes of Health. (2008). *Dietary supplement fact sheet: Vitamin D.* Retrieved June 29, 2008, from http://ods. od.nih.gov/factsheets/vitamind.asp

O'Hanlan, K. (2008). *Ten things lesbians should discuss with their health care providers.* Retrieved May 25, 2008, from http://www.glma.org/index. cfm?fuseaction=Page.viewPage&pageID=691

Organon USA. (2007). *Implanon.* Retrieved May 27, 2008, from http://www. implanon-usa.com

Oriel, K. A. (2000). Medical care of transexual patients. *Journal of the Gay and Lesbian Medical Association, 4*(4), 185–194.

Padden, M. (1999). HELLP syndrome: Recognition and perinatal management. *American Family Physician, 60*(3), 829–836, 839.

Papatsonis, D., Flenady, V., Cole, S., & Liley, H. (2005). Oxytocin receptor antagonists for inhibiting preterm labour. *Cochrane Database of Systematic Reviews,* (3), 004452.

Patient Education Page. (2005). Menstrual migraines. *Headache, 45*(1).

Paul, M., Lichtenberg, S., Borgatta, L., Grimes, D. A., & Abdalla, M. (1999). *A clinician's guide to medical and surgical abortion.* Washington, DC: National Abortion Federation. Retrieved May 27, 2008, from http://www.prochoice.org

Penney, D. S., & Miller, K. G. (2008). Nutritional counseling for vegetarians during pregnancy and lactation. *Journal of Midwifery & Women's Health, 53,* 37–44.

Pierce, J., Gaudier, F., & Sanchez-Ramos, L. (2000). Intrapartum amnioinfusion for meconium stained fluid: Meta-analysis of prospective clinical trials. *Obstetrics & Gynecology, 95*(6), 1051.

Postabortion Care Consortium Community Task Force. (2002). *Essential elements of postabortion care: An expanded and updated model* (Clinical Guidelines No. PAC in Action #2 Special Supplement). Washington, DC: National Abortion Federation. Retrieved May 27, 2008, from http://www.prochoice.org

Prendiville, W. J., Elbourne, D., & McDonald, S. (2000). Active versus expectant management in the third stage of labour. *Cochrane Database of Systematic Reviews,* (3), CD000007.

Proctor, M., & Murphy, P. (2001). Herbal and dietary therapies for primary and secondary dysmenorrhea. *Cochrane Database of Systematic Reviews, CD002124*(2), 1–11.

Pryde, P. G., Besinger, R. E., Gianopoulos, J. G., & Mittendorf, R. (2001). Adverse and beneficial effects of tocolytic therapy. *Seminars in Perinatology, 25*(5), 316–340.

Puckett, R., & Offringa, M. (2000). Prophylactic vitamin K for vitamin K deficiency bleeding in neonates. *Cochrane Database of Systematic Reviews, 4*(002776).

Reed, S., Newton, K., LaCroix, A., Grothaus, L., Grieco, V., & Ehrlich, K. (2008). Vaginal, endometrial, and reproductive hormone findings: Randomized, placebo-controlled trail of black cohosh, multibotanical herbs, and dietary soy for vagomotor symptoms: The herbal alternatives for menopause study. *Menopause, 15*(1), 51–58.

Reedy, N. J. (2007). Born too soon: The continuing challenge of preterm labor and birth in the United States (Abstract). *Journal of Midwifery & Women's Health, 52*(3), 281–290.

Renaud, M. T. (2007). We are mothers too: Childbearing experiences of lesbian families. *Journal of Obstetric, Gynecologic, & Neonatal Nursing, 36*, 190–199.

Revah, A., Hannah, M., & Sue-A-Quan, A. (1998). Fetal fibronectin as a predictor of preterm birth: An overview. *American Journal of Perinatology, 15*(11), 613–621.

Reynolds, H. (2005). *Antepartum bleeding.* Unpublished manuscript.

Rideout, S. L. (2005). Tocolytics for pre-term labor. What nurses need to know. *Association of Women's Health, Obstetric and Neonatal Nurses, 9*(1), 56–61.

Riskin, A., Abend-Weinger, M., Riskin-Mashiah, S., Kugelman, A., & Bader, D. (2005). Cesarean section, gestational age, and transient tachypnea of the newborn: Timing is the key. *American Journal of Perinatology, 22*(7), 377–382.

Rogers, R., Gilson, G. J., Miller, A. C., Izquierdo, L. E., Curet, L. B., & Quails, C. R. (1997). Active management of labor: Does it make a difference? *American Journal of Obstetrics and Gynecology, 177*(3), 599–605.

Rossouw, J. E., Anderson, G. L., Prentice, R. L., LaCroix, A. Z., Kooperberg, C., Stefanick, M. L., et al. (2002). Risks and benefits of estrogen plus progestin in healthy postmenopausal women: Principal results from the women's health initiative randomized controlled trial. *Journal of the American Medical Association, 288*(3), 321–333.

The Rotterdam ESHRE/ASRM-Sponsored PCOS Consensus Workshop Group. (2004). Revised 2003 consensus on diagnostic criteria and long term health risks related to polycystic ovary syndrome (PCOS). *Human Reproduction, 19*(1), 41–47.

Russell, L. C. (1989). Caffeine restriction as initial treatment for breast pain. *Nurse Practitioner, 14*(2), 36–37, 40.

Rust, O. A., Bofill, J. A., Arriola, R. M., Andrew, M. E., & Morrison, J. C. (1996). The clinical efficacy of oral tocolytic therapy. *American Journal of Obstetrics and Gynecology, 175*(4 Pt 1), 838–842.

Sacks, J. J., Helmick, C. G., Langmaid, G., & Sniezek, J. E. (2002). *Trends in deaths from systemic lupus erythematosus—United States, 1979–1998.* Retrieved May 27, 2008, from http://www.cdc.gov/mmwr/preview/mmwrhtml/mm5117a3.htm

Salamat, S., Ismail, K., & O'Brien, S. (2007). Premenstrual syndrome. *Obstetrics, Gynecology, and Reproductive Medicine, 18*(2), 29–32.

Salazar, S. S. (2006). Assessment and management of the obese adult female: A clinical update for providers. *Journal of Midwifery & Women's Health, 51*(3), 202.

Sanders, L. (2006). Assessing and managing women with depression: A midwifery perspective. *Journal of Midwifery & Women's Health, 51*(3), 185–192.

Saslow, D., Castle, P., Cox, J., Davey, D., Einstein, M., & Ferris, D. (2007). American cancer society guidelines for HPV vaccine use to prevent cervical cancer and its precursors. *CA Cancer Journal for Clinicians, 57*(1), 7–28.

Schrag, S., Gorwitz, R., Fultz-Butts, K., & Schuchat, A. (2002). Prevention of perinatal group B streptococcal disease. *Morbidity and Mortality Weekly Report, 55*, (RR-11), 1–22.

Schuiling, K. D., & Likis, F. E. (2006). *Women's gynecologic health.* Sudbury, MA: Jones and Bartlett.

Scott, J., Gibbs, R., Karlan, B., & Haney, A. (2003). *Danforth's obstetrics and gynecology* (9th ed.). Philadelphia, PA: Lippincott Williams and Wilkins.

Sears, W., & Sears, M. (2006). *Comparison of human milk and formula.* Retrieved December, 2007, from http://www.askdrsears.com/html/2/T021600.asp

Seidel, H. M., Ball, J., Dains, J., & Benedict, W. (2006). *Mosby's physical assessment handbook* (6th ed.). St. Louis, MO: Mosby.

Simerville, J. A., Maxted, W. C., & Pahira, J. J. (2005). Urinalysis: A comprehensive review. *American Family Physician, 71*(6), 1153–1162.

Simonsen, S. M., Lyon, J. L., Alder, S. C., & Varner, M. W. (2005). Effect of grand multiparity on intrapartum and newborn complications in young women. *Obstetrics and Gynecology, 106*(3), 454–460.

Simpson, K. R. (2007). Intrauterine resuscitation during labor: Review of current methods and supportive evidence. *Journal of Midwifery & Women's Health, 52*(3), 229–237.

Smeltzer, S., & Bare, B. (2004). In Q. McDonald, & D. McMahon (Eds.), *Textbook of medical surgical nursing* (10th ed.). Philadelphia: Lippincott Williams and Wilkins.

Smith, L. J. (2007). Impact of birthing practices on the breastfeeding dyad (Abstract). *Journal of Midwifery & Women's Health, 52*(6), 621–630.

Smith, V., Devane, D., Begley, C. M., Clarke, M., & Higgins, S. (2007). A systematic review and quality assessment of systematic reviews of fetal fibronectin and transvaginal length for predicting preterm birth. *European Journal of Obstetrics & Gynecology and Reproductive Biology, 133*(2), 134–142.

Smyth, R. M. D., Alldred, S. K., Markham, C. (2008). Amniotomy for shortening spontaneous labor (review). *Cochrane Database of Systematic Reviews,* (1).

Speroff, L., & Fritz, M. A. (2005). *Clinical gynecology, endocrinology, infertility* (7th ed.). Philadelphia: Lippincott Williams & Wilkins.

Stade, B., Bailey, C., Dzendolestas, D., & Sgro, M. (2007). Psychological and/or educational interventions for reducing prenatal alcohol consumption in pregnant women and women planning pregnancy. *Cochrane Database of Systematic Reviews,* (3).

Stap, G. (2003). Menstrual disorders in adolescence. *Best Practice and Research Clinical Obstetrics and Gynecology, 17*(1), 75–92.

Steele, L. S., & Stratmann, H. (2006). Counseling lesbian patients about getting pregnant. *Canadian Family Physician, 52,* 605–611.

Stewart, E. (2000). *The V book: A doctors guide to complete vulvovaginal health.* New York: Bantam Books.

Stokowski, L. A. (2006). Fundamentals of phototherapy for neonatal jaundice. *Advances in Neonatal Care, 6*(6), 303–312.

Stone-Godena, T. (2006). Vulvar pain syndrome: Vestibulodynia. *Journal of Midwifery & Women's Health, 51*(6), 502–509.

Summers, L., & Price, R. A. (1993). Preconception care: An opportunity to maximize health in pregnancy. *Journal of Midwifery & Women's Health, 38*(4), 188–196.

Task Force on Circumcision. (1999). Circumcision policy statement. *Pediatrics, 102*(3), 686.

Tesch, B. J. (2001). Herbs commonly used by women: An evidence-based review. *American Journal of Obstetrics and Gynecology, 1,* 89–102.

Tharpe, N. (2006). *2006–2009 clinical practice guidelines for midwifery & women's health.* Sudbury, MA: Jones and Bartlett.

Thomas, R. L., & Blakemore, K. J. (1990). Evaluation of elevations in maternal serum alpha-fetoprotein: A review. *Obstetrical & Gynecological Survey, 45*(5), 269–283.

Thompson Healthcare. (2007). *MICROMEDEX: Healthcare series.* Retrieved May 27, 2008, from http://www.micromedex.com

Thureen, P., Hall, D., Deacon, J., & Hernandez, J. (2004). *Assessment and care of the well newborn* (2nd ed.). St. Louis, MO: Saunders.

Tikkanen, M., Nuutila, M., Hiilesmaa, V., Paavomen, J., & Ylikorkala, O. (2006). Clinical presentation and risk factors of placental abruption. *Acta Obstetrics Gynecology Scandinavia, 85*(6), 700.

Turner, M. B. (2006). *Pregnancy after perinatal loss: Implications for midwifery care.* New Haven, CT: Unpublished masters dissertation, Yale University School of Nursing.

Turner, M., & Bridges, M. (2006). *Silent warmth: Midwifery management of stillbirth.* Unpublished manuscript.

United States Department of Health and Human Services. (2007). *The health consequences of involuntary exposure to tobacco smoke: A report of the surgeon general.* Retrieved May 27, 2008, from http://www.surgeongeneral.gov/library/secondhandsmoke/factsheets/factsheet6.html

United States Department of Health and Human Services. (2008). *Treating tobacco use and dependency 2008 update.* Retrieved May 26, 2008, from http://www.surgeongeneral.gov/tobacco/treating_tobacco_use08.pdf

United States Preventative Services Task Force. (2007). *The guide to clinical preventative services, 2007.* AHRQ Publication No. 07-05100. Rockville, MD: Agency for Healthcare Research and Quality. Retrieved from http://www.ahrq.gov/clinic/pocketgd07/pocketgd07.pdf

Usman, S., Indusekhar, R., & O'Brien, S. (2008). Hormonal management of premenstrual syndrome. *Best Practice and Research Clinical Obstetrics and Gynecology, 22*(2), 251–260.

Varney, H., Kriebs, J. M., & Gegor, C. L. (2004). *Varney's midwifery* (4th ed.). Sudbury, MA: Jones and Bartlett.

Vaules, M., Ramin, K., & Ramsey, P. (2000). Syphilis in pregnancy: A review. *Primary Care Updates for OB/GYNS, 7*(1), 26–30.

Vedam, S. (2004). *Eating for two.* Unpublished manuscript.

Vedam, S., Goff, M., & Nolan-Marnin, V. (2007). Closing the theory-practice gap: Intrapartum midwifery management of planned homebirths (Abstract). *Journal of Midwifery & Women's Health, 52*(3), 291–300.

Velaphi, S., & Vidyasagar, D. (2006). Intrapartum and postdelivery management of infants born to mothers with meconium-stained amniotic fluid: Evidence-based recommendations (Abstract). *Clinics in Perinatology, 33*(1) 29–42.

Von Wald, T., & Walling, A. (2002). Headaches during pregnancy. *Obstetrics and Gynecology Survey, 57*(3), 179–185.

Webb, P. M., Byrne, C., Schnitt, S. J., Connolly, J. L., Jacobs, T. W., Baer, H. J., et al. (2004). A prospective study of diet and benign breast disease. *Cancer Epidemiology Biomarkers and Prevention, 13*(7), 1106–1113.

Weed, S. S. (1985). Wise women herbals for the childbearing year. Woodstock, NY: Ash Tree.

Weinstein, L., & Ullery, B. (2000). Identification of at-risk women for osteoporosis screening. *American Journal of Obstetrics & Gynecology, 183*(3), 547–549.

Wisner, K. L., Perel, J. M., & Findling, R. L. (1996). Antidepressant treatment during breastfeeding. *American Journal of Psychiatry, 153*(9), 1132–1137.

Wolff, K., Johnson, R. A., & Suurmond, R. (2005). *Fitzpatrick's color atlas & synopsis of clinical dermatology* (5th ed.). Boston: McGraw-Hill.

Women's Health Initiative. (2002). *WHI HRT update.* Retrieved August 10, 2008, from http://www.whi.org/findings/ht/update_ht2002.pdf

Women's Health Initiative. (2004). *WHI hormone program update.* Retrieved August 10, 2008, from http://www.whi.org/findings/ht/update_ht2004.pdf

World Health Organization. (2004). *Medical eligibility criteria for contraceptive use.* Geneva, Switzerland: WHO Library Cataloguing-in-Publication Data.

Zeidenstein, L. (1990). Gynecological and childbearing needs of lesbians. *Journal of Nurse-Midwifery, 35*(1), 10–18. Retrieved May 27, 2008, from MEDLINE database.

# INDEX

**NOTES**